# Murdering to Dissect

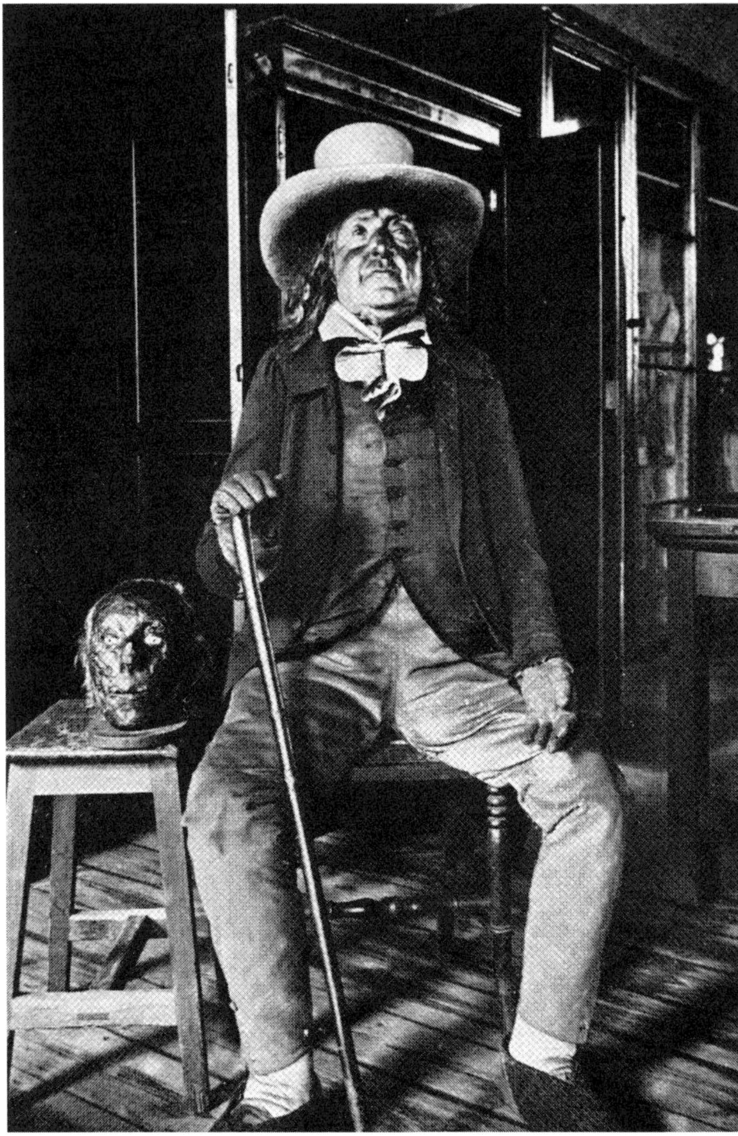

Jeremy Bentham's auto-icon.

# Murdering to Dissect

## Grave-robbing, *Frankenstein* and the anatomy literature

Tim Marshall

Manchester University Press

Manchester and New York

*Distributed exclusively in the USA and Canada by St Martin's Press*

*Published by* Manchester University Press
Oxford Road, Manchester M13 9NR, UK
*and* Room 400, 175 Fifth Avenue,
New York, NY 10010, USA

*Distributed exclusively in the USA and Canada by* St. Martin's Press, Inc.,
175 Fifth Avenue, New York, NY 10010, USA

*British Library Cataloguing-in-Publication Data*
A catalogue record for this book is available from the British Library

*Library of Congress Cataloging-in-Publication Data*
Murdering to dissect: graverobbing, Frankenstein, and the anatomy literature/Tim Marshall
ISBN 0-7190-4542-8 — ISBN 0-7190-4543-6 (pbk)
1. Shelley, Mary Wollstonecraft, 1797–1851. Frankenstein. 2. Shelley, Mary Wollstonecraft, 1797–1851—Knowledge—Crime. 3. Human disssection—Scotland—History—19th century. 4. Body snatching—Scotland—History—19th century. 5. Horror tales, English—History and criticism. 6. Medicine—Scotland—History—19th century. 7. Murder—Scotland—History—19th century. 8. Human anatomy in literature. 9. Body, Human, in literature. 10. Monsters in literature. I. Title.
PR5397.F73M35
823'. 7—dc20 95-1715
CIP 1995

ISBN 0-7190-4542-8 *hardback*
0-7190-4543-6 *paperback*

99 98 97 96 95 10 9 8 7 6 5 4 3 2 1

Typeset in Great Britain
by Carnegie Publishing Ltd, Preston

Printed in Great Britain
by Biddles Ltd, Guildford and King's Lynn

The English never wrote down their laws, they carry them about with them on their person.

Elias Canetti, *The Human Province*

For my father, Roy Stuart Marshall

# Contents

# Illustrations

# Acknowledgements

I would like to thank the following people for their help and support during my work on this book: Roger Sales, Roger Fowler, Patricia Hollis, Victor Sage, Jeanetta Pollok, Deirdre Sharpe, Ian Clarke and Richard Byford. I owe particular thanks to Anita Roy for editorial assistance; to Roy Porter for constructive criticism and a willingness to give time to my work-in-progress; and to Ruth Richardson for commenting on the book's final draft. I also want to thank Colin Clarke for his encouragement to me early in my academic career. I am grateful for permission to quote from *Crowds and Power* by Elias Canetti; copyright © Classen Verlag Hamburg 1960, English translation copyright © Victor Vollancz Ltd 1962. My greatest debt is to my family, Alison (for much help) and my son Thomas.

# Chronology of events

1752 The Murder Act of this year declares that it is necessary 'that some Terror and peculiar mark of Infamy be added to the punishment' and makes the dissection of all murderers compulsory.

1800 The College of Surgeons becomes the Royal College of Surgeons.

More than a thousand corpses a year disappear from burial grounds in England and Scotland in the first decade of the nineteenth century.

1818 *Frankenstein* appears. The first edition, a best-seller, is published anonymously.

The Patent Coffin, costing £3 10*s*., is registered and marketed as an anti-resurrectionist device.

1819 The 'Peterloo Massacre'.

In his *Hunterian Oration* John Abernethy, one of the senior surgeons of the day, recommends the use of paupers' bodies for dissection. It is the first time this idea receives public advocacy.

1823 Mary Shelley's name appears on the title-page of the second edition of *Frankenstein*, brought out in this year by her father, William Godwin.

1824 Thomas Southwood Smith publishes an article in the *Westminster Review,* in which he urges that all unclaimed bodies from hospitals and workhouses should automatically be handed over for dissection.

1825–26 The 'Great Inflation' commences: the graverobbers begin to command higher prices for the corpses they sell to the surgeons.

1826 In private correspondence with Bentham, the Home

| | |
|---|---|
| | Secretary Robert Peel indicates that the emerging moves towards anatomy reform should be conducted in secret; Bentham accedes to the request. |
| 1827 | First instalment in *Blackwood's* of Thomas De Quincey's *On Murder considered as one of the Fine Arts.* |
| 1828 | Sir Astley Cooper, President of the Royal College of Surgeons and Surgeon to the King, addresses a House of Commons Select Committee on the urgent need for legislative action to insure a supply of bodies to the surgeons. |
| 1828–29 | The Burke and Hare scandal breaks in Edinburgh. It spreads alarm waves of 'Burkophobia' fear through the country.<br>Southwood Smith's 1824 article is reprinted as a pamphlet entitled *The Use of the Dead to the Living*, and is circulated to all members of Parliament. |
| 1829 | William Burke hanged and dissected in Edinburgh.<br>The first Anatomy Bill (nicknamed 'The Midnight Bill' by its parliamentary opponents) fails in the House of Lords. |
| 1831 | The third edition of *Frankenstein* appears.<br>Copycat burkings occur in London.<br>'Burkophobia' widespread throughout the country. |
| 1831–32 | Amid the burkophobia, the Asiatic cholera arrives in England. |
| 1832 | Bentham dies on 6 June, donating his body for public dissection in a London Anatomy School.<br>The First Reform Act receives Royal Assent on 7 June.<br>Bentham's dissection is performed on 9 June by Dr Southwood Smith.<br>The Anatomy Act receives Royal Assent on 1 August. |
| 1834 | The Poor Law Amendment Act is passed. |

# Introduction: murdering to dissect

Sweet is the lore which Nature brings;
Our meddling intellect
Mis-shapes the beauteous forms of things:
We murder to dissect.

Wordsworth, 'The Tables Turned', 1798.

## The Edinburgh scandal 1828–29

When Wordsworth expressed contempt for the murderous intellect he coined an expression which certain developments thirty years later in the medical field were to revise by turning metaphor into fact. In 1828 the renowned Edinburgh anatomist, Dr Robert Knox, was popularly perceived as having connived in a series of sixteen murders in order to obtain the bodies for dissection. Knox was a brilliant teacher of anatomy, a man determined to advance his science. The killers were the subsequently infamous Irishmen, Burke and Hare, who smothered their victims in a manner that left no signs of violence on the body. The corpses were delivered to Knox's establishment via the backdoor, where payment was made. The trial of Burke and Hare in 1829 added a new word for murder to the English language: 'to burke'. Burke went to the gallows after Hare turned King's evidence and escaped prosecution. Throughout the judicial process Knox remained silent and was not charged with any crime. In the eye of the Edinburgh crowd, however, he was every bit as guilty as the killers themselves and at the execution there were calls for Knox and Hare to take the same punishment. As an Edinburgh street song of the day put it: 'Burke's the butcher, Hare's the thief, Knox the boy who buys the beef.' In 1829 the scandal was headline news all over the country. As the song said, the medical profession was murdering to dissect.

My argument in this book is that Mary Shelley's *Frankenstein*, a best-seller when it appeared in 1818, rapidly acquires new meanings through historical events taking place after first publication, the Burke and Hare case in particular. In the 1820s the science of anatomy – the science which Victor Frankenstein practises – aroused controversy and there were mounting pressures for legislation concerning it. These developments began soon after the story's first edition, as I will show. They grow in the years which span the second and third editions in 1823 and 1831 and add a specific dimension – an anatomy storyline – which could not have been fully present in the first edition.

Where Frankenstein's science is concerned, the arguments of the 1820s in favour of anatomy reform culminate in a piece of utilitarian legislation which became law just a year after the third edition of the story: the 1832 Anatomy Act. The law effected a permanent transformation of the practice and public perception of anatomy by granting anatomists access to unclaimed pauper bodies from workhouses. The reform was born in the medical, social and political culture of which Mary Shelley, as a writer, was a part. Using the perspective offered by the 1820s, I shall argue that *Frankenstein* and the Anatomy Act can be seen as identical twins – one in the world of imagination, the other in the realms of legislation. They articulate all the great themes of the era and the spirit of the age: stories of gender, of class and of living and dying. Before looking at the legislation we need to reconstruct the medical culture which fostered it.

Some of the most famous passages in *Frankenstein* concern Frankenstein's nocturnal visits to graveyards:

> I became acquainted with the science of anatomy . . . I do not ever remember to have trembled at a tale of superstition or to have feared the apparition of a spirit. Darkness had no effect upon my fancy, and a churchyard to me was merely the receptacle of bodies deprived of life [which] had become food for the worm. Now I was led to examine the cause and progress

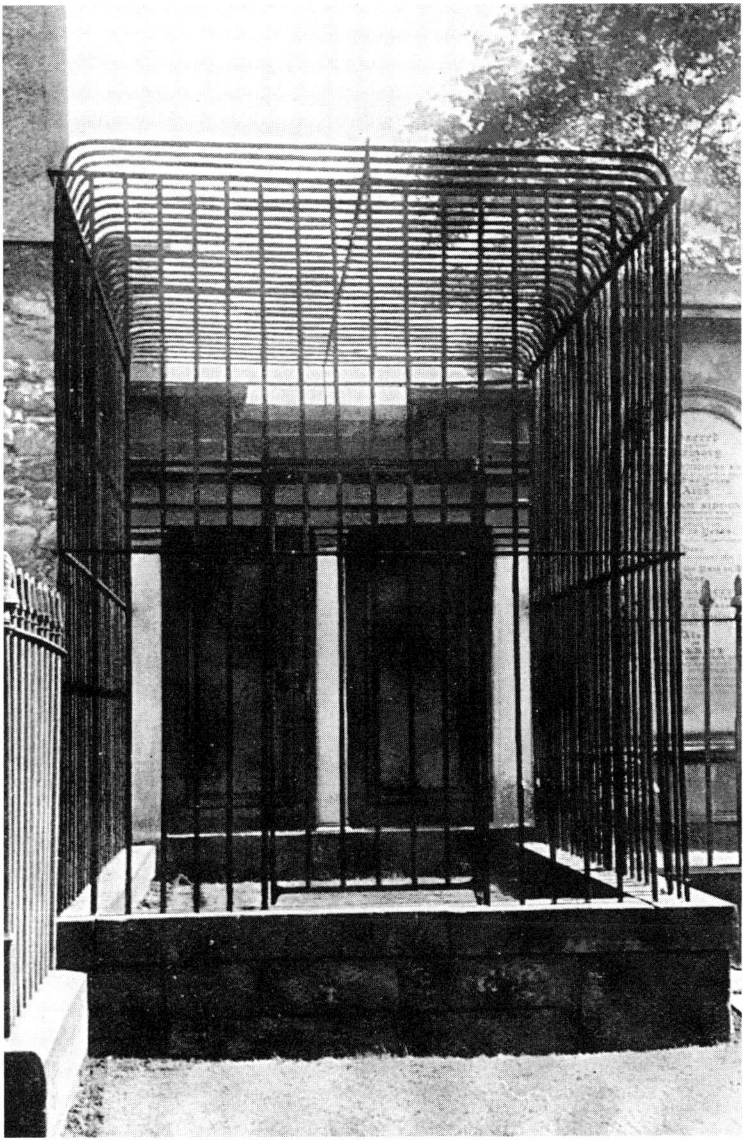

Upright mortsafe in Greyfriars Churchyard, Edinburgh. In the early nineteenth century the relatively wealthy could purchase mortsafes as protection against the graverobbers.

> of this decay and forced to spend days and nights in vaults and charnel houses . . . I collected bones . . . and disturbed, with profane fingers, the tremendous secrets of the human frame . . . The dissecting room . . . furnished many of my materials . . .[1]

As these passages show, an anatomy dimension was always in the story, for here Mary Shelley alludes to the graverobbing world as she knew it from her girlhood in Scotland.[2] The graverobbers – or 'resurrectionists' as they were called – raised newly buried bodies and sold them to the anatomists for dissection. The great scandal in 1828 saw the medical underworld turning lethal. Acting out a long predicted possibility, Burke and Hare took graverobbing to its logical conclusion: instead of digging up the dead, they accepted lucrative incentives to destroy the living.

## Galvanism

The medical profession figures in the scenario which first gave Mary the idea for her story. As is well known, the genesis of *Frankenstein* was a diversion set up by Lord Byron to engage his house guests in Switzerland in the summer of 1816. In her 'Author's Introduction' of 1831 Mary Shelley reports Byron proposing that each person present write a ghost story. The proposition was agreed and the world has been reading *Frankenstein* ever since, the story of the scientist who creates a 'monster' – as he calls it – when he restores life to dead bodies. Mary tells us she got her idea while listening to Byron and her husband, the poet Shelley, discussing the experiments of Erasmus Darwin, the famous eighteenth-century doctor and atheist:

> Many and long were the conversations between Lord Byron

[1] *Frankenstein*, 53, 56. All references to *Frankenstein* are from the 1831 edition edited by Johanna M. Smith, 1992. All dates are given in the Bibliography.

[2] Mary remains silent outside her fiction on the subject of the graverobbing. However, it was rife in Scotland in her formative years and widely reported in newspapers.

> and Shelley, to which I was a devout but nearly silent listener . . . Perhaps a corpse would be reanimated; galvanism had given token of such things: perhaps the component parts of a creature would be manufactured, brought together, and endued with vital warmth.[3]

We will never know what her few interjections were; instead, we have to read the story.

A dialogue with these famous conversations can be discerned in *Frankenstein*. It was not, and cannot have been, a wholly conscious dialogue on Mary's part, but the graveyard passages mark its appearance. Frankenstein's graverobbing exploits anchor the story in the medical realities of the day; at the same time, however, these passages reply to an implicit utopian dimension in what Byron and Shelley were talking about. What is galvanism? In their book *Patient's Progress* Dorothy and Roy Porter cite Erasmus Darwin's description of electrical shocks revivifying one of his patients:

> On a supposition that the obstruction of the bile might be owing to paralysis or torpid action of the common bile-duct, and the stimulants taken into the stomach seeming to have no effect, I directed half a score smart electric shocks from a coated bottle, which held about a quart, to be passed through the liver, and along the course of the common gallduct, as near as could be guessed, and on that very day the stools became yellow; he continued the electrical shocks a few days more, and his skin gradually became clear.[4]

The Porters comment on the significance of electrical treatment in the late eighteenth-century medical context: 'The enlargement of surgical interventions perhaps marks the first signs of a new medical Prometheanism, the belief that mechanical means could fix the misfunctioning body. The spread of medical electricity epitomised this vision.'[5] In her book on Mary Shelley, Anne

---

[3] *Frankenstein*, Author's Introduction, 1992, 22.

[4] Porter & Porter, 1989, 171.

[5] *Ibid.*

Mellor shows this 'medical Prometheanism' in action in the work of Luigi Aldini, the nephew and disciple of the physiologist Galvani, after whom the electrical treatment is named. Here is the galvanic experimentation which led Byron and Percy Shelley to discuss the possibility of reanimating a corpse:

> Galvani's theories made the British headlines in December, 1802 . . . But Professor Aldini's most notorious demonstration of galvanic electricity took place on January 17, 1803. On that day he applied galvanic electricity to the corpse of the murderer Thomas Forster. The body of the recently hanged criminal was collected from Newgate where it had lain in the prison yard at a temperature of 30 degrees Fahrenheit for one hour by the President of the College of Surgeons, Mr Keate, and brought immediately to Mr Wilson's Anatomical Theatre where the following experiments were performed. When wires attached to a pile composed of 120 plates of zinc and 120 plates of copper were connected to the ear and the mouth of the dead criminal, Aldini later reported, 'the jaw began to quiver, the adjoining muscles were horribly contorted, and the left eye actually opened.' When the wires were applied to the dissected thumb muscles they 'induced a forcible effort to clench the hand'; when applied to the ear and rectum, they 'excited in the muscles contractions much stronger . . . as almost to give an appearance of re-animation.'[6]

Aside from the experiment, this is a revealing portrait of the medical profession in the early nineteenth century. In 1803 it is barely three years since the College became the Royal College of Surgeons, an important moment in the official recognition of their science. As regards further public legitimation, however, perhaps the most intractable obstacle in the longer term was precisely the profession's association with the gallows which is explicit in Mellor's description. As we see in Chapter 1, the law since the mid-eighteenth century had permitted the bodies of

---

[6] Mellor, 1988, 105.

murderers to go to the surgeons for dissection – the more everyday scientific work conducted in the venue which we see here. Furthermore, it was the shortage of bodies from this source which led the surgeons reluctantly into league with the graverobbers; and this connection made the profession distinctly unpopular in the years before utilitarian interests manipulated the 1832 Anatomy Act into law. 'Who shall conceive the horrors of my secret toil, as I dabbled among the unhallowed damps of the grave?' asks Frankenstein.[7] The fictional doctor speaks for all the professors of anatomy before the new law ended graverobbing for good.

## Utopia and reality

The other strand of dialogue in *Frankenstein* which intersects the galvanism debate concerns the vision of the future adumbrated by Mary Shelley's father, William Godwin. The Porters tell us that 'Darwin was one of those, like Godwin, to entertain hopes of prolonged life through medical improvements'.[8] Their observations provide a lead into the anatomy text in Mary's story: 'Utilitarianism promised the victory of pleasure over pain, and utopians, like Darwin and Condorcet, pointed to a promised land not merely of longevity but of this-worldly immortality itself. *Frankenstein* was just over the horizon.'[9] The new medical Prometheanism appears in the pages of Godwin's *Enquiry Concerning Political Justice* in a section entitled 'Of Health, and the Prolongation of Human Life'. The 1831 edition of *Frankenstein* is dedicated to Godwin as the author of this volume. Godwin writes:

> If it could have been told to the savage inhabitants of Europe in the times of Theseus and Achilles that man was capable of predicting eclipses and weighing the air, of reducing to settled rules the phenomena of nature so that no prodigies should remain, and of measuring the distance and size of the heavenly

---

[7] *Frankenstein*, 56.
[8] Porter & Porter, 1988, 89.
[9] *Ibid.*

> bodies, this would not have appeared to them less incredible than if we had told them of the possibility of maintaining the human body in perpetual youth and vigour. But we have not only this analogy, showing that the discovery in question forms, as it were, a regular branch of the acquisitions that belong to an intellectual nature; but, in addition to this, we seem to have a glimpse of the manner in which the acquisition will be secured.[10]

*Frankenstein* is sub-titled 'The Modern Prometheus'. As a young man, Victor Frankenstein subscribes to Godwin's utopian scheme and dreams of delivering the promised land in the eyes of the world. Before he begins the long task of creation which culminates in a reanimated corpse, he is explicit on the point: 'Wealth was an inferior object, but what glory would attend the discovery if I could banish disease from the human frame and render man invulnerable to any but a violent death.'[11] To achieve his objective he devotes himself to the science of anatomy.

Around the time *Frankenstein* appeared a debate commenced in the medical profession concerning the need to promote the science of anatomy. In 1819 The Royal College of Surgeons was addressed by one of the most distinguished surgeons of the eighteen-teens, John Abernethy, who delivered *The Hunterian Oration.*[12] In this address Abernethy took a public initiative in the direction of anatomy reform, and for this reason his is the first voice in the cultural drama which begins just a year after Mary Shelley's story appears. He proposed the requisitioning of unclaimed pauper corpses in order to advance anatomical research. In the English context, this was the first ever[13] recommendation of this idea in a published statement:

---

[10] Godwin, 1985, 775. I am grateful to Roy Porter for pointing this statement out to me.

[11] *Frankenstein*, 45.

[12] The title of the speech refers to John Hunter, who is regarded as the father of modern anatomy. Erasmus Darwin attended Hunter's lectures in 1752.

[13] This is Ruth Richardson's finding (1989, 332–3). She notes two eighteenth-century recommendations along these lines, but Abernethy's is the first published advocacy.

> There is no short cut, nor 'royal road' to the attainment of medical knowledge. The path which we have to pursue is long, difficult, and unsafe. In our progress, we must frequently take up our abode with death and corruption; we must adopt loathsome diseases for our familiar associates, or we shall never be thoroughly acquainted with their nature and dispositions; we must risk, nay even injure, our own health in order to preserve or restore that of others. Yet if we do this, our profession will be held in the highest respect . . .
>
> Anatomical knowledge is the only foundation on which the structure of medical science can be built. Without this we should but increase the sufferings of those afflicted with diseases, and endanger their lives. Opportunities of dissection should therefore be afforded us . . . [If] the directors of hospitals, poor-houses, and prisons, were to establish it as a regulation, that the body of any person dying in those institutions, unclaimable by immediate relatives, should be given to the surgeon of the establishment for dissection, upon his signing an obligation so to dispose of it, as to give no offence to decency or humanity, I am convinced, that it would greatly tend to the increase of anatomical knowledge amongst the members of our profession in general, and consequently to the public good.[14]

In 1832, only months after the third edition of *Frankenstein*, a version of Abernethy's proposal was adopted in the Anatomy Act.

The historical record shows that on one occasion Mary Shelley appears to have owed her life to the science of anatomy. Her husband records a domestic drama which affords a glimpse of the real state of medical knowledge in Mary Shelley's time. On 16 June 1822 she suffered a miscarriage which nearly proved fatal. Two days later her husband writes to John Gisborne:

> Her situation for some hours was alarming, and as she was totally destitute of medical assistance, I took the most decisive resolutions, by dint of making her sit in ice, I succeeded in

---

[14] Abernethy, 1819, 159.

> checking the hemorrage and the fainting fits, so that when the physician arrived all danger was over, and he had nothing to do but applaud me for my boldness. She is now doing well, and the sea-baths will soon restore her.[15]

We do not have this episode in complete focus. In a recent biographer's version[16] a doctor was present 'whose efforts were mainly devoted to reducing the pain of her death which he was sure was certain . . . and it was only when Shelley made her sit in a bath filled with ice that the bleeding stopped'. The precise facts apart, it is clear that Mary was perceived to be dying as Shelley struck upon the solution.[17] And one other factor is present as this crisis is resolved – Shelley's education. Claire Tomalin observes of this episode that his 'early interest in anatomy stood him in good stead'.[18] To whom, then, after Shelley, did Mary owe her life? The answer owes nothing to utopian projections. It was Abernethy, the speaker at the Royal College in 1819. In 1811 Shelley, who at this time had ambitions to be a doctor, attended his lectures on anatomy in London, and Hogg,[19] who accompanied him, tells us that Mary's future husband walked the wards in Abernethy's hospital, St Bartholomew's.

The connection between Mary's haemorrhage crisis and Shelley's acquaintance with Abernethy's science is not definite, of course, but it is suggestive. The 1822 episode lends support to Abernethy's general point about the desirability of more advanced medical knowledge. As Tomalin is saying, Mary owed her recovery on this occasion to an educated guess. Not John Abernethy personally, but the surgeon and what he stands for in his 1819 speech is present in spirit in this domestic drama at its critical moment. Mary's survival against the odds is a powerful illustration

---

15 Cited in Feldman and Scott-Kilvert, 1987, vol. 1. p. 412.

16 St Clair, 1989, 467.

17 In her *Journal* entry for 5 Oct. 1839 Mary recalls this event and her conviction that she was about to die.

18 Tomalin, 1992, 103.

19 Hogg, 1933, vol. 2, pp. 155–6.

of what it meant in her day to benefit from – or to need – the kind of knowledge and education which was to be promoted by the 1832 Anatomy Act.[20] In 1823, a year after this episode, the second edition of *Frankenstein* appears. As Godwin wanted it, it bore Mary's name for the first time.

## *Frankenstein* and the 1832 Anatomy Act

Of course it cannot be proved that the later editions of *Frankenstein* specifically take up what Abernethy said in 1819. The claim for a connection depends upon an interpretation of the story in which certain events, and in particular each murder, appear to comment pertinently on the controversial social and political dimensions of medical culture onwards from Abernethy's 1819 pronouncement. As we shall see, the idea of handing over unclaimed bodies from hospitals and workhouses to the surgeons was vigorously argued by Thomas Southwood Smith in an article in 1824 in the *Westminster Review*. Four years later, when the Burke and Hare scandal broke, it was reprinted under the title *The Use of the Dead to the Living* and went through several editions, a copy being presented to members of both Houses of Parliament.[21] In Mary Shelley's tale, one suggestive – and provocative – scenario transforms the story into a plausible cameo of the late 1820s: the appearance of corpses which continuously turn up in close proximity to the surgeon Frankenstein, as if in delivery to him. There is a logic which governs the murderous hand in these events. The bodies in question comprise Frankenstein's family and close circle. This fact sees *Frankenstein* confirming the nationwide phobia about

---

[20] The Shelleys bear testimony to the grim medical realities of the eighteen-teens and twenties. They lose children to disease and constantly engage senior doctors in the hope of turning their fortunes. In this they are very much people of their time, living in a medical culture which precedes virtually all the major discoveries of modern medicine. In a letter to Maria Gisborne on 30 June 1821, Mary comments: 'You know how much reason we have to fear the deceitful appearances of perfect health'.

[21] This is according to Southwood Smith's granddaughter. See Lewes, 1848.

'bodysnatching' possibilities – as the fiction assembles the case to end such horrors by legislative means. The social class of these victims, however, comments on the hypocrisy which informs the anatomy controversy and its solution. The Anatomy Act was to benefit the rich and the middle classes with the prospect of improved medical education and exemption from dissection.

The arguments in favour of anatomy reform in the 1820s were an attempt to dissociate the profession from undesirable associations and to secure an invisible supply-line of corpses. In his *Hunterian Oration* the senior surgeon of the day was addressing increasingly urgent problems. For a long time in England the medical profession had been unable to acquire human corpses in sufficient numbers to enable real advances to be made in the medical field. Aside from the gallows, moreover, the graverobbing market heeded no social boundaries where the dead – or the feelings of the living – were concerned. In his speech Abernethy remained silent about this market, but the fact of its existence would have been lost on no member of his audience. However, the 1828 case (and subsequent copycat burkings) put a different complexion on these problems. As Ruth Richardson has shown in her study of the 1820s anatomy debate, the Edinburgh scandal raised a disturbing question:

> That a vocation which professed 'no object but that of conferring benefit on others' in healing the sick and the saving of human life should have been responsible for the commission of so many premeditated murders, was seen as an unspeakable paradox. 'Shall it be said', asked one practitioner, aghast, 'that we owe it to that science which professes to alleviate human suffering [that] her votaries be encouraged to encourage . . . Murder?'[22]

The materials I discuss in this book concern fables and realities of building people and destroying people, and above all the doctor/scientist as a figure of threat.[23] Victor Frankenstein is

---

[22] Richardson, 1989, 133.

[23] The remainder of this paragraph owes a debt to Roy Porter's responses to my work in draft.

emblematic of the idea of making a man; dissection in the anatomy schools symbolises destruction. However, as I will show, the relations between making and destroying are more deeply ambivalent, both in life and art. In *Frankenstein* the man who is made turns out to be a 'monster' and a destroyer of life. In the anatomy literature there is much slippage between the surgeon, the dissector, the murderer – and then the writer and artist: after all, artists have relied on anatomical dissection, and writers vicariously kill, as with Thomas De Quincey's murder fantasies in *On Murder considered as one of the Fine Arts*.

We murder to dissect, but we also dissect in order to heal. As Abernethy in 1819 was in effect saying, the dead body trade was the unacceptable face of civilisation as a rather primeval business. The most explicit suggestion in *Frankenstein* of an identity between the surgeon and the resurrectionist occurs just after Frankenstein's first encounter with 'the accomplishment of my toils', the 'monster'. The 'resurrectionist' cameo, as I shall call it, is an event in the dream which follows this sighting. It discloses Frankenstein embracing Elizabeth, his bride-to-be, as she turns into a corpse. However, her features appear to change in the next instant:

> and I thought I held the corpse of my dead mother in my arms; a shroud enveloped her form, and I saw the grave-worms crawling in the folds of the flannel. I started from my sleep with horror . . . I beheld the wretch, the miserable monster whom I had created.[24]

At the time of this dream Frankenstein's mother, Caroline Beaufort, is recently deceased. However, as it alludes to the family bereavement, this moment also recalls episodes in medical history which have seen men dissect dead members of their family in clinical detachment from their own feelings.[25] In this image the

---

24 *Frankenstein*, 58.

25 Harvey, for example, the discoverer of the circulation of the blood in 1628, dissected his father and sister *postmortem*. His discovery is alluded to in *Frankenstein* in one of Waldman's lectures.

mother, the bearer of life, remains partially hidden; but there is a further dimension of censorship as Frankenstein awakes. The violence impending on her body is displaced on to the Creature as the loaded term 'monster' appears for the first time. The resurrectionist cameo is a first intimation that members of Frankenstein's family are potential fair game as corpses for the anatomist – especially those like Caroline Beaufort and Elizabeth who retain a relationship to extreme poverty in their personal histories.

By the time of Abernethy's 1819 pronouncement targeting pauper bodies *Frankenstein* was acquiring meanings which Mary Shelley could not have foreseen. The key moment in this process is 1828, when the Burke and Hare affair put a quite new complexion on her story. In the metamorphosis of *Frankenstein* after 1818 we see how medical and legislative change plays a part in the origins of the English murder story. The Anatomy Act was a feared article of law because it threatened all poor – and potentially poor – people with dissection as an ultimate social fate. *Frankenstein* is the classic fictional account of the bodysnatching era. At the same time it is the story of the anatomy legislation, for it enacts the social meanings of the utilitarian ideology which eventually carried Abernethy's suggestion into law.

The 'anatomy literature' is certainly nothing to do with human anatomy in a technical sense. Rather, it is the literature, or a sample of it, which gives the best fictional account of the bodysnatching era, irrespective of whether the subject of human dissection is raised. Initially, the intriguing fact is the apparent reticence on the subject in early nineteenth-century texts. The silence means, however, that the question of its representation remains open to exploration. There are a number of stories – for example, Dickens' 'The Black Veil' and, later, Stevenson's 'The Bodysnatcher' – that explicitly refer to the dead body business, but these are not my particular concern in this book. Instead, I want to make the case for a much broader constituency of representation that can appropriately be called 'anatomy literature', and to explore some samples of it. The anatomy literature is essentially the literature that concerns the social ideologies which triumphed in 1832, the year of the Great Reform Bill.

The famous face in *Frankenstein* belongs to Victor Frankenstein, not the Creature. It is a masked face. At the centre of my reading of the story is the fact that Frankenstein decides to remain tight-lipped about what he knows. His death-bed narrative tells how he encountered non-stop murder and corpse after corpse: William his brother; Clerval his friend; Elizabeth his bride. On his wedding-day, moreover, this aspiring middle-class medical man, as the phrase goes, marries not for money, but where money is: he marries into aristocratic wealth. *Frankenstein* is a proleptic allegory of the 1832 political marriage between the aristocracy and the upper ranks of the middle class. Frankenstein enjoins his bride to an obligation not to ask any questions until after the ceremony of their union. His wedding-day face, in other words, has the interdictory quality which is the true face of the mask.[26]

The story of the 1832 Anatomy Act has recently been told, at least in large part, by a number of historians.[27] It is not possible for me to state the extent of my debt to the various historians whose work first informed me of this legislation. My reading of Mary Shelley's story would not have been possible without the prompting of Ruth Richardson's impressive study of the Anatomy Act in its historical context, and I am deeply indebted to her original research.

*Murdering to Dissect* derives from Foucault's and Bakhtin's writings and is my reading of their ideas. The first chapter of Foucault's *Discipline and Punish* describes the primal scene of the body-snatching era: the spectacle of the condemned man on the scaffold, the visible scene of crowds and power. And the legislative moment of 1832 reveals how a social crisis activates what Bakhtin calls the 'multi-accented' nature of the sign: that is, the capacity of language to register a diversity of social meanings. However, the nature and meaning of Frankenstein's mask is not to be found in Foucault or Bakhtin, but elsewhere. The description of the mask is given

---

[26] Canetti, 1981, 435.

[27] Richardson (1989), Fido (1988), Bailey (1991), Cole (1964), Ball (1989) and Edwards (1980) are the main authorities.

by Elias Canetti in *Crowds and Power.* Canetti won the Nobel Prize for Literature in 1981, but his study of mass psychology remains more or less neglected. *Crowds and Power* provides new concepts and has much to offer to literary and cultural studies. I have attempted to use it creatively, applying rather than summarising its ideas. *Murdering to Dissect* is my essay on Canetti. I have given him an extended say on the mastery of the body in the modern era, particularly where *Frankenstein* is concerned. Canetti's death in 1994 makes it all the more appropriate that his voice should be heard.

# Part I

# *Frankenstein*: the 1832 context

CHAPTER 1

# The dead body business

## Bentham's auto-icon

The scarecrow-like figure on the frontispiece of this book is a representation of Jeremy Bentham, the utilitarian philosopher who died in 1832, aged eighty-five. Bentham left instructions that after his death his body was to go to the surgeons for the purpose of a public dissection in a London anatomy school. His wishes in this respect went back to a will made as early as 1769, which he revised two months before his death to confirm his special request. It was his desire that his body should be used to illustrate the structure and the functions of the human body, and to promote a recognition within society of the usefulness of this kind of knowledge. It was a gesture of solidarity with the medical profession of the day and a recognition of the legitimacy of the then relatively new science of morbid anatomy.

The auto-icon, as it is called, was made as Bentham ordered it. It is a waxwork likeness of himself, dressed in his own clothes and with his walking stick in his hand; it is mounted on the skeleton which the surgeon articulated in a sitting posture. The dried head beside him is his actual preserved head, but it was felt by his close associates to be so unlike the live Bentham that a commissioned wax-head was substituted shortly after his death. The auto-icon is kept in a cabinet in the cloisters of University College, London, and is exhibited on ceremonial occasions. It is but a step from this rather strange artefact to the famous novel *Frankenstein*. The connection concerns the study of human anatomy by dissection; more precisely, it concerns the legitimation of dissection as indispensable to the advance and improvement of medical knowledge and education. Bentham's subtitle for his representation of himself was 'further uses of the dead to the living'. The figure in the glass showcase understood science in an eighteenth-century sense, that is to say, as a practical art based on empirical knowledge. In this conviction the great philosopher of utility sits in his own self-representation – disembodied, and offering his body to medical science.

The gesture is ambiguous, and the story of its ambiguity is told in *Frankenstein.* The auto-icon denies, or negates, the full reality of what has been done to the body. It is a remarkably intact-looking Jeremy Bentham who countenances the clinical dismantlement of the human body to a point beyond all ordinary recognition.

Bentham's gesture needs to be understood in its contemporary context. It is not an isolated gesture. On the contrary, it is part of a concerted but only partially successful programme of propaganda within officialdom in the 1820s which aimed to secure the legitimacy of dissection, and with it the legitimation of the medical profession. As we saw in the Introduction, the low public standing of the medical profession in the early nineteenth century was due to a large extent to its reluctant but necessary trade complicity with the graverobbers. The dead body business connection brought with it an unwelcome association with the unclean and the profane which inevitably made it next to impossible for the profession to present itself as properly scientific and in alliance with polite society.

Since the 1790s, particularly in the context of the armed forces, an urgent requirement for trained surgeons had arisen. In a sixteen-month course in surgery and anatomy every student required a minimum of three corpses to dissect. The traditional source of supply, sanctioned by royal grant, were the bodies of convicted murderers supplied by the hangman to the surgeons. This supply-line, however, as I have noted, bound the profession into an unwelcome association with the gallows. The result, as Ruth Richardson observes, was that 'the surgeon-anatomist became an executioner of the law'.[1] This was an identity which regularly earned the surgeons a hostile reception from the large crowds that attended public executions in the eighteenth century.

[1] Richardson, 1989, 34.

The 1752 Act of Parliament for 'better Preventing the horrid Crime of Murder' is an illustration of some of these difficulties. In respect of sentences for murder, it gave the Bench the discretion to order a public dissection of the criminal's body in place of a gibbeting. The move added a further punitive dimension to the punishment for murder. However, over the course of time the intention and the effect of the law placed complications in the way of the medical profession's long bid for legitimacy. By design, the law associated dissection with the punishment meted out to the worst offenders; henceforth, dissection was invested with a stigma which was difficult if not impossible to remove in the long term. The ruling elite made dissection an object of dread or superstitious fear – as the Act explicitly stated, an object of 'further Terror'.[2] The popular perception had long had reason to link dissection with punishment; and it is in this context that Bentham's opportunist donation of his own body gains its significance.

Furthermore, the gallows theatre confronted the beleaguered surgeons with their chief practical problem, for the number of corpses from this source was not equal to their requirements. It was an awkward point, but from their professional point of view there was not enough murder in society. By the 1820s several thousand bodies were required per annum, but no legal provision existed to supply them on this scale. The need to obtain corpses by some other legal source, and to end the compromising association with the hangman, is the crux of the medical profession's legitimacy problem in the early nineteenth century. Bentham's auto-icon stands as testimony to his lifelong commitment to break the popular association between dissection and murder, and with it to dissolve the stigma. It happens, indeed, that in the decade before his death Bentham devised the enduring solution to the surgeons' difficulties.

Bentham's solution was the Anatomy Act of 1832. In the national context, the legislation is a milestone in the transition to modernity that Michel Foucault describes in *Discipline and Punish*,

---

2 *Ibid.*, 37.

the story of the development of the techniques and practices of 'disciplinary' society.[3] One reader of Foucault has characterised the transition in a way that has an apt application to Bentham's proposal. Michel De Certeau comments that:

> what Foucault analyses is a chiasmus: how the place occupied by humanitarian and reformist projects at the end of the eighteenth century is then 'colonized' or 'vampirized' by those disciplinary procedures that have since increasingly organised the social realm itself. This mystery story narrates a plot of substituted corpses, the sort of game of substitution that would have pleased Freud.[4]

The historical context suggests that it is not Freud but the caste of surgeons, in fiction as well as reality, who had best reason to appreciate *a plot of substituted corpses*. A plot of this kind was in hand when the third edition of *Frankenstein* appeared in 1831. The Anatomy Act became law just months afterwards, in August 1832. It was long in design and the early stages of its inception were surrounded by secrecy. As its architect and patron intended, it achieved the utilitarian objective of obligating the dead to be useful to society. It has been commented that the auto-icon is 'the sacred relic of a secular creed'[5] which gained in stridency after 1832. The creed, utilitarianism, is one face of the middle-class hegemony which begins with the new political arrangements of the Great Reform Bill.

The class issue is central to the reading that I shall give of *Frankenstein* as an allegory of 1832. In the period preceding the legislation, grave robbery and dissection crossed class boundaries and this fact is the key to the labyrinth of the social implications of the new law. In a remarkable synchronicity of parliamentary discourse, the Anatomy Act leads a low profile, peek-a-boo existence, overshadowed by the monumental public moment of the

---

3 See Foucault, 1979.
4 De Certeau, 1986, 185.
5 Harrison, 1983, 22.

Reform Bill. The legislation – after a number of bureaucratic teething problems – delivered a reliable supply of corpses to the slab. The surgeons were granted automatic access to unclaimed bodies from the workhouse. As the chronology shows at 1832, the Reform Bill receives Royal Assent in the days between Bentham's death and his dissection, and on 1 August 1832 the Anatomy Act becomes law. The complex history of the new anatomy law is described by Ruth Richardson in *Death, Dissection and the Destitute.* The backcover summary of her book spells out the plot of substituted corpses:

> Before 1832 dissection was a feared and hated punishment for murder. The 1832 Anatomy Act requisitioned instead the corpses of the poor, transferring the penalty from murder to poverty. The Act contributed to the terrible fear of the Victorian workhouse and influences attitudes to death even today.[6]

Before 1832 the surgeons' dependency on the resurrectionist connection was usually accompanied by a barely disguised disdain for the men who provided the developing science with its materials. Sir Astley Cooper, the President of the Royal College of Surgeons, told a Parliamentary Select Committee in 1828 that the grave-robbers were 'the lowest dregs of degradation', and that he traded with them out of necessity. He observed that 'there is no crime they would not commit'.[7] This emphasis plainly anticipates murder as a logical development, as the Burke and Hare scandal later in the same year was to prove. The events in Edinburgh in 1828 were to clarify the fact that the dead body business had always been – in all but name – the medicine of murder.

## Richardson's argument in *Death, Dissection and the Destitute*

Richardson's reconstruction of the Burke and Hare scandal and the 1832 legislation in *Death, Dissection and the Destitute* deeply

---

6 I refer to the Penguin edition 1989.

7 Richardson, 1989, 117. Also quoted by Low, 1987, 91.

enriches our understanding of the society and culture of early nineteenth-century England. As a piece of major historical research, it provides opportunities to rethink the literary culture of this period; and, although it is not a work of fiction, it reads at times like Mary Shelley's compelling prose. In an early review Asa Briggs commented most appropriately that '1832 will never seem quite the same again'.[8] In this book I shall extend this compliment, for the same applies to *Frankenstein* once the anatomy legislation enters the frame of interpretation. However, even in the continuing critical appeal to the story's historical context the absence of reference to the Anatomy Act remains conspicuous.[9] Johanna Smith, for example, a recent editor of the 1831 edition, invokes the relevant scenario but omits the vital dimension of 1832, a 'double bill' in the theatre of politics:

> It is significant that the novel was re-issued in 1831, at a time when '[t]he burnings, the alarms, the absorbing politics of the day render booksellers almost adverse to publishing at all' (Letters 2.120). The 'politics of the day' to which the author refers are the increasing, and increasingly violent, public debates over a Reform Bill whose early version would have enfranchised a portion of the working as well as the middle classes. [The] former's fitness for the vote was already in question when *Frankenstein* was first published in 1818. By 1831 the issue was bitterly disputed; the propertied class feared to lose its executive legislative power to the propertyless rabble, a fear exacerbated when the working class supporters of the Reform Bill rioted each time the House of Commons voted it down.[10]

In the anatomy context, this emphasis on the escalation of public tensions and the changing political agendas between 1818 and 1831 has its most striking application in the 1829 to 1831 context. Richardson argues:

---

[8] The comment appears on the back cover of the 1989 Penguin edition.
[9] The only references I have found to the Anatomy Act by literary critics are by During, 1992, 54; and Baldick, 1987, 193.
[10] Shelley, 1992, 14.

> A close relationship between the two Bills was perceived at the time . . . It was surely not merely a coincidence that a cleverly doctored version of the Anatomy Bill which had failed in 1829 succeeded in passing through Parliament in 1832, neck-and-neck with the Reform Bill. In the interval attitudes towards the lower orders had hardened, and neither appeals to paternalist sentimentality nor fears of mob rule – which had thwarted the first Anatomy Act before – could muster sufficient parliamentary voice to prevent its passage, only a few weeks after the Reform Act. A few MPs may perhaps have been guiltily aware of their broken bargain with the working classes, but the new brutality which would be responsible for the New Poor Law two years later was in the ascendant before the Reform Act had altered parliamentary personnel.[11]

The harder attitude was always on tap, as the early editions of *Frankenstein* show. Victor Frankenstein's vocabulary is heavy with paternalist metaphor *before* he encounters his creation – and then things change. In the event, his Creature is doomed at first sight to utter condemnation. Richardson points to the decisive phase of a broad change in attitude towards 'the lower orders'. Frankenstein's dishonouring of his promise of a mate for his 'monster' is the pivot of the political allegory which his narrative constructs; the broken pledge rehearses the class betrayal which occurred on a grand scale in 1832. The reissue of *Frankenstein* in 1831 gives the story a powerfully reflective relationship to the 1820s and also to the decade of its original composition.

Johanna Smith has nevertheless rendered a valuable service to historical studies of *Frankenstein* by drawing attention to 'the characteristically double view of the Reform Bill' presented in Mary Shelley's letters.[12] On the one hand, Mary Shelley deems it 'good sense' on the part of 'the autocrats' to 'make the necessary sacrifices to a starving people'.[13] On the other hand, in another letter, she

---

11 Richardson, 1989, 262.
12 Shelley, 1992, 15.
13 *Ibid.*, 14–15.

is clearly in fear of the 'sick destructiveness' that accompanies the essentially laudable revolutionary will to quell 'tyranny'.[14] Yet: 'without [it] . . . [ie. the "sick destructiveness"], would our Land-holders be brought to reason? Yet it is very sad – the punishment of the poor men being not the least disaster attendant on it.' (*Letters* 2.122)[15] Here the punitive dimension of the anatomy legislation is plainly anticipated in Mary Shelley's language, even if it is not in her mind. Retaliative attitudes surfaced in the national reform debate around the time of these remarks, when the third edition of *Frankenstein* appeared. In my reading of the anatomy text in the story, I will cite passages that are consistent with both the fears and the sympathies in play in this correspondence. However, the priority here has to be the injunction to 'never trust the artist – trust the tale',[16] for what I am concerned with is a reading of the story as such, not the mind of the writer. In 1818, the year of the first edition, Mary Shelley was hardly to know of the events that were to occur in Edinburgh in the late 1820s.

The 'burnings' Mary Shelley refers to are undoubtedly the 'Swing' riots, the rick-burning demonstrations that swept through southern England throughout 1831,[17] and arson is a key motif in her story. However, the phrase 'the alarms' stands tantalisingly unglossed in her letter, and in Johanna Smith's commentary. It is compatible with some widely publicised developments that occurred in the wake of Burke and Hare – developments which, Richardson argues, hastened the anatomy legislation.[18] Burko-phobia versions of Burke and Hare took place in November 1831 in London, the possibilities of which had long been in the air. Indeed, murder had been predicted before the great scandal erupted.[19] The corpse was hitting the headlines when *Frankenstein*, a best-seller in 1818, reappeared in 1831.

---

14 *Ibid.*

15 *Ibid.*

16 Lawrence, 1961, 297.

17 See Hobsbawm and Rudé, 1985.

18 Richardson, 1989, 194.

19 *Ibid.*, 132.

The ideological compatibility of the Reform Act and the Anatomy Act is an integral part of the social meaning of the former measure, and much is lost without the emphasis that they are two sides of the same coin. The masking of the anatomy legislation by the Reform drama is not just a contingent irony; on the contrary, it is an effacement which lends to the Great Reform Act the character, and ambiguity, of a mask. In the contemporary working-class perceptions the terror inspired by the anatomy legislation appears as this mask's core or real shape – its least dissimulated face. 'The claim for the vote', comments E. P. Thompson, 'implied also further claims: a new way of reaching out by the working people for *social control* over their conditions of life and labour'.[20] Nowhere is the denial of this control more in evidence than in the threat imposed by the Anatomy Act, which, Richardson argues, was 'in reality an advance clause to the 1834 Poor Law'.[21] In the pre-legislative context, the case for the 'mask of 1832' is made in *Frankenstein*; but not before the story has sufficiently rehearsed the mask's meaning in the constituency of those who were to become its victims.

Richardson mentions *Frankenstein* three times in her introduction. She remarks that it was Mary Shelley's novel which first prompted her to inquire 'if the fictional doctor's researches in charnel houses bore any relationship to the historical personages Burke and Hare, and the bodysnatchers'.[22] The question led her to the 1832 anatomy legislation. Presenting her findings, Richardson comments that the topic really requires 'the necessity of a further decade's work to do the subject justice'.[23] By this she means further historical research, but her own commentary on *Oliver Twist*[24] recognises the value of literary readings in an interdisciplinary account of 1832. I shall show that the relevant texts constitute an 'anatomy' literature, a large creative statement.

---

20 E. P. Thompson, 1980, 910.
21 Richardson, 1989, 266.
22 *Ibid.*, xiii.
23 *Ibid.*, xiv.
24 *Ibid.*, 147–8.

In the literary context of the anatomy debate some of the most significant ideas in modern linguistic and critical theory come into play. The formative writings here, alongside Foucault's work on discourse and power, are Volosinov/Bakhtin's work on discourse as concrete, socio-ideological communication.[25] These writings will inform my reading of *Frankenstein*. I will introduce them here and in the next chapter. I will use references from Richardson's account, Sir Walter Scott's *Journal*, and the writings of Thomas De Quincey and Charles Dickens.

## Sir Walter Scott in Edinburgh, 1829

Richardson employs a decisive phrase that resounds through her long ideological analysis of 1832 and its antecedents. She identifies the 'successful redefinition of poverty as crime'[26] as a tactic of class warfare in the 1820s and 1830s. The transference of a stigma from criminality to poverty did not escape the attention of the Anatomy Act's potential victims, as Richardson's definition of the word 'poor' indicates:

> It signifies those who – whatever their occupation and present fortune – could never be, or never feel to be, fully sure of their distance from the workhouse. It therefore includes all working people, particularly the elderly, and much of the lower middle class, whose financial security was often only fragile. It signifies as much a state of mind as an economic reality – the pauper's funeral was an object of fear and loathing outside as well as inside workhouse walls.[27]

The popular assumption of a criminal stigma attaching to dissection remained intractable in the nineteenth century. The following extract, which Richardson does not cite,[28] from Sir Walter Scott's

---

[25] It is now virtually certain that *Marxism and the Philosophy of Language* is substantially Bakhtin's work.
[26] Richardson, 1989, 152.
[27] *Ibid.*, xvi.
[28] Richardson does use Scott's *Journal*, however (1989, 133).

1829 *Journal* acknowledges the contemporary perceptions of the stigma. Scott's observations on Burke and Hare – he attended Burke's execution in 1829 – are remarkable for their sympathetic insight into the whole consequence of the bodysnatching scandal. Scott, as Richardson says, 'understood and sympathised'[29] with the popular view that Dr Knox was an accessory to the crime of murder:

> The law which as a deeper sentence on the guilt of murder [enacts] that the body of the convi[c]ted criminal should be given up to anatomy is certainly not without effect for criminals have been known to shrink from that part of the sentence which seem[ed] to afict [*sic*] them more than the doom of death itself with all its terrors here and hereafter. On the other hand while this idea of the infamy attending the exposition of the person is thus recognised by the laws it is impossible to adopt regulations which would effectively prevent such horrid crimes as the murder of vagrant wretches who can be snatchd from society without their being missed as in the late conspiracy.[30]

Next, Scott ponders the social options and notes the susceptibilities that stand affected:

> For instance if it was now to be enacted, as seems reasonable, that persons dying in hospitals and almshouses who die without their friends claiming their remains should be given up to the men of science, *this would be subjecting poverty to the penalty of these atrocious criminals whom Law distinguishes by the heaviest posthumous disgrace which it can inflict* [italics added].[31]

And his own feelings on the matter are that:

> Even cultivated minds revolt from the exposure on an anatomical table when the case is supposed to be that of one who is dear to them. I should, I am conscious, be willing that I

---

29 *Ibid.*, 1989, 133.
30 Scott, 1972, 505.
31 *Ibid.*

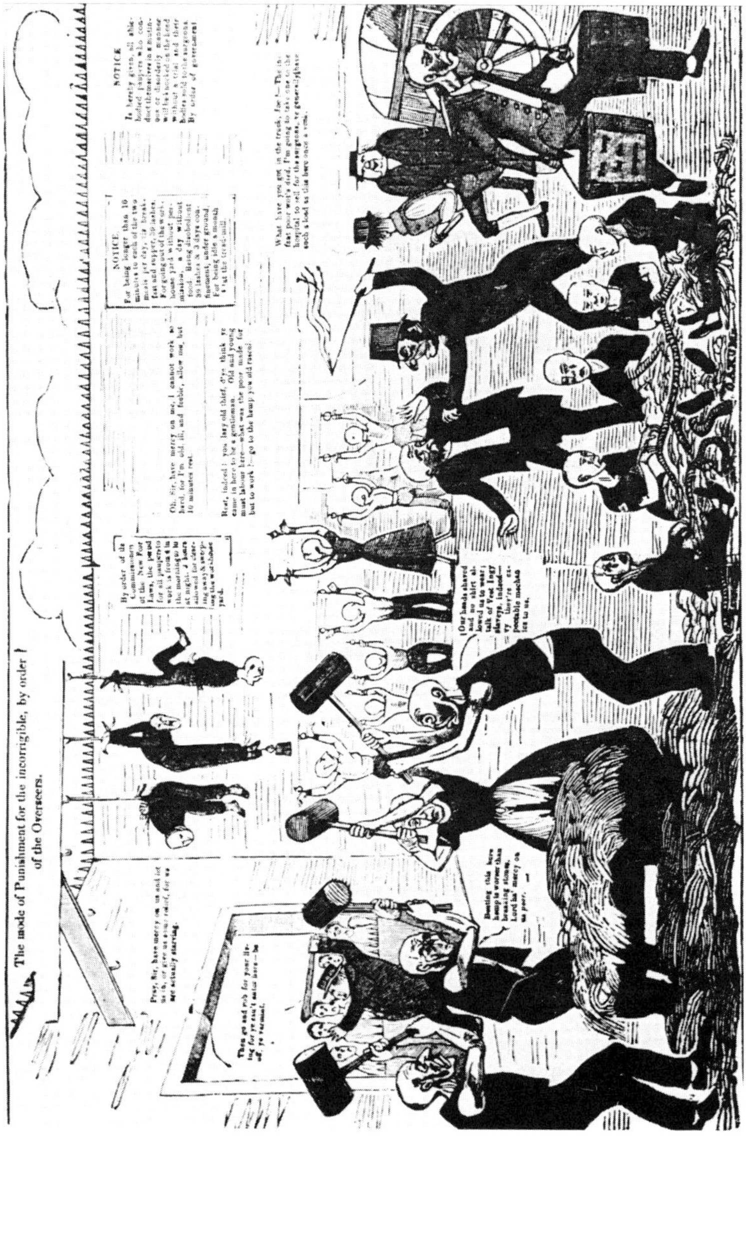
The mode of Punishment for the incorrigible, by order of the Overseers.
Pray, Sir, have mercy on us and let us in, or give us some relief, for we are actually starving.
Then go and rob for your living for ye can't starve here—be off, ye varmint.
Beating this here hemp is worser than breaking stones. Lord ha' mercy on us poor.
Oh, Sir, have mercy on me, I cannot work so hard, for I'm old, ill, and feeble, allow me, but 10 minutes rest.
Rest, indeed! you lazy old thief, d'ye think ye came in here to be a gentleman. Old and young must labour here—what was the poor made for but to work? go to the hemp you old rascal.
NOTICE
NOTICE

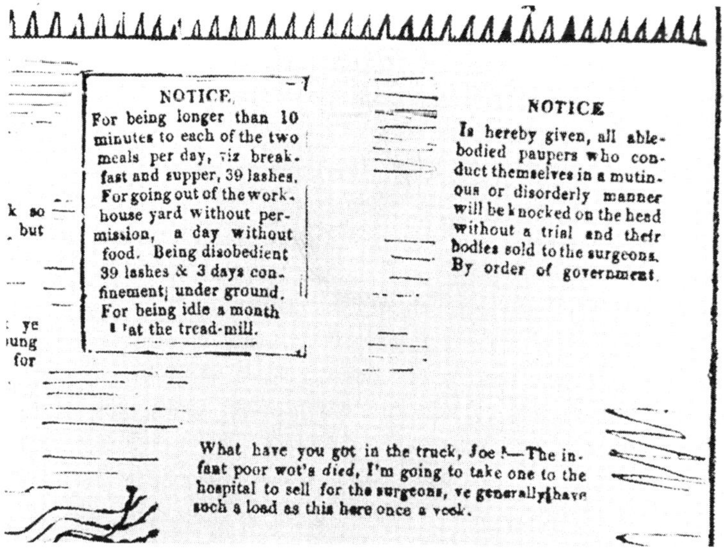


Cartoon (opposite) and detail (above) of the interior of a workhouse under the New Poor Law of 1834.

> myself should be dissected in publick if doing so could produce any advantage to Society but when I think on relations and friends being rent from the grave the case is very different and I would fight knee deep to prevent or punish such an exposure. So inconsistent we are all upon matters of this nature.[32]

In Edinburgh at the time, Scott is staring at the thin end of the wedge, for Burke and Hare did not rob from the grave – they killed the living. This witness is aware of a potential for hypocrisy where the search for solutions is concerned. As he foresees the criminalisation of poverty, Scott is saying, in effect, that one person's 'advantage' will be gained by another person's ignominious fate somewhere lower in the social scale. 'In the course of the first century of the Anatomy Act's application' comments

[32] *Ibid.*

Richardson, 'almost 57,000 bodies were dissected in the London anatomy schools alone. Less than *half a percent* came from anywhere other than institutions which housed the poor'.[33]

In the pre-1832 context *Frankenstein* rehearses the class bias – and the hypocrisy – which informs the Anatomy Act. And in a remarkable coincidence, the self-regarding middle-class anxieties of the bodysnatching era surface not long after Frankenstein and Clerval visit – of all places – Edinburgh. First, the 'resurrection' cameo in Frankenstein's retrospective account confirms his interest in the dead – his mother and his own bride-in-waiting no less; the cameo follows his use of human remains in the dissecting room. The narrative then sees the 'monster' acting out Scott's worst apprehensions: 'relations and friends' are singled out on an improvised but not arbitrary hit-list of class targets. William, the blood-relative, is the first victim. After the visit to Edinburgh, Clerval, Frankenstein's middle-class friend, is murdered and his body turns up in Ireland, Burke and Hare's original domicile. Elizabeth is the next and the last corpse to be delivered to the anatomist. This occurs on the wedding-day which marks both Frankenstein's and Elizabeth's ritual passage into bourgeois respectability. Elizabeth, notably, is a young woman who once lived in extreme poverty, and this fact is in play on the wedding-night. This fact above all, as I shall show, enables her murder to make sense in the social context I am outlining here – sense, that is to say, to the Creature himself. Elizabeth's murder is the Creature's final statement on the social and ultimately the legislative dimension of the medicine of murder.

In his *Journal* Scott gives this pen-sketch of the public's voracious appetite for the scandal:

> The corpse of the Murderer Burke is now lying in state at the College in the anatomical class and all the world flock to see him. Who is he says that we are not ill to please in our objects of curiosity? The strange means by which the wretch made money are scarce more disgusting than the eager curiosity with

[33] Richardson, 1989, 271.

> which the publick have lickd up all carrion details of this business.[34]

When the copycat killings occurred, the medical academy of the 1820s badly needed to close its front door to the public – as well as its back-door business. It is not possible to know what Mary Shelley had in mind when she refered in 1831 to 'the alarms' – but there was warrant for her choice of words. Scott, her social associate, is hearing the alarm bells as the scandal breaks around him in Edinburgh.

## The surgeon as murderer: *On Murder considered as one of the Fine Arts*

The pre-1832 public image of the medical profession in the early nineteenth century is described in two main texts of the anatomy literature: De Quincey's *On Murder considered as one of the Fine Arts* and Dickens' *Barnaby Rudge*. De Quincey's essay is a complex conceit to the effect that civilisation declines as the capacity to promote the art of murder falls into atrophy. There is one instalment of this essay prior to 1832, and two following it; the first appeared in 1827. Its usual anthology form, however, comprises the first two instalments, which are separated by a time-break of twelve years. The 1827 instalment passes off as the text of a commemoration Lecture on the state of the art delivered by an official of high standing in a clandestine Society of Connoisseurs in Murder Club. The reader is extended a vicarious membership. However, De Quincey lets it appear as if the lecture is being leaked to the public. As a 'disclosure', therefore, the Lecture on the art of murder acquires a double private-public accentuation.

The time-break division in the 1827/1839 text corresponds to a distinction drawn by De Quincey's persona in the 1839 section, where he emphatically distinguishes between *degrees* of artistry in murder. *Amateurism*, he declares, has been superseded and a

34 Scott, 1972, 514.

transition to *connoisseurship* has been achieved.[35] The first two instalments of *On Murder* rehearse an archive history of the art from its earliest origins – starting from Cain who 'tooled with his teeth'[36] – right up, as a long-delayed climax, to Burke and Hare. As I noted in the Introduction, Harc escaped prosecution by turning King's evidence, the move which secured the conviction against Burke:

> Gentlemen, we fancy Burkism to be a pure invention of our times . . . Still I have ascertained that the essential principle of the art *was* known to the ancients, although . . . it was lost in the dark ages for want of encouragement . . . By the way, gentlemen, has anyone heard lately of Hare? I understand he is comfortably settled in Ireland, considerably to the west, and does a little business now and then; but, as he observes with a sigh, only as a retailer – nothing like the fine wholesale concern so carelessly blown up at Edinburgh . . .[37]

In the 1827 'amateurism' instalment De Quincey observes the medical profession's historic association with the hangman: the surgeon as the executioner. As Peter Linebaugh has recorded,[38] around the gallows in the eighteenth century a popular charge of 'Murder' was frequently directed at the surgeons – the figures, in the crowd's view, who were completing the executioner's work. The crowd, that is to say, drew no distinction between the killer and the healer. De Quincey's example of this conflation concerns a highwayman, the 'artist' of a number of murders. The lecturer's anecdote recalls the days when the surgeons waited in the wings of the scaffold:

> I came to know who the artist was, from a celebrated surgeon, who assisted at his dissection. This gentleman had a private museum in the way of his profession, one corner of which was

35 See *Selected English Essays*, 1918, 336.
36 *Ibid.*, 349.
37 *Ibid.*, 350–2.
38 Linebaugh, 1977, 85.

> occupied by the cast of a man of remarkably fine proportions . . . 'That,' said the surgeon, 'is a cast from the celebrated Lancashire highwayman . . . At the time of his execution for highway robbery, I was studying under Cruickshank: and the man's figure was so uncommonly fine, that no money or exertion was spared to get into possession of him with the least possible delay. By the connivance of the under-sheriff he was cut down within the legal time, and instantly put into a chaise and four; so that, when he reached Cruickshank's, he was positively not dead. Mr——. a young student at the time, had the honour of giving him the *coup de grâce – and finishing the sentence of the law.*' This remarkable anecdote, which seemed to imply that all the gentlemen in the dissecting-room were amateurs of our class, struck me a good deal . . . [italics added] [39]

There is the flicker of a grimly ironic joke here about late reprieves. As Canetti observes:

> A stricken creature is given the *coup de grâce.* If it was dangerous when alive it becomes an object of hatred when it is dead . . . It is blamed for still being in everyone's way when dead; it ought not to exist at all, not even as the empty husk of a body.[40]

Richardson reports a number of instances of surgeons employing all kinds of subterfuge, often involving money, in order to secure the remains of monstrous human beings, the coveted items for the cabinet.[41] The 'collector's piece' has long possessed a proximity to the monstrous; it is in effect a fetish object, and the highwayman's remains here are the inanimate version of another kind of obscene human exhibition. In the eighteenth century, as a present-day anatomist has observed, refinement could be shown 'in the ability to entertain guests by taking them on a tour of a privately owned teratology ward'.[42] In the private-public enclosure of the

---

39 De Quincey, 1918, 325.
40 Canetti, 1981, 455.
41 Richardson, 1989, 57–8.
42 Gonzalez-Crussi, 1986, 102.

1827 Lecture on Murder, the executioner-surgeon association is explicit as the speaker indicates that 'the gentlemen in the dissecting-room were *amateurs* of our class' of murderers. Connoisseurship, in the distinction proposed, is the art of operating as murderers outside public space and away from compromising associations. The 'gentlemen' here in the 1827 text are on their way to a historic landmark in the Society's acquisition of the fine art, the Anatomy Act no less. Now the 1839 text does *not* say this explicitly. The second instalment ends with reminiscence of the Murder Club's 1838 riotous commemoration dinner – and laughter – as toasts proclaimed in Latin go up to Burke and Hare. The profession's recent legislative transformation, however, is the subtext to this salute. Burke and Hare's day is hailed as a 'sublime epoch'.[43] As underworld agents of the official State machinery, their 'revolution in the art'[44] helped to ensure that after 1832 those who could be cut up and those who were exempt from threat fell into socially distinct categories. The revellers resolve never to drink an inferior toast from the same glass.[45] In 1839 – and 1827 – *On Murder considered as one of the Fine Arts* is saying that a better health provision requires a better aesthetics of murder.

In connection with the surgeons, De Quincey's essay reads as an anticipation of Foucault's account of the transition to disciplinary society. The argument in *Discipline and Punish* has a clear-cut shape: the modern penal system came into being to replace the gallows spectacle of violent punishment with widely distributed forms of surveillance and social control. The visible indications of power precipitated a crisis of social control. The violence on the gallows required – and became the pretext for – a more economical management of signs: 'The punitive practice of the nineteenth century was to strive to put as much distance as possible between the 'serene' search for truth and the violence that cannot be entirely effaced from punishment.'[46]

---

43 De Quincey, 1918, 350.
44 *Ibid.*, 345.
45 *Ibid.*, 352.
46 Foucault, 1979, 56.

The fact that the last public execution in Britain was as late as 1868 suggests a less clear-cut state of affairs, a coexistence of spectacle and surveillance throughout much of the nineteenth century. The scene of open violence advertised a punitive power soiling its hands 'with a crime greater than the one it wished to punish'.[47] This proposal is most plausible in the pre-1832 dissection context. The crowd animus made its contribution to the reasons officialdom gave itself to eliminate capital punishment as a public spectacle of violence. In Foucault's story, humanism, or 'disciplinary' society, was born in a displacement of power into the production and surveillance of society itself. As Linebaugh has shown, the gallows crowd in the early eighteenth century frequently attempted to retrieve the body, in flashpoints of conflict with the anatomists.[48] De Quincey's highwayman anecdote is a covert acknowledgement of the popular perception that the surgeons were the 'real' murderers. But the *coup de grâce* delivered here, within the 'private' frame of the Lecture, shows the surgeons gaining distance from the angry crowd's reading of the violence. The crowd accepted no limits on its numbers; by the same token, however, the volume of protest made the case for a displacement of power.

In this connection, as early as 1755, Henry Fielding, police magistrate for Westminster – and dramatist – proposed curtailing the street procession to the scaffold and holding the executions at Newgate, thereby privatising the ritual to some degree. Drawing on his knowledge of literary device to carry his contention, Fielding argued that 'a murder behind the scenes, if the poet knows how to manage it, will effect the audience with greater terror than if it was acted before their eyes'.[49] This oddly uncircumspect use of an analogy with murder is telling. The proposal from Fielding – to semi-privatise the event within prison vicinities – was adopted in 1783. Fielding had long been uncomfortable

---

47 *Ibid.*

48 See Linebaugh, 1977.

49 Quoted in David Cooper, 1974, 99.

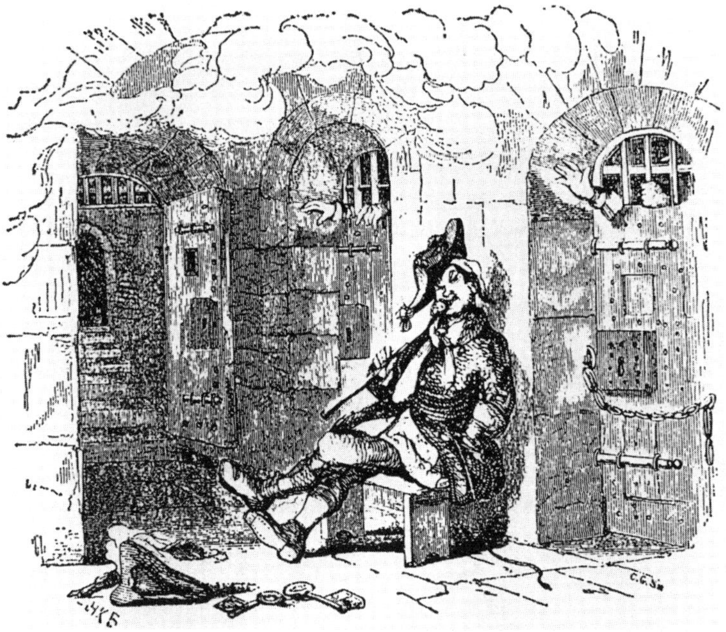

Cattermole and Brown, 'Mr Dennis the executioner' from Charles Dickens, *Barnaby Rudge*.

about the significance of a collapsing symbolism; he wanted smoother procedures. Noting the move from Tyburn to Newgate, Dr Johnson generalised that 'all the business of the world is to be done in a new way'.[50]

## The contented executioner in *Barnaby Rudge*

The illustration from *Barnaby Rudge* shows the executioner Mr Ned Dennis seated contentedly outside the cells of the men condemned to death in Newgate, as the rioting populace starts to set this hated prison on fire. In this novel, his portrait of England

[50] Quoted in Porter, 1982, 293.

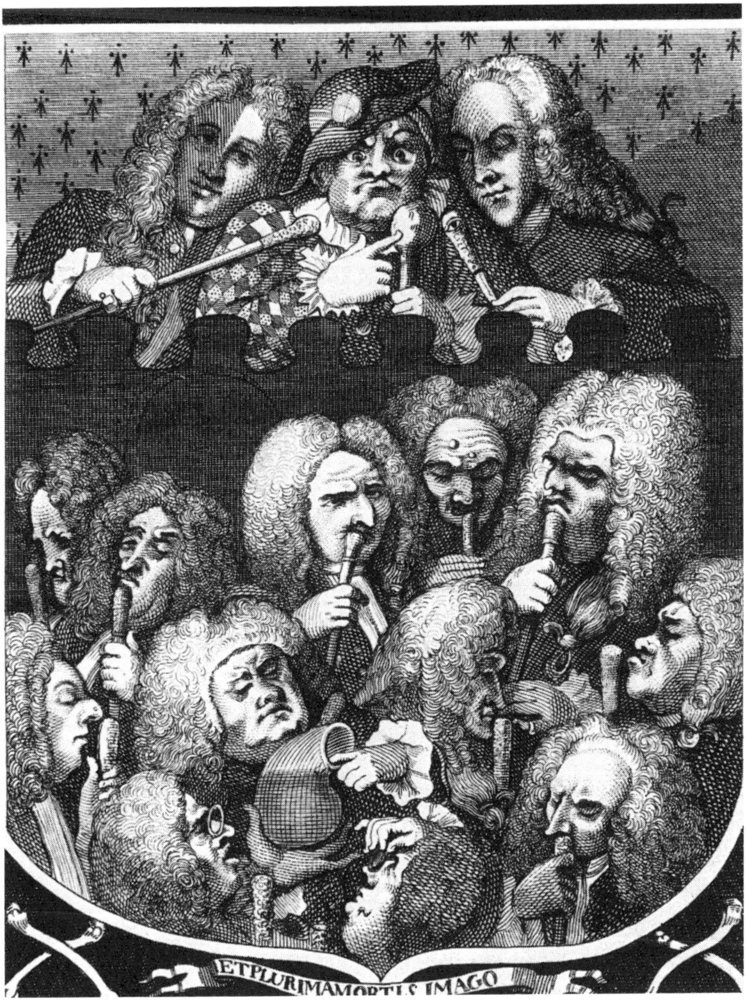

William Hogarth, 'Consultation of Physicians' or 'The Company of Undertakers' or 'Consultation of Quacks'.

in the 1780s, Dickens provides the most graphic account in the anatomy literature of the mechanisms of power which found unacceptable public form in the gallows ritual, and in particular the figure of the executioner. The illustration gains a further significance as it borrows a detail from Hogarth's 'Consultation of Physicians' (which was originally called 'A Consultation of Quacks'). Mr Dennis appears as a duplicate of Hogarth's figure of the cane-sniffing doctor in a way that corroborates the popular association of the executioner with the medical profession.

Ned Dennis is the embodiment – and the tool – of absolutism; 'this functionary of the law', Dickens calls him.[51] In a commentary in *Crowds and Power* on the giving and receiving of orders, Canetti observes that the executioner is an isolated figure who enjoys a special exemption from the command mechanisms which operate under despotic regimes.[52] Behind every command, Canetti argues, there stands ultimately the threat of death from a superior power. In the one who carries it out, the command inflicts a 'sting', a kind of cyst[53] which sinks into the person, hardening, unchanging, and never forgotten. This sting is retained indefinitely unless it can be got rid of by passing it on to an inferior. The death threat behind a command 'is almost invariably in excess of what need be used to bring about the desired action, and this is the real reason why a command leads to the formation of a sting'.[54] However, an order to a crowd, as opposed to an individual, is immediately diffused and leaves no sting behind. In the same way, individuals who accumulate stings, and who become overburdened with them, need a crowd in which to find relief from their oppression. In the 'reversal' of revolution the sting 'massifies' as the crowd turns against the sources of power and their symbols – as here in *Barnaby Rudge* with Newgate prison on fire.

But the executioner, the compliant official killer, is a special case. He alone enjoys a remarkable freedom from the oppression of stings. Canetti's analysis of the 'contented executioner' bears directly on Dickens' seated figure. In the story Mr Dennis joins the rioting crowd, but secretly maintains his real identity:

---

51 Dickens, 1987, 589.

52 Canetti, 1981, 383.

53 'Cyst' is the word Deleuze and Guattari (1988, 525) use to gloss Canetti's 'sting' metaphor.

54 Canetti, 1981, 384.

> The executioner is in the same position as anyone who submits to an order under the threat of death. But he becomes free himself from this threat by himself killing. He immediately passes on his own possible fate and so anticipates the ultimate penalty which hangs over himself. He is told to kill, and he kills . . . There is no time for a sting to form.
>
> But, even if there were time, there is no reason why a sting *should* form. An executioner passes on exactly what has been imposed on him. He has nothing to fear and so nothing remains behind in him. In his case, and in his only, the account balances; the essential nature of the command coincides with the action it brings about. Its fulfilment, moreover, is made easy for him; no obstacles are put in its way and it is unlikely that the victim will escape. All these circumstances are known to the executioner from the start. Thus he can regard the command with equanimity; he can trust it. He knows that carrying it out will change nothing in himself. It passes, as it were, straight through him, without damaging him at all. Of all men the executioner is the most contented, the least affected by stings.[55]

In the chapter in *Barnaby Rudge* entitled 'Mr Dennis enjoys himself' Dickens writes:

> here, in the heart of the building, and moreover with the prayers and cries of the four men under sentence sounding in his ears, and their hands, stretched out through the grating in the cell doors, clasped in frantic entreaty before his very eyes, it was particularly remarkable [to see a man enjoying himself]. Indeed Mr Dennis appeared to think it an uncommon circumstance, and to banter himself upon it; for he thrust his hat on one side as some men do when they are in a waggish humour, sucked the head of his stick with a higher relish, and smiled as though he would say, 'Dennis, you're a rum dog; you're a queer fellow; you're capital company, Dennis, and quite a character . . .[56]

---

[55] *Ibid.*, 383.
[56] Dickens, 1987, 589.

And he shares a vocabulary with the surgeons and De Quincey's murder artists: his victims, as he puts its, are 'subjects'.[57] 'I may call myself an artist – a fancy workman – art improves natur' – that's my motto',[58] says Dennis. Canetti comments on the commission to kill:

> killing others . . . [the executioner] frees himself from death. To him it is a clean business with nothing shocking or unnatural about it. He cannot find in himself any of the horror he awakens in others. It is important to be quite clear about this: official killers are contented in proportion as the commands they are given lead directly to death. A prison warder's life is far more difficult than an executioner's.[59]

Dickens' verbal portrait adds to the visual illustration, as it shows Mr Dennis aping the role of the prison official. The hangman 'addressed them [the condemned men] to this effect, in the tone and with the air of a pastor in familiar conversation with his flock':[60]

> Now look'ee here, you four. I'm come to take care of you, and see that you an't burnt, instead of the other thing. It's no use your making any noise . . . you'll only be hoarse when it comes to the speeches, – which is a pity. What I say in respect to the speeches always is, 'Give it mouth.' That's my maxim. Give it mouth . . . And always, when a thing of this natur's to come off, what I stand up for, is, a proper frame of mind. Let's have a proper frame of mind, and we can go through with it, creditable – pleasant – sociable. Whatever you do . . . never snivel. I'd sooner by half, though I lose by it, see a man tear his clothes a' purpose to spile 'em before they come to

---

57 *Ibid.*, 372.
58 *Ibid.*
59 Canetti, 1981, 384.
60 Dickens, 1987, 592.

> me, than find him snivelling. It's ten to one a better frame of mind, every way![61]

Here Mr Dennis projects through his counsel a statement of his own 'proper frame of mind' – his special case status. In dialogue with the illustration, Dickens comments that Dennis 'sat down on a bench in the gallery, and sucked the head of his stick with the utmost complacency, tranquillity and contentment'.[62]

The explicit links Dickens forges between Dennis and the surgeons will appear when we read the full anatomy story in *Barnaby Rudge*. My purpose here, in a supplement to De Quincey's portrait of the surgeon-executioner, is to focus what was so unwelcome – or monstrous – about the identity of the executioner as it shadowed medical efforts to advance life in the time before 1832. Commenting on the 1752 Murder Act, which added dissection to the punishment for murder, Richardson comments that those who framed it 'appear to have been concerned to a much greater extent with the infliction of punishment . . . than with incidental benefit to science'.[63] The 'sting of command' was written into the spirit and letter of the later anatomy legislation. As Bentham knew, it was a large element in the gallows stigma on dissection which persisted after 1832 as a fact of popular perception. In the next chapter I shall examine some of the ways in which the anatomy literature dramatises conflicting perceptions of the stigma – that is to say, how the literature enacts a social argument which intensifies in England in the 1820s.

---

61 *Ibid.*, 591.
62 *Ibid.*, 589.
63 Richardson, 1989, 36.

CHAPTER 2

# Multi-accentuation in *On Murder considered as one of the Fine Arts* and *Frankenstein*

## Social signs

Fielding's desire to manipulate the spectacle of punishment illustrates a more general truth about how meanings circulate in society. In the structure of language described by Volosinov/Bakhtin, the sign forms the arena of struggle between different social groups who inflect the same sign-forms with different 'evaluative accents'. That is, the same signs harbour a potential for different ideological themes. Meaning is always something temporal, provisional and contested:

> Class does not coincide with the sign community, i.e., with the community, which is the totality of users of the same set of signs for ideological communication. Thus various different classes will use one and the same language. As a result, differently oriented accents intersect in every ideological sign.[1]

The key term in this account is 'multi-accentuality'. Volosinov's theory of the sign applies to the anatomy controversy and its literature:

> This social *multiaccentuality* of the ideological sign is a very crucial aspect . . . Each living ideological sign has two faces, like Janus. Any current curse word can become a word of praise, any current truth must inevitably sound to many other people as the greatest lie. This *inner dialectic quality* of the sign comes out

[1] Volosinov/Bakhtin, 1973, 23.

> fully in the open only in times of social crises or revolutionary changes. In the ordinary conditions of life, the contradiction embedded in every ideological sign cannot emerge fully because the ideological sign in an established, dominant ideology is always somewhat reactionary and tries, as it were, to stabilise the preceding factor in the dialectical flux of the social generative process, so accentuating yesterday's truth as to make it appear today's. And that is what is responsible for the refracting and distorting peculiarity of the ideological sign within the dominant ideology.[2]

'Multi-accentuality', John Hartley explains, 'reminds us that signs do not have fixed internal "meaning", but only meaning-potentials, which are actualized in use. All signs can have their meaning potential "accented", or directed towards a particular kind of meaning, depending on the utterance, and on the speaker.'[3] And: 'Since signs are necessarily multi-accented, any discourse which seeks to "close" their potential and to prefer one evaluative accent over another is ideological: such discourses present *evaluative* differences as differences in *fact*.'[4] In our context, Bentham's auto-icon is a good illustration of the struggle to stabilise the sign in times of social crisis or controversy. Richardson's analysis of the artefact's ambiguity demonstrates the social life of the sign:

> First, by ensuring that, though dissected, his body would remain as if entire, Bentham endeavoured to endow the popular conception of dissection with an altered meaning . . . Second, there appears to have been some conflict in Bentham's intentions. For though he recognised that dissection would become stigma-free only by the elimination of popular prejudice, this in turn depended on the removal of the stigma. Bentham's own dissection was intended to allay public prejudice. However, a coercive Anatomy Bill would counter its impact, perpetuating

---

2 *Ibid.*

3 Hartley, 1985, 22.

4 *Ibid.*, 24.

> the appearance of punishment. Perhaps Bentham's hope was that his own dissection might persuade the poor to submit willingly to their fate, and thus provide immeasurable happiness to their social superiors.[5]

The stigma and its transference was a fact of social reality; it could not be conjured away by Bentham's last rhetorical gesture, nor by the law. The surgeons' historic association with the hangman was formally ended in 1832 by legislation which persecuted the poor, while benefiting the surgeons and allowing murderers to be buried whole.

## The *Note of the Editor* in *On Murder considered as one of the Fine Arts*

Before 1832 the commercial potential of the corpse meant that nobody was secure from burkers. This fact turned society into a volatile carnivalistic space of social indifferentiation – and, as De Quincey's 1827 essay appears to hint, it was a manipulable carnival. As we shall now see, there is the possibility (but no certainty) that De Quincey's essay was used by someone at *Blackwood's* to test the waters.

Two items precede and frame the Lecture on Murder. First, and by De Quincey's design, an anonymous correspondent enters a claim to have come by the text of the lecture, and to be submitting it in order to expose and incriminate the Society.[6] Next, however, a *Note of the Editor* appears, accepting the document but denying the interpretation put on it by the first voice.[7] This was an external intervention which irritated De Quincey, for he judged it to be unnecessary; nonetheless, the *Note* stayed in the text. The hand behind it remains untraceable, and De Quincey's most recent biographer states[8] – but not categorically

---

[5] Richardson, 1989, 160.
[6] De Quincey, 1918, 303.
[7] *Ibid.*, 305.
[8] Lindop, 1985, 284.

– that it was not Christopher North, alias John Wilson, the chief man at *Blackwood's*. *On Murder considered as one of the Fine Arts* appeared in 1827, on the eve of the disclosures from Edinburgh. The *Editor's Note* appears to mock the literal-minded reader, and the correspondent's submission, with a counter-assertion. Two voices contest the sign:

> *Note of the Editor.*— we thank our correspondent for his communication, and also for the communication from Lactantius, which is very pertinent to *his* view of the case; our own, we confess, is different. We cannot suppose the lecturer to be in earnest, any more than Erasmus in his Praise of Folly, or Dean Swift in his proposal for eating children. However, either on his view or on ours, it is equally fit that the lecture should be made public.[9]

The 'correspondent', as he seeks to expose the Club, is set up as a pedant. His voice is propitious nonetheless, for it accords with unease in officialdom well before 1828 as to the likelihood of criminal developments; for example, as Richardson reports, there are references to murderous possibilities in confidential and private correspondence from Bentham to Robert Peel in 1826.[10] Nevertheless, the editorial intervention here is double-edged in its allusion to Swift's satire *A Modest Proposal* – and the famous scheme to enable the children of the poor to be a benefit to the public. The *Note* renders a service to the surgeons' cause precisely by constructing the possibility of a face-value reading of De Quincey's piece, that is, an actual advocacy of murder. A backroom figure, it would appear, was reckoning the gamble-and-mischief value of a bluff. As Richardson argues, the terror spread by Burke and Hare, and their copycat successors, was co-opted by the utilitarians in Parliament into making the case for the anatomy legislation. A similar opportunism appears to inform the *Editor's Note* which found its way into De Quincey's essay. It would have been known

[9] De Quincey, 1918, 305

[10] Richardson, 1989, 132.

to somebody at *Blackwood's* that the surgeons' case stood to gain by a confusion of emphasis here, or the promotion of just such a confusion.

In the time-scheme, this rhetorical move happens to be rather neatly on cue. Without making any reference to De Quincey's essay, Donald Low in *Thieves' Kitchen*[11] reports the medical academy in Dublin admitting early in 1828 to the existence of recent rumours in the city to the effect that Irish children were being kidnapped and sold to be cut up in Scotland. Low adds that the belief may or may not have had a basis in fact.[12] Notably, this export route, via steam vessel, happens to cross the same waters that carry Victor Frankenstein to his confrontation with an angry Irish crowd, and a public charge of murder. Low even comments that the rumour 'seems to carry an echo of one of Swift's most brilliant satires'[13] – namely *A Modest Proposal*. He remarks pertinently on the curiousness of the rumours being in circulation just months before the murders committed by Burke and Hare, men who were of course Irishmen.[14] It is difficult, on the face of it, not to suspect a piece of mischief here from someone at *Blackwood's* – a retrospectively transparent move, in support of the surgeons and the proposed legislation, to exploit public horror, whether real or groundless. The timing of the allusion to Swift makes it hard to distinguish a move to play down public fear from a move to play it up. The Burke and Hare murders were not thunderbolts from the blue; however, they did sensationally confirm that murder was in the air. The art of gaining one's respectability by the promotion of terror appears, between the three editions of *Frankenstein*, to have had its sanction, and its exponents.

The anatomy literature, and *Frankenstein* in particular, exhibits a marked degree of multi-accentuation. Volosinov comments that:

The very same thing that makes the ideological sign vital and

---

11 Low, 1982, 99.
12 *Ibid.*, 100.
13 *Ibid.*
14 *Ibid.*

> mutable is also, however, that which makes it a refracting and distorting medium. The ruling class strives to impart a supraclass, eternal character to the ideological sign, to extinguish or drive inwards the struggle between social value judgements which occurs in it, to make the sign uni-accentual.[15]

Richardson's work contains relevant examples of the struggle to uni-accentuate the sign, and one in particular occurs in the same year that saw the first instalment of De Quincey's essay. She cites 'a series of lectures on human anatomy delivered by George Birkbeck at the London Mechanics Institution in the summer of 1827'.[16] By demand, a real human corpse was present in the course of the demonstrations. Birkbeck, Richardson comments, was heard appreciatively and respectfully, despite the fact that 'a superstitious and sentimental attachment to the corpse . . . formed an unspoken backdrop to the world view of each individual' in the audience.[17] Commenting on the fact that divisions in the radical community 'rendered it ineffective as a body of opposition',[18] Richardson observes: 'on the one hand there were those who believed "the march of intellect" *inherently socially progressive*, and whose awareness of issues of social class was subsumed in this belief. To them, superstition or sentiment was emblematic of ignorance, and was to be shunned' [italics added].[19] Others, on the other hand, while favourable towards anatomy and acknowledging the supply problem, were 'nevertheless sufficiently cognisant of the social relations of medicine in this period'[20] and withheld support for the proposed legislation. Richardson concludes: 'In the final analysis, the former grouping acted effectively in support of the ruling elite in the successful re-definition of poverty as crime, and the use of dissection to terrorise the poor.'[21]

---

15 Volosinov/Bakhtin, 1973, 23.

16 Richardson, 1989, 151

17 *Ibid.*, 152.

18 *Ibid.*

19 *Ibid.*

20 *Ibid.*

21 *Ibid.*

The phrasing 'inherently socially progressive' characterises an ideological stance, and in the next sentence as quoted the move to uni-accentuate the sign is apparent. In 1832 the surgeons secured the bodies, and the signs of the bodies. De Quincey's essay belongs to the ultimately successful efforts to pass off partial claims as universal interests. Only in the considerable long term did the poor stand to gain from an improved state of medical education;[22] in 1827 their bodies simply served the interests of the wealthy.

## The politics of anatomy: the voices in *Frankenstein*, 1831

Mary Shelley's story is a proleptic script that in a number of ways favours and makes the case for the impending legislation. At the same time, however, her anticipatory script is a multi-accented composition which voices the social perception that it is the surgeons who murder to dissect. By the same token, the multi-accentuation means that the story does not offer anything like the explicit nomination of agency and responsibility which informs Richardson's conclusion, as cited above. Victor Frankenstein's role as an agent and an interested party in a legislative terror design upon the poor is never stated unambiguously. The burden and secretiveness of it, especially as the violence in the story escalates, is displaced on to the 'monster' – and is for the reader to interpret. *Frankenstein*'s contemporary readers would have had cause to discern something quite topical and specific at work in this displacement.

The substitution plot – to replace the murderer's body with the pauper's body – had been thinkable, in principle, before the first edition of *Frankenstein* in 1818. However, it is contemporary history, the Edinburgh scandal – rather than the author Mary Shelley – which transforms the story into a palimpsest text: a parchment which has a second use or meaning after the original writing has been erased. The three editions stand open, in Bakhtin's sense, to accentuation from the intervening period of the body-

22 *Ibid.*, 214.

snatching era in its most intense phase.[23] The unabated national 'burkophobia' fears following the scandal would have established a context in which all the corpses in the story could appear to be left, and in effect offered, to the surgeon in the spirit of a bodysnatching commission. The 'monster' supplies the bodies, of course, but the 'doppelgänger' motif which binds Frankenstein to his Creature implies an unspeakable complicity. The Edinburgh scandal would have accentuated this complicity. The anatomist Frankenstein is progressively encumbered by a criminal association which he cannot, or will not, publicly declare – and he holds this position in common with the historical figure of Dr Robert Knox, the beneficiary of the bodysnatchers.[24] And Knox, as Scott knew, was regarded in the popular perception as the guilty agent just as much as Burke and his associate.[25]

Frankenstein effectively commences his silence as he departs from home. Ingolstadt, the graveyards, and his laboratory beckon:

> My life had hitherto been remarkably secluded and domestic, and this had given me invincible repugnance to new countenances. I loved my brothers, Elizabeth, and Clerval; these were 'old familiar faces', but I believed myself totally unfitted for the company of strangers. Such were my reflections when I commenced my journey; but as I proceeded, my spirits and hopes rose. I ardently desired the acquisition of knowledge.[26]

This 'repugnance to new countenances' prepares for the first-sight rejection of the 'monster'. Thus far the story has seen Frankenstein resolute in his will 'to penetrate the secrets of nature',[27] and destined for Ingolstadt. It is only the circumstance of his family's

---

23 But Mary did also revise the 1831 edition. In it Elizabeth is no longer Frankenstein's relative: she is a pauper but an aristocrat by birth. The full revisions can be seen in Maurice Hindle's collation of the 1818 and 1831 texts in the 1992 Penguin edition of *Frankenstein*.

24 See Richardson, 1989, 131–41 for an account of Knox's silence.

25 *Ibid.*, 133.

26 *Frankenstein*, 48.

27 *Ibid.*, 44.

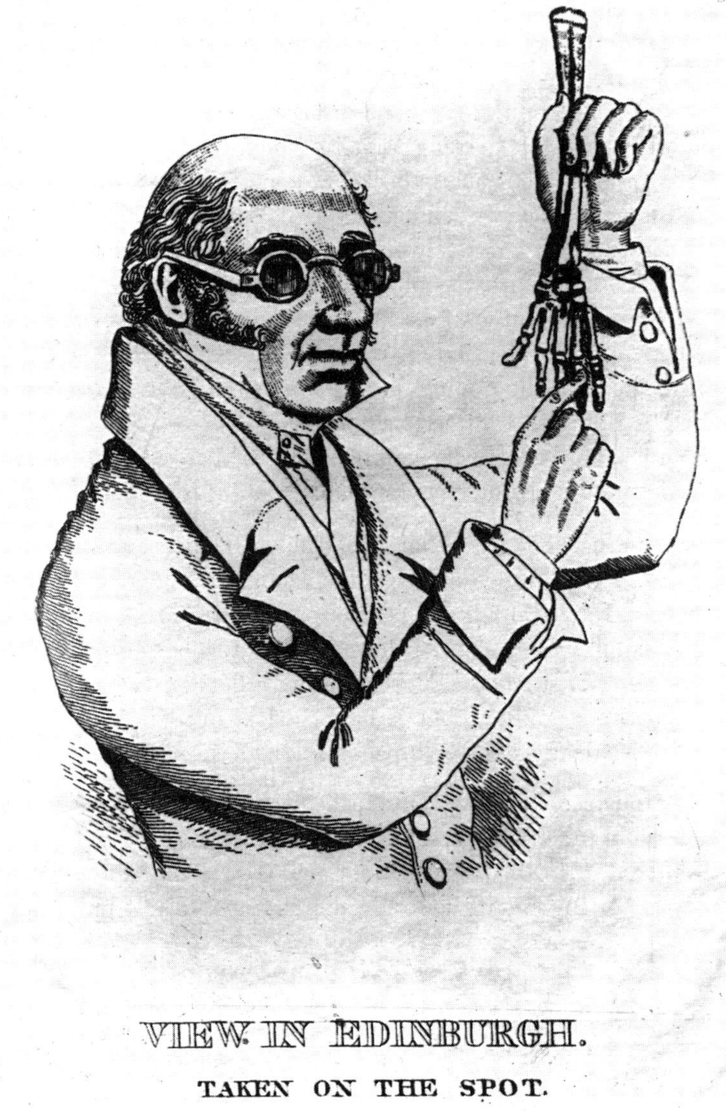


Caricature of Dr Robert Knox, the anatomist who purchased murdered bodies from Burke and Hare, *c.* 1828/9.

grief for his lately deceased mother which keeps him at home. He joins his family in mourning, albeit somewhat impatiently. The fascination with knowledge, however, is to exact a remarkable change in his emotional make-up, a repression of the heart. There is soon to be a confirmation that his true company is with the graverobbing fraternity. His part as the dutiful, grieving son undergoes transformation in the laboratory, where the dream-sequence after the creation sees him in a resurrectionist role, stealing his mother's corpse. As if to prepare for this revelation, Caroline Beaufort does not appear as a 'familiar face' of recent memory in the leave-taking reflections above.

The story turns Frankenstein's claim to be 'unfitted for the company of strangers' against him. From the creation onwards, he is constantly in the company of the publicly unknown Creature. It is, in turn, this stranger, in the part of the bodysnatcher, who sees to it that the 'old familiar faces' turn up one by one as stranger versions of themselves – as corpses. The reference is to Charles Lamb's poem 'The Old Familiar Faces' (1798), which begins 'Where are they gone, the old familiar faces?' The question recalls Scott's uneasy thought of the relation or friend lying on the anatomy table. It comments, that is, upon the difficulties of clinical detachment where the corpse is a relative or a friend, as these corpses are. The anatomist's business is with the body as a body, and nothing else. Here, however, a multi-accented sign pulls at the anatomist's professional mask and reveals the man behind it. The allusion to Lamb's poem sees Frankenstein's social conditioning speaking: that is, it catches him according a kind of aristocracy to the face where his own social caste is concerned. And as the story nears its climax, the metaphor gives way to fact. On the eve of the long deferred wedding, Elizabeth, the middle-class man's bride, metamorphosises into a wealthy aristocrat:

> Preparations were made for the event, congratulatory visits were received . . . Through my father's exertions a part of the inheritance of Elizabeth had been restored to her . . . A small possession on the shores of Como belonged to her. It was agreed that, immediately after our union, we should proceed

> to Villa Lavenza and spend our first days of happiness beside the beautiful lake near which it stood.[28]

This is the rehearsal of the great 1832 political marriage between the aristocracy and the middle class, and, as he repeatedly warns, the Creature does not accept it. As I have commented, the historic wedding of the ruling classes in 1832 effectively masked the passage of the Anatomy Act into law, and in *Frankenstein* its dress rehearsal proves to be the final provocation to the Creature.

The killing in a sequence of the blood-relative, the close friend and the fiancée enacts the suspicion and the fear that the dissection of corpses taken from graves was the thin end of a wedge in which murderers would disregard class boundaries and strike at will – and thus does the 'monster' strike. *Frankenstein* is a riot of multi-accentuality, of signs which in social crises become – like the corpses which appear in the story – inflected by different social accents and evaluations. The 'monster' is striking at social hypocrisy; but he is also provoking the power of hypocrisy. William's, Clerval's and Elizabeth's are middle-class bodies. They are the 'wrong' class of bodies for the surgeon, and the carnival of killing makes a powerful case in favour of the legislation. But it is equally true that the Creature has no permanent attachment to his murderous role and is prepared to negotiate it away. The partial acknowledgement he gains from Frankenstein is sufficient to secure him the promise of the female mate; the promise binds Frankenstein to complete partial recognition with full recognition on his Creature's own terms. The exigency on which everything turns, of course, is the fact that the violence will cease if Frankenstein honours this pledge. The Creature gives no reason to suppose that he will not in the event honour his side of the bargain and disappear far away for good. The story makes it clear that prejudice and apprehension in Frankenstein's mind are a complex of factors which undermine the promise. He, the maker, comes to fear that the 'monster' and mate will reproduce a 'race of devils' – an uncontrollable mass of offspring. This is in essence a class fear of

[28] *Ibid.*, 161. This passage was added in 1831.

a threat from below, and it plays a decisive part in breaking the binding power of the promise.

In the anatomy context, the condemnation imposed on the Creature gives him a role in *Frankenstein* identical to 'the body of the condemned man' that dominates Foucault's account of the transition to disciplinary society.[29] This 'condemned man', however, not only evades the murderer's ultimate pre-1832 punishment – the dissection – he also finally spells out to Walton that no 'unhallowed wretch', or utilitarian propagandist, will ever open his corpse. The 'monster', as readers have noted, is a multitude of bodies. For Moretti,[30] he is made up of the reunited and brought back to life limbs of the 'poor', the people 'whom the breakdown of feudal relations has forced into brigandage, poverty and death'. He is not a single corpse, but a mass-ive assemblage of corpses, a crowd.

In his study of the crowd Elias Canetti draws our attention to a very old conception – the crowd of the invisible dead. It is a mass of immense density and is usually figured as moving, and undertaking expeditions; it is often imagined as a fighting host.[31] This conception matches the socially imperceptible Creature in Mary Shelley's story and it throws some light on his role at large in society. To meet his promise, Frankenstein works in the Orkneys to assemble the Creature's mate. Fearing a propagation of 'devils', he ditches the job and dumps the half-formed female anatomy into the sea at night. He then drifts asleep in a small boat to the coast of Ireland in the early hours. Unknowingly, he is shadowed by the Creature who is one step ahead; the itinerary here invites the idea of the Giant's Causeway as a footprint. Frankenstein wakes up to confront an Irish crowd which has cause to believe he has murdered Clerval. With Clerval's murder, the anatomist is more than ever encumbered by a criminal association which he cannot declare.

---

29 See Foucault, 1979, Ch. 1.
30 Moretti, 1983, 85.
31 Canetti, 1981, 47–8.

The Ireland sequence follows Frankenstein's resolve 'to finish my labours in some obscure nook in the northern highlands of Scotland'.[32] The invisible dead, Canetti notes, figure in a compound word which derives from this locality:

> The word *gairm* means shout or cry, and *sluagh-ghairm* was the battle-cry of the dead. This word later became 'slogan'. The expression we use for the battle-cries of our modern crowds derives from the Highland hosts of the dead.[33]

In the course of his final pursuit of the Creature, Frankenstein confronts provocative 'marks in writing', 'cut in stone' and carved on tree bark, which rouse him to 'fury': 'My reign is not yet over . . .'[34] With these inscriptions the Creature serves notice that it is within his power to perpetuate the 'burking' terrors he has already committed. His victims are all throttled, a form of murder which matches the popular belief that Burke and Hare's victims died in this manner. The two men, however, became famous for having perfected a stifling technique – a 'burking' – which apparently left no signs of violence on the body. Their beneficiary, Dr Knox, acquired popular notoriety at the time of the scandal by appearing to have colluded in the deception. In the third edition of *Frankenstein* the black stifle marks left on the neck of the victims – the tell-tale signs which Frankenstein always sees first – would have spoken volumes about Knox's corrupt silence on the point as to exactly what he knew about what was going on. The bodies in the story need only be left, for the surgeon follows up each murder by turning up at the scene of the body. After Elizabeth's murder, the signs, like the corpses, threaten to inundate the public and private sphere. The mocking slogans turn up everywhere in the course of the long, futile chase.

A historic function of the crowd, as Canetti notes,[35] is to out-shout dangers: whether epidemics or enemies. People join

---

32 *Frankenstein*, 1136

33 Canetti, 1981, 49.

34 *Frankenstein*, 171.

35 Canetti, 1985, 118.

voices so that they can shout louder. It was during the cholera epidemic of 1831, when *Frankenstein* reappeared, that popular anger against bodysnatching and the doctors reached its height. The narrative in *Frankenstein*, however, is for the most part Frankenstein's voice, in the form of private, urgent disclosures which are sent back to England by Walton, the captain of the national Ship-of-State. As Frankenstein's testimony, the story is a portrait of the medical man's arrival in modern society as he projects a voice favourable to middle-class cultural hegemony. Frankenstein, that is to say, is trying to assemble a statement which is ideologically favourable to the 1832 arrangements – while lacking the legitimation which those arrangements were to confer on the medical tribe. The adjacency of the story's 1831 edition with the 1832 Anatomy Act is ironic. The story – and Frankenstein's voice – enjoyed wide circulation just months before the legislation removed the surgeons' activities from the public domain. As the profession disappeared from view, dissection, by design, remained to haunt the social imagination.

The competing voices in *Frankenstein* – Frankenstein's voice and that of his Creature – need interpretation because they each lay claim to different versions of the truth. Frankenstein makes and disowns a 'monster' whose whole existence is a will to be properly 'related'. The novel explores the ambiguities of the word 'relation'. The term encompasses speech and writing, both of which figure in the story itself, the relation of events. The Creature's first-sight rejection lies in the past when Frankenstein relates the serial murders to Walton; but, in another meaning of the word, the story makes timely reading for Walton's addressees, his relations back in England in the Saville circle – and an urgent case for the legislation. For them, as it were, the writing is on the wall. The danger the story spells for its polite readership begins from the moment the relationship between Frankenstein and his Creature is marked by non-recognition. 'Relationship' is a term for the dimension in which a human being exists in a kinship bond to others – as a relative – and is recognised as such. Frankenstein's story contains the Creature's story – his address, or appeal, to the man who does not recognise himself as the father of the being he has created. In his own words the Creature expresses his deepest desires and claims, as these dictate his perceptions and his judgement on who dies and who survives. Above all, he wants – and demands – a mate, a relation or relative, and this he is promised and then denied.

The word 'claim', as I have just used it, is a pivotal word in *Frankenstein* and in the legislation also, for a particular reason. The new law contained a notorious clause concerning the claiming of the dead pauper body. It stipulated that when a death occurred in the workhouse there would have to be proper confirmation of the *bona fide* status and identity of the relative, or relatives, who could turn up to claim the body for burial, and hence avert dissection.[36] Under new and imperfect bureaucratic arrangements, the time-period for the notification of relatives was short,[37] mainly for medical reasons. When it lapsed, the bodies which no *bona fide* relatives appeared to claim would belong henceforth to the surgeons, and by extension to the new power arrangements in society. In the 1831 edition, appearing on the eve of the legislation, Frankenstein's denial of a mate to his Creature is above all significant in this context. The broken promise in effect precipitates all the bodies which comprise 'the monster' into the impending dissection category. In the story, however, the word 'claim' is insistently multi-accented in Bakhtin's sense, and carries different social values in the narrative's two voices. In other words, an argument as to 'who belongs to who', and hence, 'who is who' is never settled, except by murder.

The two figures, above all, who are drawn into this ultimately fatal contestation are the women in the story, Elizabeth and Justine, both of whom have known extreme poverty in their childhood. The male voices – the creator and the Creature – lay conflicting 'claims' upon these two women. In the political allegory, the consequent fates of the women dramatise a specific ideology as it appears to be failing and in crisis. Elizabeth and Justine are the

---

36 Richardson, 1989, 121–2.

37 *Ibid.*, 207

products of an order of benevolent paternalism, and a philanthropic concern, which has recognised poverty to the extent of having admitted certain of its victims into the sanctity of the bourgeois home as aspiring daughters, and, in the estate of property, as acquisitions for display. Their fate, as the Creature strikes, comments on the first encounter and the later making-and-then-revoking of the bargain between the two men. The new legislative arrangements of 1832 saw the premeditated death of this ideology, as it made way for the harsher utilitarian culture.[38]

The Creature has a hand in the woman's fate in both cases. In part, their identities cede to him, and indeed 'belong' to him in ways that require a close description. He makes final claims upon them in marriage and death. As he sees them, they are versions of the mate or the 'bride' which he is promised but denied. After the condemnation imposed on him, he recognises in them who he really is. He stages Justine's criminalisation for a crowd of thousands which assembles at her trial, and he keeps his promised date in Como. The women's fates are his dramatisation of the social meaning of his condemnation in its imminent application in the anatomy context. E. P. Thompson's summary image of the age contains an unconscious reference to the legislation's most notorious clause: in 1832 'blood compromised with gold to keep out the claims of *égalité*'.[39] The anatomy literature of the early nineteenth century – and *Frankenstein* in its three editions – tells the story of this compromise as it moves up the political agenda in the 1820s.

---

[38] *Ibid.*, 267.

[39] E. P. Thompson, 1980, 902; also quoted in Richardson, 1989, 267.

# PART II

# The law made flesh

CHAPTER 3

# The instruments of law

> This machinery [of tools] transforms individual bodies into a body politic. It makes these bodies produce the text of a law . . . In changing jobs, moving from the 'application' of the law to that of surgical and orthopedic medicine, the apparatus of tools retains the function of marking or shaping bodies in the name of a law. (Michel De Certeau, 'The Scriptural Economy'.)[1]

## Intextuation

The anatomy legislation, as a deterrent to the workhouse and as the mechanism which supplied corpses to the surgeons, served disciplinary agendas in the nineteenth century. In his essay 'The Scriptural Economy' Michel De Certeau argues that juridical law, in order to be effective, imposes itself on the body via the mediation of certain kinds of tool or instrument. In *Frankenstein* the story of Justine, the young girl who is executed for a murder she does not commit, contains an inventory of these tools: the prisoner's box in court, hand manacles, the prison cell and ultimately the gallows. There is also the suggestion that her confession is extracted under torture.[2]

These tools provide key points of focus in the anatomy literature. They are the means by which the law, as the agent of social discipline, is inscribed on the body. In this scheme, the law writes the body into a text – that is, it gives it meaning and a place in the social order. De Certeau uses the term 'intextuation':

---

[1] De Certeau, 1988, 142–3.
[2] *Frankenstein*, 80. Justine is 'besieged', 'threatened' and 'menaced'.

> The intextuation of the body corresponds to the incarnation of the law; it supports it, even seems to establish it, and in any case it serves it. For the law plays on it: 'Give me your body and I will give you meaning, I will make you a name and a word in my discourse.' The two problematics maintain each other, and perhaps the law would have no power if it were not able to support itself on the obscure desire to exchange one's flesh for a glorious body, to be written, even if it means dying, and be transformed into a recognised word. Here again, the only force opposing this passion to be a sign is the cry, a deviation or an ecstasy, a revolt or flight of that which, within the body, escapes the law of the named.[3]

The metaphor is incarnation. The law made flesh, incarnated, transforms the bodies of everyone in society, including those in or close to the dissection constituency, into signifiers of the social rules.[4] The reason or *Logos* of a society 'becomes flesh' – and this in effect means that everyone carries the social rules around with them in everyday life. Furthermore, as John Fiske has pointed out,[5] De Certeau argues that the history of medicine is the story of the tools which write norms of physical and mental health upon the body. In this chapter I shall illustrate this 'scriptural economy' in the anatomy context with reference to Dickens, William Burke, *Gulliver's Travels*, *Frankenstein* and De Quincey. I also discuss the work of two senior medical practitioners of the anatomy era: Astley Cooper and John Hunter.

In *Oliver Twist* Oliver gets his surname from the parish beadle Mr Bumble, and a system:

> The beadle drew himself up with great pride, and said,
> 'I inwented it.'
> 'You, Mr Bumble!'
> 'I, Mrs Mann. We name our fondlings in alphabetical order.

[3] De Certeau, 1988, 149.

[4] I have found John Fiske's discussion of De Certeau illuminating. See *Understanding Popular Culture,* 1989.

[5] Fiske, 1989, 91.

> The last was a S – Swubble, I named him. This was a T – Twist, I named *him* . . . I have got names invented to the end of the alphabet, and all the way through it again.'[6]

Named by it, Oliver is born a *found*ling of the system of market and man. Mr Bumble, the product and servant of the system, invents his own pretences and pretexts. He of course is not *fond* of Oliver at all. Where the boy is concerned, Bumble is licensed to incarnate the work ethic with his cane, the tool that shapes Oliver's deferential body posture. Oliver's function in the story, in De Certeau's terms, is to become 'an identifiable and legible word in a social language'.[7] To this end, he has to learn a repertoire of appropriate demeanour and physical posture which intextuates utilitarian social meanings. Frequently, these postures appear in settings where the sensitivities and pretensions touched by the anatomy legislation are under review. After leaving the workhouse, the small boy stands in the undertaker's employ as 'a superb effect' – as a hired 'mute' mourner – in the proceedings of the early Victorian 'respectable' funeral.[8] In Mr Bumble's company, Oliver also assists at the equivalent ritual at the other end of the social scale, the pauper funeral.

Punishment is an integral part of the scriptural economy, and this fact is in play in Oliver's growing distance from the criminal Fagin, who is hanged at the end of the story. The small boy's eventual class distance from Fagin's world is signified by a cluster of meanings in the surname he gets from Bumble. Confounding predictions that he will end his 'twisted' criminal life on the gallows, Oliver gains a safe distance from the lethal twist of the noose. However, in a summary image, Oliver 'swoons' at the imminent prospect of Fagin's execution on 'the black stage'.[9] This swoon suggests that his essential desire is to transcend the black-decked spectacle of public execution, the stark face of utilitarian

---

6 Dickens, 1961, 31.
7 De Certeau, 1988, 140.
8 Dickens, 1961, 59.
9 *Ibid.*, 476.

ideology: his 'censor' reaction indicates a psychic need to 'twist' away from it. As Mr Brownlow's adopted son, he will, in Foucault's sense, take his discipline the gentle way.[10] The condemned man in his final hours, in the words of a prison official, is 'not a sight for children'.[11] Oliver's fainting reaction on the day in question implicitly contradicts one of Bentham's emphatic recommendations:

> Render your punishments exemplary; give to the ceremonies which accompany them a mournful pomp; call to your assistance all the imitative arts; and let the representation of these important operations be among the first objects that strike the eyes of childhood . . .
>
> scaffold painted black . . . officers . . . dressed in crêpe . . . livery of grief . . . a mask . . . emblems of his crime . . . a part of the decorations of these legal tragedies . . . terrible drama . . . serious and religious music preparing the hearts of the spectators for the important lesson . . . judges preside . . . and its sombre dignity should be consecrated by the presence of the ministers of religion.[12]

This advocacy is not easily compatible with Bentham's other efforts to break the gallows stigma on dissection. Dissection and its historic links with the gallows are not explicitly mentioned in *Oliver Twist*; but Dickens' opposition to public executions, as it informs Oliver's reaction to Fagin's impending death, is an example of social discourse which intersects with the surgeons' recent farewell to an unwelcome association.

When Dickens does comment on the medical profession of the 1830s he appropriately links their lingering image problem with a general perception of a society negotiating major cultural change. The opening description of Oliver taking upon himself for the first time 'the office of respiration' – breathing – playfully alludes

---

10 See Foucault, 1979, pt. II, Ch. 2.
11 Dickens, 1961, 473.
12 Quoted in Skillen, 1977, 141.

to the 1832 political settlement. The 'office' marks the distance Oliver eventually secures from the English 'Bastille' within the constituency of political rights:

> The fact is, there was considerable difficulty in inducing Oliver to take upon himself the office of respiration – a troublesome practice, but one which custom has rendered necessary to our easy existence; and for some time he lay gasping on a little flock mattress, rather unequally poised between this world and the next, the balance being decidedly in favour of the latter. Now, if during this anxious period, Oliver had been surrounded by careful grandmothers, anxious aunts, experienced nurses, and *doctors of profound wisdom*, he would most inevitably and indubitably have been killed in no time. There being nobody by, however, but a pauper old woman, and a parish surgeon, *who did such matters by contract*, Oliver and Nature fought out the point between them. Oliver breathed, sneezed, and proceeded to advertise to the inmates of the workhouse . . . that very useful appendage, a voice [italics added].[13]

It is an uncertain, unassisted individual struggle to commence breathing – that is to say, this is breathing in the new *laissez-faire* culture – and Oliver is up to it. The half-pun on the 'orifice' in 'office' comments on the proximity of politics to breathing. It recalls the utilitarian voices in Parliament which made breathing freely possible once again – and 'burking', the art of stopping the windpipe, a thing of the past. In this passage Dickens directs heavy sarcasm against the mentality which now runs the national 'office of respiration'. His inventory acknowledges the pieties, the anxieties, the financial power and the medical expectations of an emergent middle class which is now in possession of a significant political voice. The description remains silent about dissection, and the claiming of the body by relatives – but not entirely silent. Given the 'Bastille' workhouse context, this portrait of familial solicitude recognises the ready proximity of relatives as a feature of the new

---

[13] Dickens, 1961, 23.

class culture. Dickens' tilt against the parish surgeon is the first of many scathing remarks in the story about the medical profession.[14] To judge from what is said, their homicidal image evidently still sticks, even with the bodysnatching era in recent eclipse.

## Public and comparative anatomy

In the early nineteenth century the norms of class- and gender-based social power are intextuated into the everyday body of the individual as they are into the body politic of society. The medical profession's enhanced legitimation after 1832 gives it a role in this process, and a more authoritative voice. Increasingly, the doctor identifies and polices lines of potential resistance, particularly among the young, the poor and women. In *Frankenstein*, for example, at the crisis-juncture of the story the Creature's bid for a mate flounders on Frankenstein's fear that the female may prove to be outside all social and sexual control.[15] In this context, as an episode in her *Journal* shows, Mary Shelley herself was a witness to the sexual politics of the medical culture of her day. In 1820 the author of *Frankenstein* was a passing spectator of 'public' anatomy. Her *Journal* entry in January of this year records a visit to an Italian museum which housed a famous collection. The *Journal*'s editors describe the scene:

> The Gabinetto Fisico was a museum of natural history, chiefly celebrated for its collection of wax models of the human anatomy, some of which were extremely gruesome. 'This awful region, which should be sacred to men of science, is open to all. Nay, the very apartment where the gravid uterus and its processes is unveiled, is a favourite lounge of the ladies, who criticise aloud all the mysteries of sex.' (Forsyth, 1813)[16]

---

[14] For example, in a sardonic passage, Ch. 5 of *Oliver Twist* sees the surgeons cutting up the bodies of children who have been starved to death.

[15] *Frankenstein*, 140.

[16] Quoted in Feldman and Scott-Kilvert, vol. 1, p.306.

Victor Frankenstein is one such man of science; and he retracts his promise to create a mate for his Creature after he fantasises about her promiscuity and inclination to breed – the gravid uterus, to be precise. Joseph Forsyth, the authority cited here by Feldman and Scott Kilvert, was a writer who visited the museum in 1803 and who wrote up his trip in 1813. His emphasis on the proper male preserve of anatomy was probably known to Mary Shelley. According to her *Journal*, she read Forsyth's volume in April 1819, in preparation for her visit to the famous wax models.[17] In the same year – as we saw in my Introduction – John Abernethy in the *Hunterian Oration* publicly declares the need to requisition pauper bodies. In the contemporary accentuation that *Frankenstein* acquires during the 1820s the murderous Creature eludes the law and therefore escapes automatic dissection: that is to say, he refuses the incarnation of middle-class utilitarianism upon the body. By the same token, his subversion makes a case for the legislation which substituted the workhouse inmate for the murderer on the anatomist's table – and for the class hegemony which sanctioned improvements in social medicine after 1832.

As the artificial product of the dissecting room, the Creature's multi-bodied frame in *Frankenstein* is an early version of the transplant body of modern 'spare part' surgery.[18] When the boundaries between self and other disappear, Frankenstein's Creature is inside all of us. As De Certeau points out, the instruments of the scriptural economy sculpt the transplant body:

> The identification of the pieces and their operations makes it possible to substitute artificial parts for those that wear out or have some defect, and even to construct automatons. The body can be repaired. It can be educated. It can even be fabricated. The panoply of orthopedic instruments and means of treatment expands in proportion to what one can henceforth take apart and repair, cut off, replace, take out, add, correct, or straighten.

---

[17] *Ibid.*, 257.

[18] See Helman, 1991, 19–28 'The Body of Frankenstein's Creature'. Helman makes no reference to the Anatomy Act.

> The network of these tools becomes more complex and extensive.[19]

Cecil Helman's recent discussion of the 'transplant body' in *Frankenstein* has an application to the legislative substitution plot. 'Capitalism', remarks this contemporary anatomist, 'demands the notion of replaceable parts, as well as replaceable people'.[20]

In 1829, all the voices that contested the anatomy question intersected in one execution spectacle. William Burke, 'a Monster' according to contemporary broadsheets,[21] was hanged, and then dissected in a closed session. Afterwards (as we have seen Scott commenting in his *Journal*) the corpse was publicly re-exhibited, and on the trial judge's instruction the skeleton was preserved in memory of his crimes. 'Burke's dissection,' Richardson comments: 'represented the apotheosis of a punishment to fit the crime. But it also represented a medical, judicial and political paradox, whereby the punishment worked ultimately to prompt further crimes of the same type.'[22]

By subjecting William Burke to an exemplary anatomisation the law reaffirmed the criminal stigma on dissection. In this complexly accented spectacle, officialdom's need for corpses speaks just as loudly as the dimension of punishment. The popular perception of the surgeons as the murderers was once again sanctioned. Burke's condemned, dissected body advertised the shortfall and the better asking prices which could be obtained from the surgeons. The copycat burkings followed soon afterwards. Like Burke and Hare, Bishop and Williams, the London 'burking' killers of 1831, also left no marks of violence on their victims; and they were more prolific and skilful operators. As I have noted, the 1831 edition of *Frankenstein* gains in historical accentuation in this context, for the black throttle-marks pointedly left by the Creature on his victims – for the eye of the surgeon – are signs which comment not only

[19] De Certeau, 1988, 142.
[20] Helman, 1991, 26.
[21] See Richardson, 1989, 142.
[22] *Ibid.*, 143.

on Burke and Hare but also on their imitators. Only months after the third edition of *Frankenstein* the law was used to move anatomy, and dead bodies, out of public space.

Early in the nineteenth century there occurred a spectacular and rare moment in the history of 'public' anatomy. An event took place involving Astley Cooper, a long-term colleague of Abernethy's and, in due course, an outspoken exponent of the surgeons' legislative cause. In 1801, Cooper, a self-confessed client of the resurrectionists, dissected the carcase of an elephant from the Tower Menagerie, outside his house in the City of London.[23] The elephant 'articulation' took place in front of a large crowd. Cooper was hard pressed to acquire a sufficient daily supply of human subjects for his knife; he regularly anatomised animals in order to make inferences about human structure. This is comparative anatomy, the foundations of which were laid in the eighteenth century by Cuvier, who died in 1832; it was widely practised by anatomists in the pre-modern era. Alongside many surgeons of the early nineteenth century, Victor Frankenstein is a comparative anatomist: 'One of the phaenomena which had peculiarly attracted my attention was the structure of the human frame, and indeed, *any animal* endued with life [italics added].'[24]

'The slaughter-house', he tells us, 'furnished many of my materials'.[25] Cooper's virtuoso outdoor performance of comparative anatomy illustrates and comments upon the surgeons' early century legitimacy-and-respectability crisis, for it is heavy with shades of the fairground spectacle, a distinctly un-bourgeois cultural space. Cooper at work on the elephant is the archetypal pre-1832 surgeon, a professional in want of his materials. This spectacle precedes the modern medical and disciplinary world of naturalised, invisible norms which the Anatomy Act helped to bring into existence. The out of sight supply-line of bodies to the surgeons after 1832 accords with De Certeau's general argument that cultural

---

23 See Bailey, 1991, 62.

24 *Frankenstein*, 53.

25 *Ibid.*, 56.

norms work most effectively and gain credibility when they do not draw attention to themselves:

> The *credibility* of a discourse is what first makes believers act in accord with it. It produces practitioners. To make people believe is to make them act. But by a curious circularity, the ability to make people act – to write and to machine bodies – is precisely what makes people believe. Because the law is already applied with and on bodies, 'incarnated' in physical practices, it can accredit itself and make people believe that it speaks in the name of the 'real'. It makes itself believable by saying: 'This text has been dictated for you by Reality itself.' People believe what they assume to be real.[26]

Cooper, sensitive to the legitimisation of his profession, would have understood the proviso that completes this argument. Throughout the late 1820s, as he called for legislative help for the surgeons, Cooper countenanced the use of the body to intextuate and incarnate the law: 'but this "reality" is assigned to a discourse by a belief that gives it a body inscribed by the law. The law requires an accumulation of corporeal capital in advance in order to make itself believed and practiced.'[27] In 1821 Cooper received a knighthood for removing a tumour from the top of George IV's head. The success of the operation, alongside luck, owed a great deal to his experience as a comparative anatomist.[28]

*Gulliver's Travels* is an enormous resource in the eighteenth-century constituency of anatomy literature. A surgeon by trade, Gulliver – when he can – cuts up some of the massive animals and insects in Brobdingnag in a rudimentary role as a comparative anatomist; but he has cause to rue the fact that he left his dissection knife proper back aboard ship.[29] As it pits the English surgeon against enormous, live creatures, Swift's satire mocks Gulliver with Rousseau's insight that 'the study of animals is useless without

---

[26] De Certeau, 1988, 148.
[27] *Ibid.*
[28] Low, 1987, 88.
[29] Swift, 1966, 118.

anatomy.'[30] The 'comparative anatomy' episode in the second voyage sees Gulliver visited by a monkey:

> After some time spent in peeping, grinning, and chattering, he at last espyed me; and reaching one of his paws in at the door, as a cat does when she plays with a mouse, although I often shifted place to avoid him; he at length seized the lappet of my coat (which being made of that country silk, was very thick and strong) and dragged me out. He took me in his right fore-foot, and held me as a nurse doth a child she is going to suckle; just as I have seen the same sort of creature do with a kitten in Europe: and, when I offered to struggle, he squeezed me so hard, that I thought it more prudent to submit. I have good reason to believe, that he took me for a young one of his own species, by his often stroaking my face very gently with his other paw.[31]

Gulliver then describes 'the greatest danger I ever underwent' in Brobdingnag. In this image the medical man is a spectacle for the crowd:

> In these diversions he was interrupted . . . whereupon he suddenly leapt up to the window . . . and thence upon the leads and gutters, walking upon three legs, and holding me in the fourth, until he clambered up to a roof that was next to ours . . . the palace was all in an uproar; the monkey was seen by hundreds in the court, sitting upon the ridge of a building, holding me like a baby in one of his fore-paws, and feeding me with the other, by cramming into my mouth some victuals he had squeezed out of the bag on one side of his chaps, and patting me when I would not eat; whereat many of the rabble below could not forebear laughing.[32]

This is one of the higher primates who have abandoned the trees

---

[30] Rousseau, 1981, 114.
[31] Swift, 1966, 127–8.
[32] *Ibid.*

for the ground. As the monkey takes flight, it displays the faculties it has retained from life in the trees – the environment where the hand originated. The passage comments on the monkey's strength of grasp, a function, in the human context, which Gulliver has already had good cause to observe in this land of giants: on his arrival in Brobdingnag, for example, he is grasped tight in the farmer's enormous hand. The grasp function is the reason why the monkey and Gulliver do not fall in the course of the very rapid movements described here. The paragraph after this passage sees the monkey gaining speed, but letting go of Gulliver on to 'a ridge-tyle' five hundred yards above the ground, from whence he is rescued.[33] The animal was not 'able to make speed enough with his three legs'[34] and needed the unhindered use of his limbs to gain full acceleration.

## Trading

In a discussion of the monkeys' faculties, Canetti draws attention to the partnership of the hands in consecutive stages of grasping and letting go:

> While the one hand is reaching for a new branch, the other holds fast to the old one. This holding fast is of cardinal importance for it alone prevents a fall. In no circumstances must the hand from which the weight of the body is suspended loosen its hold, and this teaches the hand a tenacity of grip which is quite different from the older grip on prey. In addition, as soon as the second hand has grasped the new branch, the first hand must loosen its grip on the old one. Unless this is done quickly the climbing creature cannot proceed. The hand thus acquires a new faculty: the ability to let go of something instantly. Prey was never relinquished except under extreme pressure and against all the habits and desires of the holder.[35]

---

[33] *Ibid.*, 129.
[34] *Ibid.*
[35] Canetti, 1981, 247.

Nor is there any indication that the frolicsome primate in Brobdingnag regards Gulliver as prey. The spectacle of Gulliver in the clutches of the climbing monkey seems a long way from the bodysnatching era and its notorious revelations, but the monkey's nimble movements here cast some light on a coded reference in De Quincey's essay to the trade in bodies. Canetti points to the human occupation which most clearly recalls the monkey's two hands in partnership, as it were, with each other:

> The essence of trading is the giving of one object in exchange for another. The one hand tenaciously holds on to the object with which it seeks to tempt the stranger. The other hand is stretched out in demand towards the second object, which it seeks to have in exchange for its own. As soon as it touches this, the first hand lets go of its object; but not before, or it may lose both. The crudest form of cheating, when something is taken from someone without any return being made, corresponds, translated into the context of climbing, to falling from the tree. To prevent this the trader remains on his guard during the whole transaction and scrutinises every movement of his opposite number. The profound and universal pleasure men take in trading is thus partly explained by the fact that trade is a translation into non-physical terms of one of the oldest movement patterns. In nothing else today is man so near the apes.[36]

The temptation offered to the stranger is sketched in the 1839 instalment of *On Murder considered as a Fine Art* where a trading encounter involving human remains is described. From a post-1832 vantage point of respectability, the Lecturer in Murder indulges a reminiscence of the bodysnatching days. The subtext between De Quincey's speaker and his addressee, Christopher North, is evidently the corpse trade:

> A good many years ago you may remember that I came forward in the character of a *dilettante* in murder. Perhaps *dilettante* may be too strong a word. *Connoisseur* is better suited to the scruples

[36] *Ibid.*, 248.

> and infirmity of public taste. I suppose there is no harm in *that* at least. A man is not bound to put his eyes, ears, and understanding into his breeches pocket when he meets with a murder. If he is not in a downright comatose state, I suppose he must see that one murder is better or worse than another in point of good taste. Murders have their little differences and shades of merit as well as statues, pictures, oratorios, cameos, intaglios, or what not. You may be angry with the man for talking too much, or too publicly (as to the too much, that I deny – a man can never cultivate his taste too highly); but you must allow him to think, at any rate . . .[37]

The speaker continues: 'and you, Doctor – you think, I am sure, both deeply and correctly on the subject, Well, would you believe it? all my neighbours came to hear of that little aesthetic essay which you had published'.[38] This appears to be a reference to 'Noctes Ambrosianae XIX'.[39] As Martin Fido has commented,[40] John Wilson – alias 'Christopher North' – 'made no secret of his belief that Knox had consciously bought murdered bodies'. The speaker recalls the public murmuring:

> and, unfortunately, hearing at the very same time of a Club that I was connected with, and a Dinner at which I presided – both tending to the same little object as the essay, viz, the diffusion of a just taste among Her Majesty's subjects, they got up the most barbarous calamities against me. In particular, they said that I, or that the Club, which comes to the same thing, had offered bounties on well-conducted homicides – with a scale of drawbacks, in case of any one defect or flaw, according to a table issued by private friends.[41]

---

37 De Quincey, 1918, 337.
38 *Ibid.*
39 *Blackwood's Magazine*, Edinburgh, March, 1829.
40 Fido, 1988, 130.
41 De Quincey, 1918, 337.

As we have seen, the case for a switch from *dilettante* to *connoisseur* artistry became persuasive when the Burke and Hare murders reminded the public about the ongoing commerce in corpses. Implicit in the proposition above – that one murder is discernibly better or worse than another – is a mock, hindsight parade of scruple about the murderous end of the resurrectionist market in the days before 1832. The 'breeches pocket' comment is pertinent. In the dilettante phase, the beneficiary of the murder was 'bound to put his eyes, ears, and understanding into his breeches pocket' – as he dug for the money to pay, or to commence the bargaining. In this image the surgeon is reluctantly drawn into the trade encounter with any Tom, Dick or Harry who turns up with a body. The word 'bound' is appropriate: it comments on the necessary evil of the trading and the graverobbers' (and potentially the burkers') power to extort large payments, according to demand. The image also sees the surgeon concealing a first show of interest as he presents the poker face, the face closed off to scrutiny but active in the scrutiny of the other.

These postures comment on a fact which was not lost on higher officialdom in the bodysnatching era. In the decade spanning the first three editions of *Frankenstein* the price of the corpse was subject to inflation.[42] As Frieda Sandwith observes: 'Licences were not required for anatomy schools; they were not limited in numbers, so that keen competition between teachers played right into the hands of unscrupulous gangs'.[43] (The question of a gang's rise in wages, to be paid by the anatomists, comes up in the conversation of the resurrectionists in *Barnaby Rudge*.)[44] Noting the wrong sort of public talking, De Quincey's murder connoisseur mimes the troublesomeness of rumour and scandal. But here, close to the end of the second instalment, he is on the verge of dropping the mask and celebrating Burke and Hare by name. As we have seen, the Irishmen are invoked as the 'artists' whose

---

42 See Fido, 1988, Ch. 5, 'The Great Inflation'.

43 Sandwith, 1960, 42.

44 Dickens, 1987, 181–2.

work clinched the transition to connoisseur murder and, into the bargain, the legislation.

Astley Cooper, who was nicknamed 'The King of the Resurrectionists', was well versed in the details of 'the understanding', as De Quincey puts it, for he too had the inevitable arguments about the price.[45] In 1828 Cooper, as the Sergeant Surgeon to the King, was a star witness when he bluntly told a Commons Select Committee that: 'if you have none but ignorant medical men, it is you who will suffer from it; and the fact is, that the want of subjects will soon lead to your becoming the unhappy victims of operations founded and performed in ignorance.'[46] He added: 'There is no person, let his situation in life be what it may, whom, if I were disposed to dissect, I could not obtain . . . The law only enhances the price, and does not prevent the exhumation.'[47]

John Hunter's work requires a longer analysis. A cameo of Hunter at work is given in William Hazlitt's 1821 essay 'The Indian Jugglers'. Hazlitt sketches the father of modern anatomy performing comparative anatomy:

> John Hunter was a great man – *that* anyone might see without the smallest skill in surgery. His style and manner showed the man. He would set about cutting up the carcase of a whale with the same greatness of gusto that Michael Angelo would have hewn a block of marble[48] [Hazlitt's emphasis].

As with Astley Cooper dissecting the elephant, individualism is here turned into spectacle. Nothing could be further from either man's energies than a social ideology of shared distribution, a large slaughtered animal divided by numbers of men working together. Performing solo, Hunter articulates and transforms the marble with an intimidating ease of power. In addition, the reference to Michael Angelo in Hazlitt's compliment reminds us that art has long been

[45] For details of the cheating, see Cole, 1964, Ch. 1.
[46] Quoted in Low, 1987, 90.
[47] *Ibid.*
[48] Peacock, 1918, 249.

twinned with anatomy: the artist and the surgeon alike study the human form.[49] To explore the full range of Hazlitt's compliment, we must turn to an instance of Hunter's work – or art.

## The surgeon as artist: John Hunter and Mrs Martin Van Butchell

One other contemporary anatomist has noted a number of cultural agendas in John Hunter's work. F. Gonzalez-Crussi comments:

> In the West, embalming and greed seem to have been wedded from the beginning. [In 1775] John Hunter, younger brother of the Scottish anatomist, came across an exceptional opportunity to employ his brother's methods. A wealthy woman, Mrs Martin Van Butchell, under motives obscure and indecipherable, wrote a peculiar will. It was her intention, duly legalised by seals and signatures, that her surviving husband should have control of her fortune only for as long as she would remain above ground. Upon her demise, her husband acted with a determination all the more admirable for being mixed with grief. John Hunter was summoned to the homestead. Mrs Van Butchell's remains were injected intra-arterially with fluids of recent invention, and the lady ended up, fashionably clad in her best finery, inside a glass-lidded container, before which she received friends and relatives.[50]

In *Patient's Progress* Dorothy and Roy Porter point out that the medical man did not always hasten to the homestead when the end was nigh.[51] Doing so often forced an illustration of impotence. It was not always the case, as it is in Jane Austen's *Sense and Sensibility* that 'Hope . . . entered' with the doctor in attendance.[52] *Patient's Progress* carries an ironic allusion to Bunyan as it details

---

[49] A point made by Helman, 1991, 118.
[50] Gonzalez-Crussi, 1986, 2.
[51] D. & R. Porter, 1989, 145.
[52] See *Sense and Sensibility*, Ch. 43.

a progression towards the medicalisation of death, the taking of the traditional notion of 'the good death' out of the control and choice-range of the dying.

Mrs Martin Van Butchell puts a rather different complexion upon death and social choice, as does her husband. Sontag observes that, 'etymologically, patient means sufferer' and 'it is not suffering as such that is most deeply feared but suffering that degrades'.[53] In Mrs Butchell's self-presentation all traces of any suffering have been effaced. Dying in 1775, Mrs Butchell stands removed in time from Bentham's auto-icon and the contradiction-prone propaganda which aimed to remove stigmatic associations on dissection in the 1820s. Her upright figure projects – it literally bodies forth – a social ideology of confident, assertive selfhood. Choice and medicalisation appear to pose no conflict in this case, for Gonzalez-Crussi implies that her husband holds her express will as his rationalisation to secure the money. As she finally puts her money where her body is, Mrs Martin Van Butchell is evidently worth a call to John Hunter.

Discussing the 'machinery of representation' in the scriptural economy, De Certeau identifies two main operations:

> The first seeks primarily to *remove* something excessive, diseased, or unaesthetic from the body, or else to *add* to the body what it lacks . . . From the inside or the outside, they correct an excess or a lack, but in relationship to what? As in the case of removing the hair from one's legs or putting mascara on one's eyelashes, having one's hair cut or having hair reimplanted, this activity of extracting or adding is carried out by reference to *a code*. It keeps bodies within the limits set by the norm. In this respect clothes themselves can be regarded as instruments through which a social law maintains its hold on bodies and its members, regulates them and exercises them through changes in fashion.[54]

---

[53] Sontag, 1990, 37.
[54] De Certeau, 1988, 147.

Hunter would have added a good colour to the cheeks, removing the appearance of emaciation. The object of Gonzalez-Crussi's gentle irony, of course, is Mrs Van Butchell's mentality, the greyer matter within. Not many women had the art of exercising control over their husbands down to quite so fine a point. Mrs Martin Van Butchell is making 'cultural capital' out of her body. In his book *Distinction*, the sociologist Pierre Bourdieu describes a metaphor at work in society: cultural capital, he argues, underwrites economic capital.[55] The metaphor refers to cultural processes as though they were economic. The dominant classes, like Mrs Butchell, attempt to control culture for their own interests as effectively as they control the circulation of wealth. Mrs Butchell, adding art to nature, is striking precisely because she presses the claims of the metaphor so hard. Her composure is the very image of exclusivity, of power ideally exerted.

There is a configuration of power even in her posture. Canetti has shown that human postures in daily life retain a primary kind of significance that comes into play 'at the core of everything that we – rather vaguely – call power'.[56] He observes:

> The *standing* person seems autonomous, as though standing for himself alone and as though still having the possibility of any decision. The *sitting* man exercises a pressure, his weight presents itself to the outside, arousing a sense of permanence. The way he sits, he cannot fall; he becomes larger when he stands up.[57]

In my frontispiece photograph, Bentham, another showcase figure, retains a magisterial membership of 'the society of the erect',[58] as Canetti calls it. Mrs Butchell stands upright: she is a symbol of what it is to belong to the world of the fully adult. In this society the first real contacts usually take place standing, as rituals of respect and, less explicitly, as measurements of oneself against others.[59] As

---

[55] Bourdieu, 1984, 116, 120, 303; Fiske, 1987, 18.

[56] Canetti, 1987, 14.

[57] *Ibid.*, 14–15.

[58] Canetti, 1981, 456.

[59] *Ibid.*, 451.

such Mrs Butchell stands; and with the sting in her will it is as if she stands for the first time without fear or concealment. The advantages of standing imply the value of personal independence; but equality within the social group remains a valuable social fiction.[60] Canetti – who speaks only in general terms – can help us to see one form of this figure's cultural capital. 'Standing', he observes, 'is the central position, from which every other position can be directly reached and any movement initiated';[61] 'we tend, therefore, to ascribe a relatively high degree of tension to anyone who is standing, even when he himself does not in fact feel it.'[62] Following the metaphor, like the standing which precedes walking, there is a suggestion of energy or power – or capital – yet to be used. Hunter's work on the corpse involved a partial dissection and a fee of around 100 guineas.[63] The anatomist Cecil Helman comments:

> In the dissecting room we come to realise the true paradox of anatomy. For the real agenda of dissection is the taming of Death, or rather the fear of Death. Because of this, we are asked to perform impossible alchemies. We must turn the cadaver into a three-dimensional textbook, a limited edition of tissues and organs. To do this, we must transform a dead body into the creation of a living body. The cadaver must become raw clay or pigment, the medical student a special type of performance artist. Our task is to create, or rather re-create, the body as a public sculpture, or as a series of sculptures. We must give to the body a posthumous life, through the rebirth of its parts. They must be reborn as objets d'art, as named, labelled, living commodities.
>
> But in turning the body into a soft book, we are doomed to be copyists. We are fakers who can only reproduce in cut flesh the abstract aesthetic of the anatomy book, with its lonely limbs

---

60 Ibid.
61 *Ibid.*, 450–1.
62 *Ibid.*
63 Noted by Litten, 1991, 48.

and organs. Our signatures must remain hidden away, somewhere inside ourselves. In taming death, we have also tamed the anomalies of life.[64]

The high compliment that Hazlitt pays Hunter, as the Michaelangelo of the public sculpture, is laced with a rhetorical move to promote the father of modern anatomy out of the company of copyists. When he calls Hunter 'a great man', Hazlitt is in effect calling him a 'creative genius'. The approbation implicitly carries the full ideological weight of the term 'genius' in romantic philosophy. As Bourdieu observes, the genius enjoys truly human creativity:

> Art is called upon to mark the difference between humans and non-humans: artistic experience, a free imitation of natural creations, *natura naturans,* whereby the artist (and through him, the beholder) affirms his transcendence of *natura naturata* by producing 'a second nature' subject only to the laws of creative genius, is the closest approach to the divine experience of *intuitus originarius*, the creative perception which freely engenders its own object without recognising any rules or constraints other than its own.[65]

## Aesthetics and murder

Bourdieu argues that 'what is at stake in aesthetic discourse, and in the attempted imposition of a definition of the genuinely human, is nothing less than the *monopoly of humanity*'.[66] At the basis of it is a capacity for sublimation, or a 'disgust at the facile':

> 'Pure' taste and the aesthetics which provides its theory are founded on a refusal of 'impure' taste and of *aisthesis* (sensation), the simple, primitive form of pleasure reduced to a pleasure of the senses, as in what Kant calls 'the taste of the tongue, the

64 Helman, 1991, 117–18.

65 Bourdieu, 1984, 491.

66 *Ibid.*

> palate and the throat', a surrender to immediate sensation which in another order looks like imprudence . . . it could be shown that the whole language of aesthetics is contained in a fundamental refusal of the *facile*, in all the meanings which bourgeois ethics and aesthetics give to the word; [as in] . . . facile music, or a facile stylistic effect, but also 'easy virtue' or an 'easy lay'. The refusal of what is easy in the sense of simple, and therefore shallow, and 'cheap', because it is easily decoded and culturally 'undemanding', naturally leads to the refusal of what is facile in the ethical or aesthetic sense, of everything that offers pleasures that are too immediately accessible and so discredited as 'childish' or 'primitive' (as opposed to the deferred pleasures of legitimate art) . . . Pure taste [on the other hand] demands respect, the distance which allows it to keep its distance.[67]

The loss of distanciation, Bourdieu argues, is the basis of a kind of 'horror' and 'disgust'.[68] In Kant's aesthetic, 'disgust discovers with horror the common animality on which and against which moral distinction is constructed'.[69] This discovery explains the impact the female Creature's sexuality has on Frankenstein while he creates her body, for he fantasises about her 'easy virtue'. He says she may turn 'with disgust'[70] from the Creature to lust after 'the superior beauty of man' – but actually the word applies more appropriately to his own mounting horror, and fascination, with her appetite for sensual pleasure.

As I showed in Part I, De Quincey's famous proposal to view murder 'aesthetically, as the Germans call it, that is, in relation to good taste'[71] accommodates an argument in favour of the surgeons' cause in the pre-1832 era. The speaker in *On Murder considered as one of the Fine Arts* extends compliments – which are ironic up to a point – to 'artists' who respect their audience. The Lecturer,

---

67 *Ibid.*, 486.
68 *Ibid.*, 489.
69 *Ibid.*
70 *Frankenstein*, 140.
71 De Quincey, 1918, 306.

an English Kantian, calls for higher standards of murder in public and private life – and reviews the surgeons' long-standing popular reputation as murderers. From the surgeons' point of view, the 1832 legislation transformed the art, as civilised society started to obtain the bodies at a safe remove from the public hangman. The distance gained from public, despotic power was 'prudent' in Bourdieu's sense of the word. The reviled anatomists had long known, as they waited in its wings, that the aesthetics of the gallows ritual was regularly threatened with the possibility of a violent, popular upset.

At one point in De Quincey's second instalment, the members of the Murder Club are provoked to protest at the recidivist attachment of one of their number to 'facile' gratification. Reminiscing with Christopher North in the 1839 instalment the senior dignitary of the Society recalls the blackballing of his own nephew from the premises. The speaker mimics the club members' objections:

> If we were to elect him, why, the next thing we should hear of would be some vile butcherly murder, by way of justifying our choice. And what sort of a concern would it be? You know, as well as we do, that it would be a disgraceful affair, more worthy of the shambles than of an artist's *atelier*. He would fall about some great big man, some huge farmer returning drunk from a fair. There would be plenty of blood, and *that* he would expect us to take in lieu of *taste* [italics added], finish, scenical grouping. Then, again, how would he tool? Why, most probably with a cleaver and a couple of paving stones: so the whole *coup d'oeil* would remind you rather of some hideous Ogre or Cyclops, than of the delicate operator of the nineteenth century.[72]

These voices belong to the club's more prudent members, who, as members and audience, demand to be treated with more respect. 'Pure taste', Bourdieu notes, 'expects the work of art, a finality

---

72 *Ibid.*, 339.

with no other end than itself, to treat the spectator in accordance with the Kantian imperative, that is, as an end, not a means'.[73] What it means to have 'taste', as De Quincey uses the term here, is illustrated in a statement by Kant, which Bourdieu quotes in *Distinction.* 'Pure taste', or 'taste of reflection' equates with 'the conscious expectation of the future': 'This capacity for facing up in the present to the often very distant future, instead of being wholly absorbed by the enjoyment of the present, is the most decisive mark of the human's advantage.'[74]

The nephew, a regressive pleasure-seeker, arouses the other members' disgust as well as their censure. 'Pure' or legitimate taste can come about only through social training and discipline, and, as De Quincey well knows, it is the key to civilised behaviour. The nephew remains incapable of heeding any kind of 'don't' injunction where murder is concerned. In the members' eyes, he is 'common' in the sense of being 'vulgar' – 'a quality', as Kant puts it, 'everywhere to be met with – which by no means confers credit or distinction upon its possessor'.[75] Kant's definition of 'the 'human's advantage' would not have been lost on any self-aware surgeon bidding for social legitimation before 1832. The first two instalments of *On Murder* stand either side of the year which saw the Anatomy Act come into force. The first, in 1827, belongs to the 'dilettante' phase of the art; the second, in 1839, belongs to the 'connoisseur' phase. That is to say: the former stands to the latter as the 'present moment' stands to the 'distant future' in Kant's scheme. The speaker in the 1839 text has achieved 'the future' – the legislation – and from this vantage point he parodies the progress of Vice:

> For if once a man indulges himself in murder, very soon he comes to think very little of robbing; and from robbing he comes next to drinking and Sabbath-breaking, and from that to incivility and procrastination. Once you begin upon this

---

[73] Bourdieu, 1984, 488.

[74] *Ibid.*, 598.

[75] Quoted by Bourdieu, 1984, 489.

> downward path, you never know when you are to stop. Many a man has dated his ruin from some murder or other that perhaps he thought little of at the time. *Principiis obsta* [Check the beginning] – that's my rule.[76]

This is nostalgic, ironic and stamped with learning. The sequence in the parody attributes the same order of priorities to the bodysnatcher and the surgeon alike, as did the public perception in 1828. The legislation in 1832, as it guaranteed the future, enabled the profession to present a less back-to-front set of priorities, and to emerge from the resurrectionist-man's shadow.

De Quincey's essay constructs a discursive alliance between the medical profession and romantic aesthetics. 'Pure' taste, as Bourdieu puts it, 'is pre-disposed to become a symbol of moral excellence, and the work of art a test of ethical superiority, an indisputable measure of the capacity for sublimation which defines the truly human man.'[77] In *Frankenstein* the disinterested contemplation of the aesthetic belongs above all to Henry Clerval, who, quite early in the story, is released from a career in commerce. The relationship between Frankenstein and his friend dramatises a De Quinceyian alliance between knowledge and aesthetics. The two men travel across Europe to England, and north into Scotland via the Lake District. As they travel, Frankenstein extols his companion's romantic being – 'his overflowing soul',[78] and 'imagination . . . chastened by the sensibilities of his heart'.[79] In the Lake District, Clerval finds 'in his own nature' even 'greater capacities and resources'[80] – the story here sketches the alliance in a pastoral setting. Clerval, a sexless, intellectual figure, is the free man:

> The opposition between the tastes of nature and the tastes of freedom introduces a relationship which is that of the body to

76 De Quincey, 1918, 340.
77 Bourdieu, 1984, 491.
78 *Frankenstein*, 133.
79 *Ibid.*
80 *Ibid.*, 137.

> the soul, between those who are 'only natural' and those whose capacity to dominate their own biological nature affirms their legitimate claim to dominate social nature.[81]

Moreover: 'The culture which results from this magical division is sacred. Cultural consecration does indeed confer on the objects, persons and situations it touches, a sort of ontological promotion akin to a transubstantiation.'[82] In these terms, Henry Clerval, Frankenstein's benign double, is the 'genuinely human man'. He is murdered not long after the two men visit Edinburgh, from whence they separate – forever, as it turns out. The aesthetic, as we have seen, marks the difference between the human and the non-human – and, as he attacks Clerval, the 'monster' draws the social basis of this difference into greater prominence in Frankenstein's language. With Clerval dead, Frankenstein loses 'the image of my former self'[83] and henceforth talks a more strident language of antagonism and reprisal against his Creature. That is to say, he employs a version of the rhetoric which assisted the passage of the Anatomy Act into law.

The social basis of the opposition between 'taste of reflection' and 'taste of sense' is apparent when Frankenstein first encounters his 'monster':

> how can I delineate the wretch whom with such infinite pains and care I had endeavoured to form? His limbs were in proportion, and I had selected his features as beautiful. Beautiful! . . . the beauty of the dream had vanished, and breathless *horror and disgust* filled my heart [italics added].[84]

The word 'disgust' recurs when the Creature looks at the portrait of Caroline Beaufort, Frankenstein's middle-class mother. He has just murdered William, her youngest son, and he meets her gaze: 'She whose resemblance I contemplated would, in regarding me,

---

81 Bourdieu, 1984, 491.
82 *Ibid.*, 6.
83 *Frankenstein,* 135.
84 *Ibid.*, 58.

have changed that air of benignity to an expression of disgust and affright.'[85] As Bourdieu concludes, the antithesis between the 'taste of freedom' and the 'taste of nature' is 'rooted in the opposition of the bourgeoise and the people'.[86] In the Kantian scheme, the opposition between the social classes is constructed 'as stages in an evolution . . . the progress from nature to culture'.[87] This evolution is present in *Frankenstein* as the story charts the aspirations of Justine and Elizabeth to rise from poverty to middle-class status. When the 'monster' intervenes and exacts their fates, Justine and Elizabeth are respectively realigned with criminality and poverty: Justine is executed, and Elizabeth is denied a consolidation of respectability. In death they are reclassified as lower-class, lower-order people.

As she stands in the frame of Bourdieu's cultural capital metaphor, Mrs Butchell is a perfect replica of the distanciation that is central to the economy of the bourgeois body. In death and behind glass she stands, the nascent bourgeois subject. In the uprightness of her non-being, and, in Kant's sense, taking 'the human's advantage', she looks to the long distant future. This figure belongs, however, to the era of public anatomy: she could be viewed by prearrangement throughout her husband's life. Her husband died in 1814 and his son removed his mother from the public gaze by presenting her to the Curio Room at the Royal College of Surgeons in 1815, three years before *Frankenstein* appeared.

One other detail about Mrs Martin Van Butchell must be observed. Dead and on her feet, she receives friends and *relatives*. In this respect the figure in the glass illustrates the key 'claiming' clause in the eventual anatomy legislation. In Gonzalez-Crussi's pen-sketch, the relatives surround the body. 'Bentham's chosen constituency', Richardson observes,[88] 'would be all those who died in poverty with no relatives to bury them, and those whose relatives were too poor to do so'. There were strands of euphemism

[85] *Ibid.*, 123.
[86] Bourdieu, 1984, 490.
[87] *Ibid.*
[88] Richardson, 1989, 110.

and ambiguity in the legislative drafting that stayed attached to the term 'unclaimed',[89] and the bureaucratic mechanisms of contacting the relatives remained rather vague.[90] Outside nearest known relatives, '*bona fide* claimants in any ordinary sense'[91] were not recognised. Frankenstein's Creature is a man who desperately seeks a mate – in the event, however, he is condemned to exist without 'real' claimants in either sense. I discuss the 'claiming' vocabulary in *Frankenstein* in the next chapter.

---

89 *Ibid.*, 121–9.
90 *Ibid.*, 207.
91 *Ibid.*, 234.

CHAPTER 4

# The death command, anatomy and the law, 1750–1850

## The gibbet

The anatomy question has a historical timetable which commences around the 1750s. As we have seen, in 1752 an Act of Parliament was passed which enabled the judiciary to add dissection to capital punishment for murder; the new law required that, following execution, murderers should either be hung in chains or anatomised. The murder sentence thus acquired an extra punitive dimension. The dissection was adopted as a way to differentiate the punishment for murder from the executions routinely ordered for a large number of other crimes, mainly offences against property. The subsequent attempts to destigmatise dissection reveal the power of exemplary spectacle to concentrate the mind. In the previous chapter, for example, we saw Bentham expressly recommending the gallows for 'the eyes of childhood'. A comparable example is given by Wordsworth in *The Prelude*, the 1805 poem in which he describes the 'growth' of his mind. Wordsworth recalls from his boyhood a solitary encounter with a gibbet. The gibbet – another tool of the scriptural economy – was an encasement in which the murderer's corpse was hung in chains and exhibited as a warning to others. Wordsworth's account indicates the power of this apparatus to disturb and haunt the mind. He recalls a danger that is sensed before it is actually seen:

> I remember well
> That once, while yet my inexperienced
> hand
> Could scarcely hold a bridle, with proud hopes
> I mounted: and we journeyed towards
> the hills:

> An ancient solitary of my father's house
> Was with me, my encourager and guide:
> We had not travelled long, ere some mischance
> Disjoined me from my comrade;
> and, through fear
> Dismounting, down the rough and stony
> moor
> I led my horse, and, stumbling on, at
> length
> Came to a bottom, where in former times
> A murderer had been hung in iron chains.
> The gibbet-mast had mouldered down, the bones
> And iron case were gone; but on the turf,
> Hard by, soon after that fell deed was wrought,
> Some unknown hand had carved the murderer's name.
> The monumental letters were inscribed
> In times long past; but still, from year to year,
> By superstition of the neighbourhood,
> The grass is cleared away, and to this hour
> The characters are fresh and visible:
> A casual glance had shown them, and *I fled*,
> Faltering and faint, and ignorant of the road
> [italics added][1]

'The gibbet', comments Richardson:

> with its creaking human-scarecrow corpse occupied an important place in popular imaginative apprehension of 'justice' and judicial retribution. As an exemplary punishment it was exceeded in power only by dissection. The intention of both punishments was to deny the wrongdoer a grave.[2]

The popular view of dissection after 1832 sustained the association with the murderer and execution, the final resort mechanism to command obedience. As I have noted, the despectacularisation of

---

1 Wordsworth, *The Prelude*, bk XII, 230–48.
2 Richardson, 1989, 36.

power is one of the main ways in which effective norms, in De Certeau's sense, are established and maintained. In contrast to a dissection conducted away from the public eye, the gibbet was a potentially counter-productive spectacle and its use was abolished in 1834. Towards the end of the eighteenth century, according to Foucault, many actions previously regarded as criminal, and specific to individuals, began to assume political meaning as protests against the existing state of society. The developing threat to social order was most in evidence at the ritual gallows spectacle of violence. The excess of this spectacle became the preponderant reason for the threatened disintegration of the sovereign's power to command obedience. *Discipline and Punish* tells the story of how the guardians of the new order heeded the fact that once a command ceases to exact obedience and recognition, it is better not to try to revive it.[3]

In principle, a command is meant to be obeyed; it is, after all, the nature of an order to admit of no contradiction.[4] Foucault's account was anticipated in a commentary on command given by Canetti in *Crowds and Power* that does much to suggest the menace carried by dissection in the eighteenth and early nineteenth century. Canetti was concerned above all to clarify what comes into play in a command to secure obedience, and the anatomy timetable either side of 1832 provides a corroboration of his analysis. The generality of Canetti's basic premise notwithstanding, it is not difficult to see in his proposal a description of the role of commands and power in modern Western society. His commentary on command describes two scenarios, the second of which is a reversal or a domestication of the first. Command, Canetti argues, is a social phenomenon, the earlier and more striking forms of which can be traced back to the original, fundamental use of power, a command to flee:

> The basic situation in nature arises from the fact that many animals feed on other animals. Those they feed on belong,

---

[3] See Foucault, 1979, chs 1 and 2; and Harland, 1987, 164.

[4] See Canetti, 1981, 352.

> however, to species different from their own, and thus most animals feel threatened by creatures of a different kind; it is strangers and enemies who command them to flee.[5]

The substance of every command draws on the 'arche-command' to flee sent out by the stronger animal threatening to kill the weaker one. The power of the human command derives from a death sentence, against which flight is the final and only appeal.

The passage above from *The Prelude* is apposite in this context, for Wordsworth affirms that the scene of the gibbet-mast caused him to flee. The command-character of the threat embodied in the gibbet is vestigial, but it is somehow powerfully present to the mind as the human figure is compelled into flight.[6] The flight is not merely a reaction against the command; rather, it is a simultaneous part of it, the other face of the death sentence.[7] Canetti's clarification is that commands are a *suspended* threat of death. There is no clearer testimony to this social fact than the State's appropriation of anatomical subjects after 1832, as the role of commands and power underwent a social transformation that was legislative in the first instance and a domestication of command in the longer term. The gallows stigma was transferred to the world of poverty and its potential victims, and hence retained.

## *Frankenstein*: the arche-command

The Creature in *Frankenstein* literally embodies the signs of power. Canetti hypothesises that all command derives from an original flight-command, an arche-command:

> The original command results in *flight*. Flight is dictated to one animal by a stronger animal, by something *outside* itself. Flight only appears spontaneous; danger always has a shape and no

5 *Ibid.*, 355–6. See also Barnouw 1983.

6 The same configuration, the gibbet which compels flight, is described by Dickens at the end of Ch. 1 of *Great Expectations*.

7 This point is made by Deleuze and Guattari in their commentary on *Crowds and Power* in *A Thousand Plateaus*, 107.

> animal flees unless it discerns it. Disparity of strength between the two animals involved is inherent in the nature of flight. The stronger proclaims its intention to hunt and eat the other, and thus flight is a matter of life and death. Whether in fact it is pursued or not, the weaker is compelled by the 'command' to flee. It flees from the threat alone, *from the eyes, the voice, the whole terrifying shape* . . . Flight is the final and only appeal against a death sentence [italics added].[8]

The most famous moment in *Frankenstein*, the nocturnal first encounter between Frankenstein and his Creature, shows this 'command' in action. The second appearance of the Creature, which soon follows the first appearance, is sufficient to compel Frankenstein into terrified flight. The second sighting commences as he awakes – recumbent and defenceless – from the dream in which he figures as a resurrectionist preying on his mother's grave, but dream and reality continue to merge at a juncture prior to full wakefulness. The vision repeats and intensifies the first wakeful apprehension. The eyes and the voice enter into 'the whole terrifying shape':

> I started from my sleep with horror: a cold dew covered my forehead, my teeth chattered, and every limb became convulsed; when, by the dim and yellow light of the moon, as it forced its way through the window shutters, I beheld the wretch – the miserable monster whom I had created. He held up the curtain of the bed; and his *eyes*, if *eyes* they may be called, were fixed on me. His jaws opened, and he muttered some inarticulate sounds, while a grin wrinkled his cheeks. He *might have spoken,* but I did not hear; one hand was stretched out, seemingly to detain me, but I escaped and rushed downstairs. I took refuge in the courtyard belonging to the house which I inhabited, where I remained during the rest of the night, walking up and down in the greatest agitation, listening attentively, catching and fearing each sound as if it were to announce the approach

[8] Canetti, 1981, 351–2.

> of the demoniacal corpse to which I had so miserably given life [italics added].[9]

The arche-command is a bestial threat of incorporation. In this first meeting with his creation, Frankenstein encounters the configuration of the command as naked force and threat. Relatively late in the historical timetable of the anatomy question, he encounters in the spectacle the terroristic death-command sanction that is openly wielded by the absolutist State. The teeth have already been sighted; subsequently, it is always the eyes as first encountered which haunt Frankenstein. He remains henceforth a figure in flight, haunted by the association with absolutist power which the surgeons needed to expunge from their public image. As the story proceeds, this power also shadows the 'monster', for in the historical context his crimes qualify him for dissection, were he to face the law. When *Frankenstein* appeared in 1831 the law was only months away from transposing this extra dimension to the punishment for murder on to the world of poverty. In this first encounter, the Creature's condemnation, announced by the first appearance of the word 'monster', establishes him as an 'at large' version of 'the body of the condemned man' which figures prominently in Foucault's account of the transition from despotism to 'disciplinary' society.[10] The 1832 anatomy legislation marks the point at which the command mechanism undergoes its social transformation. In this transformation, however, the command stands as a suspended death sentence, for dissection was popularly perceived to be nothing but the punitive violence originally reserved for the body of the condemned man.

There are moments in *Frankenstein* where the bestial threat recurs. In one instance, the Creature threatens to 'glut the maw of death until it is satiated' with the blood of Frankenstein's remaining friends.[11] In another example the child William, 'as soon as he beheld my form', fears a cannibal: 'you', he says in

---

[9] *Frankenstein*, 58.

[10] See Foucault, 1979, Ch. 1.

[11] *Frankenstein*, 90.

terror, 'wish to eat me and tear me to pieces'.[12] Where William is concerned, the Creature entertains a hope that in the companionship of so young a person he will cease to be an object of outright rejection. The story implies, of course, that recognition would assimilate the Creature into human identity. However, where recognition is concerned, the formal terms in the impending law concerning claims on pauper bodies begin to appear in the Creature's discourse after the William episode. The demand he imposes on Frankenstein sees him trying to secure what was to become the only mechanism of escape from the dissection constituency recognised by the new law: the claim of a relative. Furthermore, as we have seen, in the eyes of the law only relatives as such, as opposed to *bona fide* claimants, were deemed to qualify. Richardson has shown that while the crucial wording in the legislation on this point remained loose, it was this stricture in particular, the non-recognition of *bona fide* claimants, that often prevailed in practice.[13] In this context the Creature's revenge killing on Frankenstein's wedding-night expresses his own exclusion from – and his desire for – legally sanctioned union.

## Claiming

The initiative to assemble the second creation comes from the Creature himself and he demands it 'as a right'[14] – which means a political right. The security of Frankenstein's family depends on his acceding to the demand. As he works, reluctantly, on the female creation Frankenstein's preoccupation continues to be his own security – should the Creature come 'to claim his companion'.[15] Here – as I noted in Chapter 2 – is an example of the pivotal verb 'to claim' surfacing in the story. Following the broken promise, the murders of Clerval and Elizabeth are mediated by

12 *Ibid.*, 140.
13 Richardson, 1989, 234–5.
14 *Frankenstein*, 124.
15 *Ibid.*, 140.

the fact that the Creature cannot establish requisite status in the strict terms of reference. By contrast, Frankenstein speaks of 'the one reward I promised myself from my detested toils'. It is 'the prospect of that day when I . . . enfranchised from my miserable slavery . . . might claim Elizabeth'.[16] The wedding-night assignation is to turn the bride into a corpse, a forensic exhibit.

The extent to which the famous first encounter turns on misperception on Frankenstein's part is often remarked on by readers of the story.[17] Frankenstein's reaction apart, the Creature moves to elicit recognition and initiate a claim. The Creature 'might have spoken', apparently, but only 'some inarticulate sounds' are heeded by the figure in flight. The Creature, from his own subsequent report, acquires language later. But, as noted, the context here is a dream, or a waking nightmare, which has subjective validity for Frankenstein himself. The sight of the jaws opening is perhaps the key moment in the encounter. Frankenstein, when fully awake, has already seen the Creature's phalanx of 'pearly white' teeth. This second glimpse, however, sees the Creature demonstrating the mouth's double function: Frankenstein encounters the intimate, unceasing blend of language with the parts of the mouth – the lips, teeth, tongue and throat – used for eating.[18] He, after all, has made this Creature; he is familiar, as only an anatomist can be, with the incorporation process inside the body. The moment confronts him with the indissoluble connection between culture and the animal digestive process – but he declines to look the connection fully in the face. In the report of his escape, intelligible speech on the Creature's part is neither denied nor affirmed: 'he might have spoken, but I did not hear'. Where this 'monster' is concerned, it is not easily conceded that language shares the same

---

[16] *Ibid.*, 131.

[17] See, for example, Victor Sage (1988, 167–73); Chris Baldick (1987, 48.)

[18] My reading of this passage owes much to Canetti's note in *The Human Province*: 'does this intimate blend of all the sounds that we form, with lips, teeth, tongue, throat, the very parts of the mouth that serve eating – does this blend express the fact that language and food must forever be connected . . . ?' See Canetti, 1985, 106. See also Piel, 1987.

orifice with eating. From this moment on, the Creature is condemned to remain outside human culture, until he acquires the language which the dream scheme accommodates here.

In contrast, as the encounter ends, Frankenstein himself effects the transition from nature to culture as he gains the asylum of the courtyard. The transition sees him fully awake and alert, 'catching and fearing each sound', as if it presages the reappearance of the Creature. There is a larger implication to be drawn from this famous scene. Contrary to Frankenstein's desire, when in flight from his 'monster', to keep nature and culture apart, the encounter suggests that nature and culture in certain respects coexist. The utilitarians who designed the anatomy legislation were in effect constructing a fiction of clear lines of demarcation. They were, after all, attempting to dissociate the new social arrangements of 1832 from the realm of predatory violence. Their problem with the stigma on dissection involved them in contradiction, however, for the source of the stigma was of course the death-command which they wrote into the law – and into civilisation. In a recent essay on *Crowds and Power* Edgar Piel has commented pertinently that the emphasis in Canetti's account of authority in modern society is 'that civilisation is by no means simply a wonderful antithesis to the realm of bestiality and natural violence, [and] nor does culture as such represent the conquest of the jungle'.[19] As Piel explains, Canetti deliberately erases a firm line of demarcation in order to concentrate on transition and transformation:

> Taken together, the interlinked, merging processes of seizure, incorporation and digestion constitute . . . that process which is fundamental to the copiousness of Man's psychic, spiritual, and social being, and also to his culture. Through continually renewed transfers, transpositions of this one process into other spheres, beyond Nature (which was out to devour Man) into Man's own flexing of teeth, muscles, and nerves, and thence into the psychic, social and political realms – through all of this

---

[19] Piel, 1987, 150.

> adaptation and metamorphosis of a single paradigmatic process, the pre-human creature became Man.[20]

Frankenstein, the moment his work is complete, flees an exhibition – a flexing – of the teeth. As readers of the story have observed, the Creature cannot metamorphose because he is doomed to be 'complete' from the outset.[21] He is excluded at first sight from the impending political settlement of 1832, while ever more desperately seeking admission. Not long after he acquires language, but unable to effect the transformation he craves, he turns murderous, commencing with William's death.

The encounter scene, as Frankenstein flees, contains the first sign of the Creature's efforts to gain accommodation: a representation, on the Creature's part, by means of his hand. In a discussion of what he calls 'the entrails of power', Canetti comments on the interplay of body and word:

> One could say that objects in our sense, objects which have value because we ourselves have made them, first existed as signs made by hands. There seems to be an immensely important turning point where the nascent sign language for things first comprehends a desire to shape them oneself, long before this is actually attempted. What man, with the help of his hands, enacted, was only *made* long afterwards, when it had been enacted often enough. *Words* and *objects* are accordingly the emanations and products of a single unified experience: *representation by means of the hands*. Everything that a man can do, everything that represents his culture, he first incorporated into himself by means of transformation. Hands and face were the instruments of these transformations and their significance, compared with the rest of the body, became increasingly great. The specific life of the hands, in this its earliest sense, still retains its pristine force in gesticulation.[22]

---

20 *Ibid.*, 152.

21 However, as I show in Ch. 9, the Creature is capable of transformations which enable him to evade capture.

22 Canetti, 1981, 254.

As we have seen, the full dimension of the Creature's first gesture eludes Frankenstein. To him it remains equivocal whether the hand movement is accompanied by words or not. As the hand beckons – 'seemingly to detain me' – Frankenstein flees because he construes a predatory design. It escapes him that the gesture, in Piel's terms, is a demonstration of 'psychic, spiritual and social being' – and a claim on him. The first meeting between the creator and his 'monster' shows the 'father' disowning the claims of the 'son'. The *donné* of the story is that Frankenstein, by any fair reckoning, *is* the Creature's father – that is to say, an immediate relative. In language which prefigures the Anatomy Act's vocabulary Frankenstein – as he begins to assemble the Creature – imagines himself as the 'father' laying 'claim'[23] to his child's gratitude. But the by-pass of human biology in the creation gives him a let-out clause where the impending law's operative terms of reference are concerned. The encounter, in other words, rehearses the legislation's controversial 'unclaimed' clause in terms of the possibility, already noted, that real claims – perfectly *bona fide* claims – stood to be ignored where the strict letter of the law was applied. This scene is the *locus classicus* in the anatomy literature of the impending 'claiming' ritual under the law; and it enters the caveat that Frankenstein is the Creature's father.

A similar equivocation recurs in the honeymoon scene as the Creature faces Frankenstein and gesticulates:

> I felt a kind of panic on seeing the pale yellow light of the moon illuminate the chamber . . . and with a sensation of horror not to be described, I saw at the open window a figure the most hideous and abhorred. A grin was on *the face* of the creature; he *seemed* to jeer, as with his fiendish finger he *pointed* towards the corpse of my wife [italics added].[24]

The figure at the window has by this time acquired and used language to make himself and his needs known to Frankenstein.

---

[23] *Frankenstein*, 55.
[24] *Ibid.*, 164.

In the event, only one occasion can ultimately suffice to symbolise all the transformations – that is, the Creature's entire cultural potential – which are denied to him by the broken promise of a mate: his creator's wedding-night. In a hands-and-face appearance, he despairingly enacts a 'claiming' ritual in the relevant sense of the word. Elizabeth is the bride *he* has lost as well as the bride whom Frankenstein has just gained: she is bride to two 'claimants'. The Creature's pointing is a 'hands off' gesture directed at Frankenstein, but he relinquishes the corpse as he eludes Frankenstein's pistol shot. Using the wedding-night to act out his loss, he appears at the window gesticulating in an oddly equivocal way. The report that 'he seemed to jeer' does not affirm an actual verbal remonstrance. The billingsgate violence of the gesture has a curious dumb-show dimension. But by pointing to Elizabeth, whom he has murdered, the Creature alone remains the figure who silently indicates the ultimate predatory dimension of Frankenstein's desire for professional legitimacy – the fact that it does not stop at their mutual bride. The murder, moreover, occurs on the special day of Frankenstein's social, and professional, respectability. On this day, the Creature is pointing at the surgeons, who murder to dissect.

## 1832: the domestication of command

In Canetti's account of the command, the death threat can never be entirely eliminated from power if it is to anticipate success: 'beneath all commands glints the harshness of the death sentence'.[25] As the Creature's pointing finger on the wedding-night indicates, the retained threat in 1832 was the stigmatic dissection sanction. Canetti's broader argument in *Crowds and Power*, however, concerns the transformation of unacceptably explicit command into commands apparently rendered harmless. This transformation takes place in the legislative move to break the association of the surgeons with the gallows. Canetti describes a denaturing of the biological command to flee; in a significant formula, command is described

[25] Canetti, 1981, 352.

as becoming *domesticated*.[26] Social evolution has seen to it that virtually nothing remains of the original threat or message to flee. Quite the reverse:

> A master calls his slave and the latter comes although he knows he will receive an order. A mother calls her child and it does not invariably run away; although she rains orders of all kinds on it, it continues on the whole to trust her . . . The same is true of a dog: it stays near his master and comes at once when he whistles.[27]

The explanation of this development towards domestication 'lies in the fact that . . . a kind of bribery is practised'.[28] In a scenario-reversal, the command, instead of operating through a bestial threat, is transformed into a guarantee of food:

> a close link grows up between commands and the giving of food . . . Domesticating the command means linking it with the promise of food. Instead of being threatened with death and thus put to flight, some creature is promised what all creatures most want; and this promise is strictly kept . . . This adulteration of the original flight-command trains men and animals for all kinds and degrees of voluntary captivity, but it does not entirely change the nature of commands in general. Every command still contains the same threat. It is a modified threat, but there are stated penalties for non-compliance and these can be very heavy. The heaviest of all is the original penalty, which is death.[29]

There is a warning in *Frankenstein* about the strict keeping of promises: when the famous promise is not kept, the Creature speaks of a revenge 'dearer than light or food'[30] – and takes it.

In *The Great Transformation* the economic historian Karl Polanyi

---

26 *Ibid.*, 355–7.
27 *Ibid.*
28 *Ibid.*
29 *Ibid.*
30 *Frankenstein*, 142.

describes the moves towards a full market economy in the 1830s. Polanyi comments on the political and social importance of the utilitarian application of the domesticated command principle, as it was applied in the world outside the workhouse:

> the Parliamentary Reform of 1832 achieved a peaceful revolution. By the Poor Law Amendment of 1834 the social stratification of the country was altered, and some of the basic facts of English life were reinterpreted along radically new lines. The New Poor Law abolished the general category of *the poor*, the 'honest poor,' or 'labouring poor' . . . The former *poor* were now divided into physically helpless paupers whose place was in the workhouse, and independent workers who earned their living by labouring for wages. This created an entirely new category of the poor, the unemployed, who made their appearance on the social scene. While the pauper, for the sake of humanity, should be relieved, the unemployed, for the sake of industry, should *not* be relieved. That the unemployed worker was innocent of his fate did not matter. The point was not whether he might or might not have found work had he only really tried, but that unless he was in danger of famishing with only the abhorred workhouse for an alternative, the wage system would break down, thus throwing society into misery and chaos.[31]

The main reason why the workhouse was regarded as abhorrent was undoubtedly the Anatomy Act. Bentham, the patron of the anatomy reform, also exercised an influential voice in the arguments before 1832 that pressed the case hard for a full market economy, specifically on the subject of the abolition of outdoor relief. The newly constituted Parliament moved fast to see to it that the hungry would work for the crust, and discipline themselves in the process. Polanyi puts the central issue:

> That this meant penalising the innocent was recognised. The perversion of cruelty consisted precisely in emancipating the

[31] Polanyi, 1980, 224.

> labourer for the avowed purpose of making the threat of destruction through hunger effective. This procedure makes intelligible that dismal feeling of desolation that speaks to us from the works of the classical economists. But to lock the doors safely upon the supernumeraries who were now caged in the confines of the labour market, government was put under a self-denying ordinance to the effect that – in Harriet Martineau's words – to provide any relief to the innocent victims was on the part of the state a 'violation of the rights of the people.'[32]

The anatomy legislation, and the fear of it, is implicit in Polanyi's observation that 'the demand for popular government was the political source of the tension'.[33] And as Polanyi also comments, the element of provision in the domesticated command culture means economic growth:

> Not before the working class had passed through the Hungry Forties and a docile generation had emerged to reap the benefits of the Golden Age of capitalism; not before an upper layer of skilled workers had developed their unions and parted company with the dark mass of poverty-stricken labourers; not before the workers had acquiesced in the system which the New Poor Law was meant to enforce upon them was their better paid stratum allowed to participate in the nation's councils. The Chartists had fought for the right to stop the mill of the market which ground the lives of the people. But the people were granted rights only when the awful adjustment had been made.[34]

The separation of the people from power over the economic conditions of their lives in the 'Hungry Forties' meant that effective political opposition to the anatomy legislation was rendered impossible. In the reversal that was accomplished in the course of domesticating the command, the threat of dissection was retained as the harshest of sanctions. (In my Conclusion I discuss the portrait

---

32 *Ibid.*

33 *Ibid.*, 225.

34 *Ibid.*, 226.

of working-class militancy and the anatomy story-line in Mrs Gaskell's *Mary Barton*.)

## The coach scene in *Oliver Twist* and *Frankenstein*

The most famous request for food in the anatomy literature is made inside the workhouse: 'Please, sir,' says Oliver Twist, 'I want some more.'[35] This request needs to be understood in the light of the distance – the ideological as well as the actual distance – which Oliver eventually achieves from the English 'Bastille', the source of the corpses. Like *Frankenstein*, *Oliver Twist* comments on how 1832–34 is a key period in the domestication of command, the transition from absolutism to an early phase of a consumer-orientated society. In the figurative sense of the term, nurture in *Oliver Twist* is an ideological construction, a desert rather than a right. The ideological change of climate around the time in question can be focused in two scenes from the literature, one from *Oliver Twist* and one from *Frankenstein*. In both texts the scene concerns a coach and a human figure on the roadside. This is the episode in Dickens' story where Oliver, who is famished, is begging:

> He waited at the bottom of a steep hill till a stage coach came up, and then begged of the outside passengers; but there were few who took any notice of him, and even those told him to wait till they got to the top of the hill, and then let them see how far he could run for a halfpenny. Poor Oliver tried to keep up with the coach a little way, but was unable to do it, by reason of his fatigue and sore feet. When the outsides saw this they put their halfpence back into their pockets again, declaring that he was an idle young dog and didn't *deserve* anything; and the coach rattled away and left only a cloud of dust behind [italics added].[36]

---

[35] Dickens, 1969, 36.
[36] *Ibid.*, 81.

Richardson comments on this scene:

> During the period the Anatomy Act was being formulated and Dickens was writing, an older, more paternalist view of help to the needy was compounded and in some quarters almost eclipsed by the morally loaded qualification of '*desert*'. Helping only the 'deserving poor' involved the imposition of social and political value judgements on the distribution of poor relief. Because Oliver could not perform the feat they expected of him, the travellers abused him, and mutually agreed that he was beneath their consideration, despite the child's evident need.[37]

As Richardson adds, the new attitude easily legitimised the view that 'poverty somehow reflected moral shortcomings';[38] and it accommodated some long-standing Malthusian arguments which recommended withdrawing all forms of assistance, backed by the deterrent of the workhouse. The older paternalist view of help to the needy is apparent in *Frankenstein* in the accommodation given to Elizabeth by the benign figure of Caroline Beaufort, Frankenstein's mother. By contrast, Frankenstein's first-sight rejection of the Creature – as the hand, 'seemingly to detain me', beckons – is an example of the harder attitude in action. In reply, on the politically symbolic wedding-night, the propertyless 'wretch' provocatively acts out the moral shortcomings imputed to poverty.

The coach episode in *Frankenstein* occurs on the morning after the great rejection scene. In contrast to the encounter with the 'monster', it contains intelligible speech, another hand gesture which this time is unambiguous and reference to relatives. Unlike the *Oliver Twist* passage, this episode involves a meeting which is perceived to be between two social equals. Here Frankenstein is more than ready to be 'detained':

> I remained some minutes with my eyes fixed on a coach that was coming towards me . . . and on the door being opened, I perceived Henry Clerval, who, on seeing me, instantly sprung

37 Richardson, 1989, 147–50.
38 *Ibid.*, 148.

> out. 'My dear Frankenstein,' exclaimed he, 'how glad I am to see you! How fortunate that you should be here at the very moment of my alighting!'
>
> Nothing could equal my delight on seeing Clerval; his presence brought back to my thoughts my father, Elizabeth, and all those scenes of home so dear to my recollection. *I grasped his hand*, and in a moment forgot my horror and misfortune; I felt suddenly, and for the first time during many months, calm and serene joy [italics added].[39]

The coincidence remarked by Clerval is evidently a kind of wish-fulfilment where Frankenstein is concerned. The early morning encounter with the 'wretch' has brought on strong heart palpitations in Frankenstein. The firm handshake with Clerval dispels them; immediately, all memory of the work of creation and the first encounter evaporates. As the anatomy legislation brings benevolent paternalism to an end in 1832, this passage in *Frankenstein* is the ideological inverse of the coach scene in *Oliver Twist.* The irony in the episode is that Clerval, Frankenstein's double, is a benevolent version of Frankenstein as he might have been and never again can be – that is, minus the 'monster' he has just spurned. In due course, the corpses of William, Clerval and Elizabeth turn up in delivery to the anatomist.

Nor was the medical academy quite the same again after the murders in Edinburgh brought the 'monster'[40] William Burke to public attention. Where the 1831 edition of *Frankenstein* is concerned, the encounter scene between Frankenstein and his Creature yields a pointed comment on the 1828–29 scandal. As Frankenstein says, the Creature's hand beckons, 'seemingly to detain me'. This is an ambiguous formula. In one sense, as we have seen, the gesture is a 'claim' upon the parent figure in the relevant sense of the word. In the waking dream nature of the moment, however, Frankenstein senses a predatory design. The moment of first touch, Canetti comments, belongs to the entrails of power:

---

39 *Frankenstein*, 59–60.

40 Richardson, 1989, 142.

> Contact through the other senses, sight, hearing, and smell, is not nearly so dangerous. With them there can be space between the attacker and the victim and, as long as this space exists, there is still some chance of escape . . . The design of one body on the other becomes concrete from the moment of touching. Even at the lowest levels of life this moment has something decisive about it. It contains the oldest terrors; we *dream* of it, we imagine it, and civilised life is nothing but a sustained effort to avoid it [italics added].[41]

The bodysnatching contribution to civilised life ended in 1832, as the surgeons jettisoned their criminal connections. Moreover, the criminal context adds a further dimension to the hand image under review here. As I commented in the second chapter, the figure in particular who obtrudes into a historicised reading of *Frankenstein* is Dr Robert Knox, the anatomist beneficiary of Burke and Hare. In the context of the late 1820s a pertinent irony informs Frankenstein's move to evade the Creature's outstretched hand. Canetti observes:

> The touch to which one resigns oneself because all resistance appears hopeless – and particularly so as regards the future – has, in our society, become the *arrest*. The feel of the hand of authority on his shoulder is usually enough to make a man give himself up without having to be actually seized. He cowers and goes quietly. He maintains an appearance of composure, even though it is not everywhere that this is justified by what is likely to happen to him subsequently.[42]

The popular opinion in Edinburgh in 1828–29 was that Robert Knox was an accomplice to the crime of murder.[43] However, the crowd at Burke's hanging called in vain for the distinguished anatomist to take the same punishment. In the encounter scene in *Frankenstein* the Creature looms as an accusing popular policing

---

41 Canetti, 1981, 238.
42 *Ibid.*
43 Richardson, 1989, 138–141.

group, but his hand cannot 'detain' – or arrest – Knox. In Bakhtin's sense, this 'citizen's arrest' image gains accentuation in the 1831 edition of the story, for it carries a larger charge of inherent injustice against the legislative moves which immediately impended.

## Dickens' executioner

The injustice in question, the stigma and social inequality written into the 1832 anatomy reform, is commented on in Dickens' *Barnaby Rudge*. This novel, published in 1841, has a special relationship to the changing command culture under review: the story doubles as a representation of the two historical phases either side of 1832, absolutism and domesticated command. The portrait of the Gordon Riots of 1780 merges with some dictation from Thomas Carlyle on the evils of Chartism in 1839. However, the portrait of Chartism does not directly concern us here. The significant figure, as I noted in Chapter 1, is Mr Dennis the executioner. Dickens links this man to the surgeons and to two other characters who act out the story's anatomy debate: Hugh Maypole and Simon Tappertit. In Mr Dennis, Dickens portrays the executioner-surgeon association which is at the root of the medical profession's unpopularity throughout the pre-legislative phase of the anatomy timetable. It is now appropriate to look at this figure in more detail.

Dickens' executioner is a tool of the Bloody Code[44] and, into the bargain, a vocal defender of the law even as he foments the rioting. He dresses in the clothes of his victims. His connection with the surgeons is captured in its essence at the height of the riots, as he accompanies Hugh Maypole and Sim Tappertit. He takes a question about his job:

---

[44] As J. A. Sharpe (1990, 30) puts it: 'After 1688 the English Parliament passed a long series of laws which, by 1800, had placed some 200 capital offences, many of them property crimes, on the statute book.' These laws were known as the 'Bloody Code'.

'I'm of as gen-teel a calling, brother, as any man in England – as light a business as any gentleman could desire.'

'Was you 'prenticed to it?' asked Mr Tappertit.

'No. Natural genius,' said Mr Dennis. 'No 'prenticing. It come by natur'. Muster Gashford knows my calling. Look at that hand of mine – many and many a job that has done, with a neatness and dex-terity, never known afore. When I look at that hand,' said Mr Dennis, shaking it in the air, 'and re-member the helegant bits of work it has turned off, I feel quite molloncholy to think it should ever grow old and feeble. But sich is life!'

He heaved a deep sigh as he indulged in these reflections, and putting his fingers with an absent air on Hugh's throat, and particularly under his left ear, *as if he were studying the anatomical development of that part of his frame*, shook his head in a despondent manner and actually shed tears.

'You're a kind of artist, I suppose – eh!' said Mr Tappertit.

'Yes,' rejoined Dennis; 'yes – I may call myself an artist – a fancy workman – art improves natur' – that's my motto.'

'And what do you call this?' said Mr Tappertit taking his stick out of his hand.

'That's my portrait atop,' Dennis replied; 'd'ye think it's like?'

'Why – it's a little too handsome,' said Mr Tappertit. 'Who did it? You?' [italics added] [45]

At this point in the story the executioner is in effect masked, for Hugh Maypole does not yet know what Dennis' job actually is, or whose orders he follows. The man speaking here is the em-bodiment of the death-command culture. The job description has strong onanistic overtones: the face on the stick-handle was carved by one of his many 'worked off' victims, as Dennis likes to put it. Mr Dennis himself, however, is doomed to eventual execution and his stick figures in his desperate bid for a personal reprieve. There is some lettering on it which finally discloses the paternal link between John Chester, the aristocrat who manipulates the

[45] Dickens, 1987, 372.

riots to gain personal ends, and Hugh Maypole, the anatomical 'subject' of Mr Dennis' gaze here. Before the link comes to light, Sir John muses on the prospect of Hugh's dissection:

> 'They will be a singular party,' said Sir John, leaning his head upon his hand, and sipping his chocolate; 'a very curious party. The hangman himself; the centaur; and the madman. The centaur would make a very handsome preparation at Surgeon's Hall, and would benefit science extremely. I hope they have taken care to bespeak him. – Peak, I am not at home, of course, to anybody but the hairdresser.'[46]

In fact, Hugh escapes dissection, as does Barnaby, the 'madman', who is reprieved. Following Hugh's execution, an inscriptionless coffin in a midnight burial is accompanied by the sole figure of the legitimate brother that 'the centaur' never knew – Edward Chester. Nevertheless – in a gesture which recalls the rejection scene in *Frankenstein* – when John Chester learns he is Hugh's father the news brings no retraction of the attitude that is coldly spelt out here. The 'centaur' nickname suggests a link to comparative anatomy; Hugh is the Frankensteinian 'monster' in *Barnaby Rudge* and another image of the coveted physical specimen. In a description which recalls De Quincey's conceit, Hugh, 'of muscular and handsome proportions . . . might have served a painter for a model'.[47] 'Perfect musculature', as Martin Fido comments,[48] 'ranked second only to deformity or disease in attracting the anatomist's notice.' Old John Willet, a self-appointed spokesman for the death-command culture, describes Hugh as 'an animal',[49] and he thoroughly approves of the government's policy of hanging such people as Hugh's mother for passing forged notes.

The reference to anatomy in the exchange between Dennis and Tappertit is a key detail. It compounds the executioner with the

---

46 *Ibid.*, 671.
47 *Ibid.*, 138.
48 Fido, 1988, 76.
49 Dickens, 1987, 140.

surgeon in a way that exactly corresponds to the popular perception of the surgeons. De Certeau observes:

> for Kant and Hegel, there is even no law unless there is capital punishment, that is, unless in extreme cases the body signifies by its destruction the absolute power of the letter and of the norm – a questionable assertion. However that may be it remains that the law constantly writes itself on bodies.[50]

His motto 'art improves natur' notwithstanding, Mr Dennis does not have an art, or a hand, that bears cultivating – and his is the shadow which falls across the medical profession's long bid for legitimation before 1832.

## *Barnaby Rudge* and *Frankenstein*: the sting of command

As we saw in the first chapter, Mr Dennis enjoys the executioner's special exemption from the sting of command. The executioner, acting under orders, passes on the sting, the lethal threat contained in the command, to his victim. As a result, no sting is left inside him. As Canetti observes, no other recipient of a command is ever privileged in this way. The sting debases and wounds its victim; it must be passed on to a social inferior and got rid of:

> A command is like an arrow . . . An arrow remains sticking in the flesh of the man it hits and he has to pull it out in order to free himself of the threat it carries. When a command is passed on it is as though a man pulled out an arrow which had hit him, fitted the same arrow to his bow and shot it again.[51]

Dennis' exchange with Tappertit illustrates the analogy. Hugh serves as the executioner's victim, and, as Dennis fingers Hugh's 'anatomical development', the passage links the executioner with the medical profession. It is ironic and fitting that it should be

---

50 De Certeau, 1988, 139–40.
51 Canetti, 1981, 357.

Tappertit who confronts the surgeons' worst version of themselves in this exchange, for Tappertit has a role in the novel's implicit debate about the 1832 anatomy legislation. In the course of the events concerning this young man the same passing-on mechanism is exemplified in a way that concerns Miggs, the servant in Gabriel Varden's house. In Simon Tappertit Dickens dramatises some other ideological voices which carried influence and sway in the anatomy argument, the voices in particular of Francis Place and Carlyle.

The historian J. W. M. Mackenzie comments on Francis Place in a way that underlines Place's achievement:

> Politically, the mob began to decline with the invention of the urban police in the 1820s; but it had been a dangerous beast, easily provoked, easily exploited, but difficult to kennel – 'the beast with many heads', 'the mutable rankscented many'. Yet somehow James Mill and Francis Place had managed by 1830 to find intermediaries, and to create at least a show of revolutionary organisation good enough to frighten the establishment into a Whiggish show of revolution.[52]

Richardson's analysis of the persuasion exercised by Place during the publicly controversial phase of the proposed anatomy legislation provides a clear instance of the passing-on mechanism operating within Place's ideological objectives. It offers a remarkable glimpse of the 'milk and water Radical' because the episode in which he declares his views puts into question Place's claim to the moral high ground in the transformation of the working class. Richardson highlights Place's skilful and opportunist use of laughter to promote the case for the working man's exemption from dissection. In February 1832 Place addressed a large meeting of the National Political Union on the subject of the anatomy legislation and the question of exemptions. Place, Richardson observes, 'championed only the 'respectable' portions of the working class',[53] and he

52 Mackenzie, 1975, 152.
53 Richardson, 1989, 152.

spoke to his audience to counter any assumption 'that the Bill could affect members present':[54]

> 'The members of this Union,' he declared, 'are not "the poor", pride and ignorance may call them "the lower classes" but I say they are not "the poor". Whose bodies are to be given up?' he asked rhetorically, and answering his own question, replied:
>
> 'None but such as no-one will claim, none but such as no-one will bury, and is this the case with the members of the union? Certainly not. Is there a member who does not belong to a benefit club, which will pay for a decent funeral, for him or his wife; have not most of them the ready means either through the club or from his own savings, to provide the means, and is there a near relative of such a man for whom a decent funeral would not be provided? Surely not. The Bill has then no reference to the members of the Union in this respect much more than it has to the rich.'[55]

The passing-on mechanism is apparent in the timing and the tone of the performance from Place that followed:

> Having flattered the social aspirations of all those present, lulled them into a sense of security, and invited them to join him in forgetting about the real poor (who in any case had hitherto been 'buried in a way, truly disgusting'), Place changed his tack, and trivialised the proceedings by describing how as a tailor he took the measurements of female clients without any hint of 'indelicacy'. Drawing a parallel with dissection, Place assured his audience that dissection likewise showed no indelicacy, even to the bodies of 'the most delicate females'. The sexist wit with which Place both emphasised his kinship with the world of toil, and his support of the Bill, was decisive. His humorous remarks about female anatomy provided light relief to a grim discussion, and were greeted with laughter and cheers. The upshot was a

54 *Ibid.*, 156.
55 *Ibid.*

> petition to Parliament from the council of the NPU in support of Warburton's Bill.[56]

This rhetorical success, Richardson argues, exemplifies a divide-and-rule tactic which informs the social meaning of the impending law.[57] Place's objective was to ally the labour aristocracy with respectable society and diminish sympathy for the improvident poor.

Gabriel Varden's house in *Barnaby Rudge* is a symbol of the British Constitution. At the outset of the story Tappertit has a provisional footing within its pale so long as he faithfully sustains the work ethic in his part as an apprentice locksmith. By virtue of his daytime work, that is to say, Tappertit has the key to a secure position in civil society in his own hands. Miggs, too, hopes to gain security for herself: Tappertit has given her his word that they will marry at some point in the future. In the story this arrangement lapses; the young, work-shy apprentice is drawn into the mass riot, in the course of which he dishonours his promise to Miggs. Tappertit's word matters to Miggs, for she too exists just within the margin of regular employment under Varden's roof (and does not join the rioting). Tappertit's eventual betrayal of Miggs, and her attitude to it, is indicated early in the story in the brief seconds when she sees him illicitly slipping away from Varden's house at night:

> 'Why I wish I may only have a walking funeral, and never be buried decent with a mourning coach and feathers, if the boy hasn't been and made a key for his own self!' cried Miggs. 'Oh the little villain!'[58]

From her window vantage-point the servant woman thus delivers the imagery which spells out her own perception of her potential social fate. The distinction she draws between a pauper and a

---

56 *Ibid.* Henry Warburton was the utilitarian MP who piloted the anatomy legislation through Parliament.

57 *Ibid.*, 265–6.

58 Dickens, 1987, 120.

respectable funeral is particularly significant in the post-1832 context. The two kinds of funeral conspicuously exemplified the social distance between the victims and the beneficiaries of the anatomy reform. Francis Place's reference to burial clubs is also relevant here. Aside from respectable society, burial club payments – made possible by prudential financial habits – enabled poor people 'to be buried decent', as Miggs puts it. Ironically, the unhappy outcome of her suit for Tappertit's hand is in effect sealed as she makes these observations. Tappertit here is heading off to his dissolute night-time fantasy life as the king-figure at the head of the 'Prentice Knights. The Knights are a low but numerous company of fellow apprentices who notch up reprisals against their superiors in the form of black crosses marked against names, and who in due course join the riots to exact their revenge.

During the nocturnal antics of the Knights, Tappertit, wearing military uniform, officiates at the induction of one Mark Gilbert. Gilbert has been punished for casting eyes at his employer's daughter when he should have been attending to his work.[59] This apprentice mirrors Tappertit's own desires for Gabriel Varden's daughter. The lust which he entertains for Dolly Varden is the fantasy component of a larger desire to rise in the social scale without earning anything through effort, self-respect and sobriety. Sim Tappertit, in other words, yields to all the easy inclinations and habits which Place, over a long period of advocacy, thought were disastrous to the best interests of working men. Place's famous remark that for the urban poor in the late eighteenth century sex and drinking were the only pleasures of life, and of the two, 'drunkenness is by far the more desired',[60] is actually true of Tappertit, for whom the bottle is a regular and ready substitute for Dolly Varden.

Prior to the rioting, the night-time alleyway world is the setting for a revealing piece of street-theatre which Tappertit and the blind man Stagg act out together. As they do so, they are secretly

---

[59] *Ibid.*, 114.
[60] Quoted in Golby and Purdue, 1984, 49.

observed by the hidden figure of Barnaby's father, Rudge, the murderer. This episode is, I think, the novel's moral equivalent of Place's rhetoric to the National Political Union. Tappertit, notably, is dressed in his general's uniform, his riot carnival-costume:

> The light came to the level of the pavement . . . and a man ascended, bearing in his hand a torch. This figure unlocked and held open the grating as for the passage of another, who presently appeared, in the form of a young man of small stature and uncommon self-importance, dressed in an obsolete and very gaudy fashion.
>
> 'Good night, noble captain,' said he with the torch. 'Farewell, commander. Good luck, illustrious general!'
>
> In return to these compliments the other bade him hold his tongue, and keep his noise to himself; and laid upon him many similar injunctions, with great fluency of speech and sternness of manner.
>
> 'Commend me, captain, to the stricken Miggs,' returned the torch bearer in a lowered voice. 'My captain flies at higher game than Miggses. Ha, ha, ha! My captain is an eagle, both as respects his eye and soaring wings. My captain breaketh hearts as other bachelors break eggs at breakfast.'
>
> 'What a fool you are, Stagg!' said Tappertit, stepping on the pavement of the court, and brushing from his legs the dust he had contracted in his passage upward.
>
> 'His precious limbs!' cried Stagg, clasping one of his ankles. 'Shall a Miggs aspire to these proportions! No, no, my captain. We will inveigle ladies fair, and wed them in our secret cavern. We will unite ourselves with blooming beauties, captain.'
>
> 'I'll tell you what, my buck,' said Mr Tappertit, releasing his leg; 'I'll trouble you not to take liberties, and not to broach certain questions unless certain questions are broached to you. Speak when you're spoke to on particular subjects, and not otherways. Hold the torch up till I've got to the end of the court, and then kennel yourself, do you hear?'
>
> 'I hear you, noble captain.'

> 'Obey then,' said Mr Tappertit haughtily. 'Gentlemen, lead on!' With which word of command (addressed to an imaginary staff or retinue) he folded his arms, and walked with surpassing dignity down the court.[61]

The duo act here accords a dominant role to Tappertit in which every word of his is either an 'injunction' or a 'command'. Stagg takes the part of the 'voice' that extrapolates the predatory nature of those famous legs – in a mockery of Tappertit's sexual narcissism. The blind man replies to the reprimands he invites with a stream of sexual innuendo concerning Miggs and Dolly Varden. In their complicity and banter the two men construct between them in fantasy a multi-accented 'carnival' of the woman's body in which both Miggs and Dolly receive praise and abuse at the same time.[62] The claims of 'the stricken Miggs' on Tappertit – 'Shall a Miggs aspire to these proportions?' – are given a cruel sexual slant and are turned into a pretext to humiliate her erotically. A violent version of Stagg's laughter will later be heard from Hugh Maypole, when Tappertit promises to let Hugh have Miggs as a sexual trophy (this is a fate which Miggs escapes). The fantasies in play in the alley are solicited by Tappertit and negatively acknowledged. They have a direct bearing on the callousness he eventually shows to Miggs, when, in a drunken performance, he spurns and abuses her in Gabriel Varden's presence. When this humiliation occurs, Miggs manages a reasoned plea to Tappertit to beware the consequences for himself of his intoxicated behaviour. As she sustains her plea, however, she exhibits the 'symptoms of the acutest mental suffering'.[63] Thus does she take the rejection which carries with it the danger of a fall into Place's category of 'the poor'.

The riots are Tappertit's salvation and damnation. He has put up with twelve years of subordination under the firm but patient Varden, during which time, as he sees it, he has received and

---

[61] Dickens, 1987, 197–8.

[62] I have found Colin Mercer's essay 'Complicit Pleasures' helpful on the politics of carnival. See Bennett *et al.*, 1986, 50–68.

[63] Dickens, 1987, 472.

stored up command after command, order after order, without an outlet to get rid of them. He is not the only one in this position, however. Hugh Maypole's emotional identification with his executed mother indicates the harsher social dis-ease which needs relief. *Barnaby Rudge* demonstrates that the stings of command are potentially volatile. They make possible the abuse and the manipulation of real needs into destructive crowd energies. Gordon, a celebrity-seeker variant on the mob-orator, is only important in the formative stage of the crowd. A mere slogan suffices to relieve the stings of inequality and isolation, igniting the multitude of the victims of the death-command culture into a violent crowd. Hugh, in an illiterate slip, amends 'No Popery' to 'No Property'. Tappertit, hating his locksmith's work, joins what Canetti calls the 'open' crowd: 'The open crowd . . . does not recognise houses, doors or locks and those who shut themselves in are suspect. "Open" is to be understood here in the fullest sense of the word; it means open everywhere and in any direction.'[64] The relief 'is temporary and, as it is not concerned with the causes of the social illness, illusory'.[65] Hugh Maypole, out of control, is well under control, as John Chester knows. The spirit of the 'open' crowd quickly puts Tappertit into Chester's pocket and in due course it draws his latent hostility towards Miggs to the surface.

Tappertit's top-ranking military uniform tells the story of his desire. The general's uniform exemplifies the process of *promotion* inside a hierarchy. Promotion is the process which provides the opportunity to get rid of the stings of command in oneself by passing them on to inferiors: 'Promotion is . . . the public manifestation of something more profound which remains secret, if only because the way it functions is never understood by more than a very few. Promotion is the outward manifestation of the hidden workings of the stings of command.'[66] This process is apparent in the street-theatre exchange between Tappertit and Stagg, as

---

64 Canetti, 1981, 17.

65 This is Dagmar Barnouw's phrasing. See 'Mind and Myth in *Masse und Macht*', *Modern Austrian Literature*, 16, 1983, 65–79.

66 Canetti, 1981, 365.

Tappertit's stings come out into the open as commands. Tappertit's abuse of the top-rank uniform is a manifestation of his desire to rise within the ranks and rewards of civil society without discipline or effort – without, in other words, the obligation of a step-by-step progression up the ladder. As Canetti observes, promotion, the power to use the stored up stings of command, is a secret form of discipline within the social hierarchy. This fact figures in the anatomy debate in *Barnaby Rudge* – but it also has an application to Place's successful joke to the National Political Union. The uniform, as worn by Tappertit in the scene with Stagg, and throughout the riots, is the index of a fantasy that is under rehearsal long before Tappertit's covert attitude to Miggs becomes explicit. Miggs, who remains single, eventually takes a job as a turnkey in a woman's prison. By her self-help efforts, therefore, she stays just outside the category of the improvident poor.

Close to the end of Dickens' story there is a scene in which Sim Tappertit is conspicuous by his absence. It is set in 'the bright household world'[67] of Varden's house and concerns the table laid out in honour of the impending marriage of Dolly Varden and Joseph Willet, the successful soldier in the story. The food, set out 'in rich profusion', is Dickens' construction of the domesticated command culture. One person is conspicuous by his absence: Tappertit is not at the table.

Where the domestication of command is concerned, one other voice can be heard in *Barnaby Rudge*. In his 1839 essay 'Chartism' Carlyle identified what he saw to be the worker's struggle for 'justice'. He linked the worker's right to be properly recompensed with his right to be properly governed:

> It is 'for justice' that he struggles; for 'just wages,' – not in money alone! An ever toiling inferior, he would fain (though as yet he knows it not) find for himself a superior that should lovingly and wisely govern: is not that too the 'just wages' of his service done? It is for a manlike place and relation, in this world where he sees himself a man, that he struggles. At bottom,

[67] Dickens, 1987, 714.

> may we not say, it is even for this, that guidance and government, which he cannot give himself, which in our so complex world he can no longer do without, might be afforded him?[68]

In this version of 'justice' the divide-and-rule tactic in the anatomy context is complete, for in Carlyle's notorious rhetoric the problem of pauperism called for the rat-catcher and the workhouse. Carlyle never says so explicitly, but the 'man-like place and relation in the world' includes exemption from dissection.[69] The pathetic figure of Tappertit at the end of *Barnaby Rudge* is an inversion of Carlyle's famous formula. He emerges from the riots with both legs broken and amputated, and begging Varden for relief from 'utter destitution'[70] – in Place's reiterated phrase, one of 'the poor'. The final image of Tappertit sums up a workshy existence. He obtains from the surgeons some wooden replacements for his legs which the woman he eventually marries is prone to confiscate, leaving him to the derision of the street.

The sting is an unchanging irritant which lives within the self. Canetti emphasises that it only results from the carrying out of a command; moreover, when a command functions normally there is nothing to be seen of the damage it leaves behind in the mind and the body. The sting sinks into the person who obeys, remaining hidden and immutable: the 'exact image'[71] of the order is 'imprinted'[72] with a degree of impression which depends upon the superiority of the source of the command, and its actual content. In phrasing that has surgical overtones, it is 'an implant',[73] 'a foreign body lodged in the flesh'[74] and:

> however long it lodges . . . it is never assimilated, but remains a foreign body . . . The sting is an interloper who never settles,

---

68 Carlyle, 1987, 166.

69 But he is abreast of the anatomy question. See *Selected Writings*, 1987, 97.

70 Dickens, 1987, 734.

71 Canetti, 1981, 380–1

72 *Ibid.*

73 *Ibid.*

74 *Ibid.*

> an undesirable one wants to get rid of. *It is what one has done* and has, as we have seen, the exact shape of the command given to one. It lives within its host as an alien, not subject to his authority, and thus does not cause him any feeling of guilt. He does not accuse himself, but the sting; this is the true culprit, whom he carries with him everywhere.[75]

In this formulation the passing-on mechanism puts dissection, and the threat of it, on to a wider disciplinary agenda. An example of this process is given in Richardson's history, and it demonstrates that dissection retained stigmatic associations after the passing of the legislation. In December 1832 one Polly Chapman,[76] a prostitute, was found drowned and was dissected. This woman was used by male authorities (the male pronoun in Canetti's description is appropriate) to set a disciplinary example; the coroner, Richardson notes, appears to have used the stigma in a retributive move. The 'nearest known relative' rule in the law was applied; it prevented Chapman's associates – '*bona fide* claimants in any ordinary sense'[77] – from averting her fate. Chapman's occupation marked her out as a fit target for the penalties for social non-compliance to come into play.

Victor Frankenstein's story of his 'monster' bears out Canetti's description of the latent life of the sting inside its host. There are two different ways in which freedom from the sting can be achieved. There is the passing-on mechanism; or there is the process of paying back to superiors what has been suffered and stored up from them. *Frankenstein* shows this second possibility in action. The sting remains in the recipient, but it seeks opportunities to surface and fully emerge. In the story it surfaces – or erupts – after William's murder: that is, after the Creature's utter condemnation at first sight. It is therefore inflected with *his* perception of arbitrary justice, for the sting 'is the hidden replica of the command he received and could not immediately pass on'.[78] It is immutable:

---

75 *Ibid.*, 386.
76 Richardson, 1989, 234–5.
77 *Ibid.*
78 Canetti, 1981, 360.

> The content of the command – its force, range and definition – was fixed for ever in that moment in which it was first promulgated, and this, *or rather its exact image in miniature*, is stored up . . . and may remain submerged for years or decades before it comes to light again [italics added].[79]

In *Frankenstein* it surfaces as the literally *miniature* portrait of the philanthropic mother which the Creature places on Justine as the 'frame' which is decisive in condemning her to the noose.[80] This particular 'surfacing', however, needs to be seen in the light of the emphasis carried by the word 'exact' in Canetti's commentary:

> [the sting] is preserved unaltered until he himself produces it again. But the occasion must be there; the new situation which releases the command must be the exact replica of the situation in which it was received. This reproduction of earlier situations, but *in reverse*, is one of the chief sources of energy.[81]

Exact reversal is the *only* thing the sting can recognise;[82] it is what the sting waits for. This too is the Creature's emphasis to his creator: 'I will watch with the wiliness of a snake, that I may sting with its venom. Man, you shall repent of the injuries you inflict.'[83] In the vocabulary of power relevant to the anatomy legislation, 'injury' and 'sting' are cognate terms; they both invoke the stigma on dissection. The Creature has indicated his willingness to accept a subservient position in society[84] if Frankenstein will provide him with a mate. The narrative which culminates in his demand shows him adopting self-improvement habits and working selflessly for others. For example, he chops and stacks the firewood for the de Lacey family: this imagery points to the Creature as a potential member of England's labour aristocracy.

---

79 *Ibid.*, 354.
80 *Frankenstein*, 124.
81 Canetti, 1981, 355.
82 *Ibid.*, 354.
83 *Frankenstein*, 142.
84 *Ibid*, 90.

The words 'sting' and 'injury' appear as he confronts the unexpected development which precipitates him into Francis Place's loaded category of 'the poor': Frankenstein's revoking of his promise. With his subsequent victims – Clerval the middle-class man, Elizabeth the aristocratic bride – the condemned man repays the class hierarchy. 'The body of the condemned man' comments Foucault, proclaims 'the 'lack of power' with which those subjected to punishment are marked'.[85] The fictional Creature's social kinship with the unsung Polly Chapmans of the anatomy era commences when his claim upon a mate ceases to be honoured, for henceforth he stands outside the letter of the impending law. 'Polly Chapman' comments Richardson, 'was not "unclaimed". The Anatomy Act alone made her so.'[86] There are occasions, Canetti observes, where commands, multiplying and repeated over time, can combine in a body in such a way that 'the sting loses its clear outline and develops into a monster which endangers life'.[87] The monster cannot find an appropriate outlet and remains deeply burdensome to its host. In this eventuality, the only means of possible liberation from the sting is within a crowd.[88] In Chapter 2, I noted Franco Moretti's observation that the monster is a crowd, a reanimated assemblage of the historic remains of 'the poor'.[89] What materialises in the vast, sting-riddled body which Frankenstein brings to life is a mass of bodies long bound over to proclaim the truth of crime and power.

---

[85] Foucault, 1979, 29

[86] Richardson, 1989, 235.

[87] Canetti, 1981, 380–1.

[88] *Ibid.*

[89] Moretti, 1983, 85.

# Part III

# The eighteenth century

CHAPTER 5

# The medical gaze and popular culture

In this chapter I shall describe the rise of the science of anatomy in the eighteenth century and the popular hostility to the surgeons. In addition, I will show how *Frankenstein* recalls one particular ritual form of opposition to the anatomists, the 'gallows wedding' drama.

## Hogarth's 'The Reward of Cruelty'

Hogarth's 1751 illustration 'The Reward of Cruelty', which features a dissection at the Company of Surgeons, is a famous visual document in the history of modern medical science in England. In a lecture in 1817 Hazlitt singled out Hogarth's work by remarking that 'Other pictures we see, Hogarth's we read'. I shall now 'read' 'The Reward of Cruelty' as it comments on the Company's aspiration towards formal and wider cultural legitimation. The aspiration was not fulfilled until well into the second half of the nineteenth century. Victor Frankenstein's narrative is an early nineteenth-century instance of a voice which lacks the longer-term legitimation conferred on the profession by the 1832 Anatomy Act, and in the 1831 edition his voice is shadowed by the Burke and Hare scandal. Frankenstein's difficulty, however, is a problem with a history of hindrances and milestones. As we have seen, the unwelcome connection with the gallows was severed in 1832, but Hogarth is commenting on it as early as the 1750s. Also, six years before 'The Reward', a milestone was passed when the Company ceased to be formally associated with the barber's trade, a link which for years had saddled surgery with a low status in the medical hierarchy. Hogarth, however, also indicates that the Company's

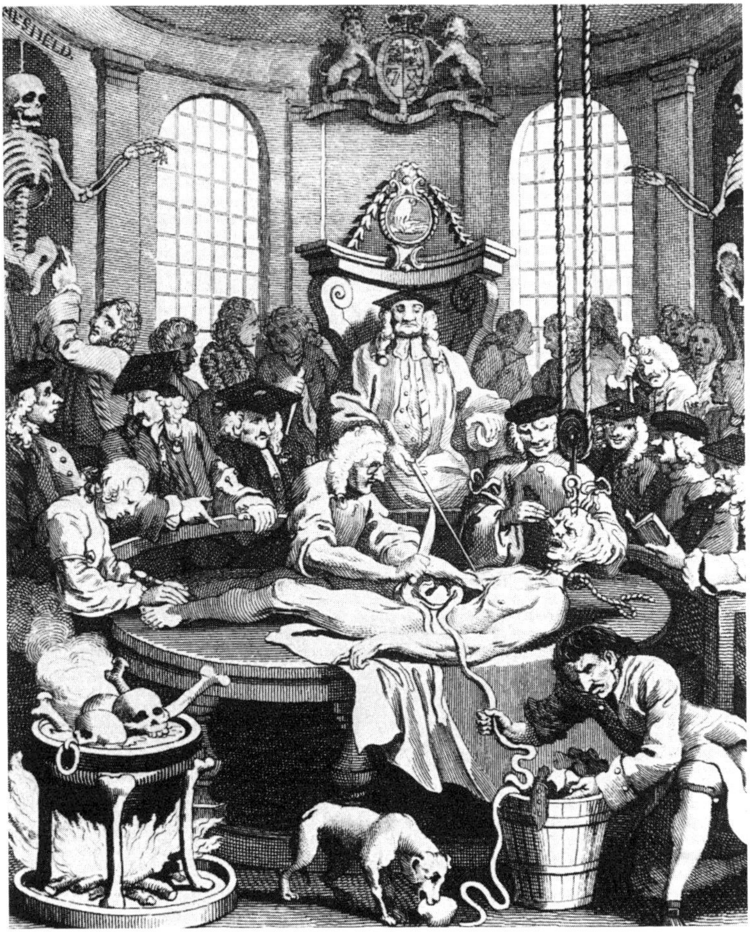

IV THE REWARD OF CRUELTY

Behold, the Villain's dire disgrace
  Not death itself can end:
He finds no peaceful burial-place;
  His breathless corse, no friend.

Torn from the root, that wicked tongue
  Which daily swore and curs'd!
Those eye-balls from their sockets wrung,
  That glow'd with lawless lust.

His heart, expos'd to prying eyes,
  To pity has no claim;
But, dreadful! from his bones shall rise
  His monument of shame.

case for greater social recognition is grounded in significant changes in medical perception and practice. I shall begin with this aspect of Hogarth's statement.

There is a sense in which the illustration is aware of an audience. Hogarth's commentary starts not with the working surgeons but the expensively robed figure at the back on the left pointing with his index finger upwards to the mounted skeletons. This figure enjoys, or is attempting to enjoin, an eye-contact relationship with the picture's reader; no one else is privy to or aware of his solicitation. He belongs not to the foreground theatre of surgery but to the more detached group behind the Company President's high chair. This man's gesture heralds the dawn of a new medical epistemology. The body in the theatre is a construct of the eyes which are being trained to constitute it. The object of vision is not pre-given; it is created by a historical variable, the act of seeing, and is not apparent to the untrained eye. It is the knife in the hand which carves the object. In 1828, Sir Astley Cooper spoke in the following terms when he addressed a House of Commons Select Committee on the need for legislative action to secure a supply of subjects: 'A knowledge of anatomy consists not in being acquainted with the names of things, but with their relative situation, and relative situation cannot be taught by casts or by models in *papier mâché*.'[1] These remarks exemplify a sense in which the body is the discursive construct of a medical perception which is not neutral. In Foucault's writings the term 'discourse' denotes 'the combination of a practice and a certain way of speaking'.[2] In this case, the practice – pathological anatomy – promotes a way of speaking in terms of separate internal organs. It is this discursive creation of an 'object' which belies humanism's official mythology of an advance out of ideology to science. In his account of modern science Foucault identifies and attacks a teleology: a claim upon the 'truth' which effectively relegates all past discoveries and knowledge to an anticipatory script, a lesser degree of enlightenment.

---

[1] Quoted in Low, 1987, 90.

[2] Harland, 1987, 103.

The new medical gaze also threatens alternative cultural constructions of the body. Implicit in Hogarth's anatomy of the criminal – the social 'other' – is a wider axis of contempt for the corpse as it exists in popular perception. The verse caption is more concerned with retribution than scientific advance. In Surgeon's Hall at least, this 'villain' has 'no Friend' – but even this emphasis tacitly recognises a cosmology of popular concern for the corpse. In the eighteenth century there still existed in the popular culture context a complex world of bereavement ritual which expressed a superstitious respect for the corpse. One ritual was the practice of 'watching' the dead body in the period between death and burial in the belief that it possessed some form of sentience.[3] (Later in this chapter we shall see 'corpse-watching' in action in *Frankenstein*.) In Hogarth's image the central act of violence is charged with disregard for all such perceptions. The question – what is a corpse? – is a question which medical science seeks to monopolise, as Richard Harland puts it, by 'turning the human body into an object for being objective about'.[4] Thus, for example (as I noted in the Introduction), in the seventeenth century William Harvey had sufficient clinical detachment, and distance from superstition, to cut up his father and sister *post mortem*.[5] Harvey's discovery of the circulation of the blood, published in 1628, is alluded to in *Frankenstein*[6] in a lecture by Waldman which Frankenstein listens to in a spellbound state of mind.

'The Reward of Cruelty' long precedes another, albeit relatively small, milestone in the Company's history, the 1778 Charter. This Charter had a number of effects. For the first time the surgeons could be said to have gained a status equivalent to that of the physicians who had become a Royal College in 1681. But even in 1751 Hogarth is noting the scale of the Company's longer-term objectives and alliances. As is apparent, several discourses participate in the conscription of the body into ideology. The elevated ceiling

---

3 See Richardson, 1989, Ch. 1

4 Harland, 1987, 103.

5 See Richardson, 1989, 31.

6 *Frankenstein*, 51.

invites an idea of ecclesiastical architecture. Richardson[7] points out that the role of the corpse in popular culture involved many beliefs and ritual observances in which the established Church played little if no role. In the Hogarth, established religion accommodates and is drawn into complicity with the 'march of the intellect'.[8] Hogarth nevertheless seems to comment with a touch of irony on the expediency of this alliance with imposingly visible power, for the emphasis falls on the central group's inturned concentration of attention.

The older royal dispensation of criminal corpses to the surgeons is commented on by the throne-like seat of the law. It is as if the king is present in person, granting permission for the body to be opened. In the early decades of the eighteenth century, however, the provision of felons' bodies from the king fell far short of the quantity the surgeons required. As a result the gallows frequently became a scene of violent conflict between the crowds and the surgeons, as each claimed final possession of the body. The most prominent sign of the Company's longer-term objectives is the legal apparatus in the picture. The massive, raised chair is the pinnacle of cultural and judgemental superiority. In it, wearing the sable hat, sits the hanging judge who is also the Company President. As judge and President double with the king, the Old Bailey doubles as the operating theatre. The law's 'scriptural' claim on the body – to recall De Certeau's metaphor – is made by the instrument – is it a knife or a writing implement? – guided by the hand of the diligent, scribe-like figure in profile at the subject's feet. The 1752 Act of Parliament for 'better Preventing the horrid Crime of Murder', which extended dissection to all murderers and replaced Henry VIII's small provision of six bodies annually, is only a year hence from Hogarth's portrayal. As Peter Linebaugh comments: 'Although the Parliament's sole interest in the law was

---

[7] Richardson, 1989, gives a full account of 'official' and 'folk' theology existing in 'a state of simultaneous conflict and symbiosis' in the eighteenth and early nineteenth centuries.

[8] This is a contemporary phrase, gathering currency in the early nineteenth century.

in making the death sentence terrifying, the Company of Surgeons [was] happy at this coincidence between the interests of criminal deterrence and its own.'[9] The 1752 Act effectively brought the unruly conflicts around the gallows to an end. Hogarth anticipates this advance. Within these walls things are as they ought to be: there is no crowd to contest the proceedings.

However, as Linebaugh also notes, after 1752 the surgeons could get 'on a regular basis'[10] only the bodies of felons sentenced under the new law. In the long term, and up to the time of *Frankenstein*, the supply proved inadequate, and the shortage produced the scandal-prone resurrectionist trade which figures in Mary Shelley's story. In this context the royal Hanoverian heraldic coat-of-arms at the top of the portrait acquires an ironic forward-looking dimension, for it comments on charters and advances in prestige yet to come in the Company's history. For example, it was not until 1800 – forty-nine years later – that the Company became the Royal College of Surgeons. By adding the royal coat-of-arms, Hogarth signals the Company's aspiration to a broader, hegemonic legitimation, which in 1751 was at least a century away. The only remaining trace of the public theatre of the gallows in the picture is the noose around the subject's neck. As the picture's title hints, the future 'reward' within the Company's historic purview is the removal of the gallows association from their activities.

Where this association is concerned, Hogarth implicitly addresses some earlier proposals for the law to requisition the criminal body. In 1725 Bernard Mandeville called for all hanged criminals to be anatomised following the Dutch legislative example:

> But suppose that many of our common Thieves were not to be buried at all, and some of them made Skeletons; and that several parts of others, variously prepared, should be preserved for the Instruction of Students? What if it was a Disgrace to the surviving Relations of those, who had lectures read upon their Bodies, and were made use of for Anatomical Preparations?

---

9 Linebaugh, 1977, 77.
10 *Ibid.*, 102.

> The Dishonour would seldom reach beyond the Scum of the People; and to be dissected can never be a greater scandal than to be hanged. The University of Leyden in Holland have a power given to them by the Legislature to demand, for this purpose, the Bodies of ordinary Rogues executed within that Province; but, with us, it is the general Complaint of all Professors of Anatomy, that they can get none to dissect: Where then shall we find a readier Supply; and what degree of people are fitter for it than those I have named? [11]

As Janet Semple notes, Mandeville here is callously indifferent to the feelings of the poor, who widely regarded dissection 'as a cruel and unnatural punishment fit only for murderers'.[12] This perception was in place well before the 1752 Murder Act; it derives from the earlier royal permission for the murderer's corpse to be anatomised. There is, however, a sense in which the eventual 1832 Anatomy Act delivered a version of Mandeville's advocacy, for people generally, rather than murderers, were targeted in Bentham's legislative design. The 1832 repeal of the association with the gallows ultimately required a broad projection of criminality on to all social groups whose common fear throughout the nineteenth century was to die unclaimed in the workhouse. In the Anatomy Act the surgeons were given recognition not least because their dreaded ministry enabled authority to cast a widening arc of surveillance across society.

The finger pointing up at the skeleton in 'The Reward' is laying claim to a scientific version of the human body which gains in currency during the anatomy timetable. The robed figure gestures towards the truth, as if to dispel ignorance and superstition. However, in Foucault's account in *The Birth of The Clinic* 'superstitious' medicine is accorded respect as a discourse of a different syntactical complexion.[13] In *Superstructuralism* Richard Harland explains:

---

[11] Mandeville, 1964, 26–7.
[12] Semple, 1993, 66.
[13] Foucault, 1989, 195.

> According to Foucault, the old 'superstitious' medicine made perfectly good sense of disease – but in terms of a discourse which has since been banished and forgotten. This discourse framed disease against a dominant assumption of life; and against a dominant assumption of life, disease showed up as a counter-life, an evil, a negative force. Disease was always the invisible 'other' of the visible human body. But in the new discourse emerging around the end of the eighteenth century, disease shows up not as a negative force but as a positive object for a positivist science to study. Disease is no longer the invisible 'other' of the visible human body, but something visible right *inside* the human body.[14]

Only in death can organic dependences and pathological sequences be clearly seen. In *The Birth of the Clinic* Foucault graphically describes death as 'the great analyst . . . [that] bursts open the wonders of genesis in the rigour of decomposition'.[15] Death is conceptualised as the apex of a triangle in which life and disease are the other two terms. In this cosmology death is 'the concrete *a priori* of medical experience'.[16] This scheme is implicit in Astley Cooper's demand in 1828 for an informed knowledge of separate internal organs. 'The object that modern medical science studies', comments Harland, 'no longer appears as something natural and obvious; on the contrary, it has to be carved literally or mentally out of the body, by an unnatural act of violence against the body.'[17] Visible and legible, death is the enabling presupposition of the new medical gaze.

In Mary Shelley's story Victor Frankenstein departs from his family and moves into a historically new kind of institutional space. He crosses the epistemological threshold which Foucault is describing. The charnel houses and churchyards visited at night are ports of call on the way to the clinic, via the dissecting-room of

---

14 Harland, 1987, 102.
15 Foucault, 1973, 144.
16 *Ibid.*, 196.
17 Harland, 1987, 103.

'filthy creation'. The key threshold, as Waldman indicates – 'if your wish is to become really a man of science, and not merely a petty experimentalist'[18] – is from the lecture hall into the laboratory.[19] Frankenstein's tutor, Waldman, knows that the new science requires dead bodies. In a quickly complete academic *rite de passage,* he escorts Frankenstein into the laboratory, 'instructing me as to what I ought to procure'.[20] Foucault also notes that towards the end of the eighteenth century the doctor gains in status – above those who dispense everyday medical care – by virtue of expertise: the new figure would possess theoretical knowledge in the natural sciences as well as medical theory. Victor Frankenstein has such a *curriculum vitae,* and the certainly of belonging to an elect group.

## Unhallowed wretches

In *Hospital Life in Enlightenment Scotland* Guenter Risse comments on the didactic role of the autopsy in the eighteenth-century hospital and on the difficulties of obtaining subjects where the feelings of the deceased's relatives were concerned. His observations establish the historical precedent for the eventual 'unclaimed' clause in the 1832 legislation:

> In one of his clinical lectures delivered in 1772 Cullen noted: 'It is not improperly said that the earth hides the faults of physicians. If every patient that dies were opened, it would too often discover the frivolity of our conjectures and practice.' . . . Private practice had hitherto discouraged most attempts to dissect those who died. The statement 'my patients being numerous and situated at a great distance from each other, I had no opportunity of obtaining permission to open the body,' was representative of conditions faced by most eighteenth-century British practitioners. Even where the rare occasion of real need

---

18 *Frankenstein*, 52.

19 Foucault, 1973, 146.

20 *Frankenstein*, 52.

> arose, it was difficult to secure consent for an autopsy, given the nature of the private patient-physician relationship.[21]

However:

> Hospitals, on the other hand, seemed to create favourable conditions for the performance of postmortem dissections. Patients belonged to a lower social class than private patients and were indebted for the free medical care received. Many of them were newcomers to the city, living alone *without relatives*. Under those circumstances, requests for autopsies were frequently unnecessary [italics added].[22]

Where autopsy is concerned, the Creature in *Frankenstein* withholds his body from scientific objectification and, via Walton, addresses officialdom in no uncertain terms. He speaks as one for whom the broken promise of a mate entails an existence without relatives: 'I shall collect my funeral pile and consume this miserable frame, that its remains may afford no light to any curious and unhallowed wretch who would create such another as I have been.'[23] This, his final riposte to the surgeons and their problems, would have gained in pertinence in each edition of the story up to 1831: 'Unhallowed wretches' is a blunt counter-evaluation which alludes to graveyard sacrilege. And in a late eighteenth-century context, the term 'curious' accurately characterises the scientific inquiringness which led surgeons like John Hunter to seek the remains of medically interesting human beings.[24]

---

21 Risse, 1986, 261.
22 *Ibid.*
23 *Frankenstein*, 184.
24 The Creature's intention to secure his own sea-burial safely away from the anatomists has one remarkable precedent in the late eighteenth-century context. In 1783 the ailing 'Irish Giant' Charles Byrne (or O'Brien) gave instructions for his own burial at sea in an anxious bid to escape John Hunter's grasp; however, he failed in his obsession to elude the famous surgeon. His remains can still be seen today in the Royal College of Surgeons. In his lifetime Byrne enjoyed commercial success, billed as a giant, on a tour of the British Isles. See Richardson, 1989, 57–8.

By evading the law, the massive figure in *Frankenstein* lives 'at large' in a number of senses. He is out of custody, unaccommodated, poor – and a 'monster' of capital crime, the enemy of all. Existing at large, he embodies the growing shortfall in the legal provision of bodies for the slab. By the mid-1820s the search for a legislative solution to the problem is gathering pace; and so is the understanding that the solution will entail criminalising the poor. In this decade, the years which span the first three editions of *Frankenstein*, the shortfall is placing the pauper body on to an agenda of social utility. In another sense, however, the 'monstrosity' of Frankenstein's nameless Creature – despite his constitution as a mass of reanimated corpses – arises from the fact that he has no relatives. The 'monster' therefore 'qualifies' as unclaimable, and he thus directly answers the strict letter of the 'unclaimed' clause in the eventual 1832 law. As I have commented, the use of the verb 'to claim' in *Frankenstein* is prophetic. It appears when the abandoned Creature recalls his early bewilderment:

> But where were my friends and relations? No father had watched my infant days, no mother had blessed me with smiles and caresses; or if they had, all my past life was now a blot, a blind vacancy in which I distinguished nothing. From my earliest remembrance I had been as I then was in height and proportion. I had never yet seen a being resembling me or who *claimed* any intercourse with me. What was I? [italics added][25]

Logically, to contest the 'unclaimed' clause – or to press it all the harder – the 'monster' must appear to target all of Frankenstein's family.

Quite early in the anatomy timetable, Hogarth's famous picture comments on a transformation in the perception of punishment. Behind the academic figures wearing mortar-boards is another group of observers whose relation to the proceedings is more discrete. These onlookers stand level with the President; they evidently are figures of officialdom. Their presence is a sign that

---

[25] *Frankenstein*, 107.

the new medical perception has ideological applications elsewhere in society. As we have seen, in the eighteenth century the gallows violence inflicted by the king on the criminal rubbed off on the surgeons in popular perception. With only the noose remaining, Hogarth retains a trace of the older asymmetry of power, but, as noted, he eliminates the gallows crowd. The shadowy figures in conclave behind the great seat of power – whoever they are – are an audience-outside-the audience; they contemplate not the immediate theatre so much as its symbolic value within a wider design of administrative and political power. They are to the theatre as producers to actors, its managerial interests. With the surgeon's exceptional violence centre-stage, the double audience in the picture foregrounds a production and manipulation of signs from which certain lessons can be drawn. Hogarth, as he recalls the gallows violence, is anticipating – or provoking – reformist moves towards more 'humane' punishment. Here is Foucault's version of the reward of cruelty:

> The principle of moderation in punishment, even when it is a question of punishing the enemy of the social body, is articulated first as a discourse of the heart. Or rather, it leaps forth like a cry from the body, which is revolted at the sight or at the imagination of too much cruelty. The formulation of the principle that penality must remain 'humane' is expressed by the reformers in the first person.[26]

There is a clue here to the illustration's implied spectator, as constructed by the eye-contact which is sought by the figure on the left:

> It is as if the sensibility of the speaker were being expressed directly; as if the body of the philosopher or theoretician had come between executioner and victim, to affirm his own law and impose it finally on the entire economy of punishment . . . In fact, it bears within it a principle of calculation. The body, the imagination, the pain, the heart to be respected are not, in

[26] Foucault, 1979, 91.

> effect, those of the criminal that is to be punished, but those of the men, who, having subscribed to the pact, have the right of exercising against him the power of assembly.[27]

The assembly is apparent in the picture, with the picture's viewer solicited as a member. The offended sensibility implements a 'humane', economic regulation of power which, for Foucault, is constitutive of 'disciplinary' society:

> Beneath the humanisation of the penalties, what one finds are all those rules that authorize, or rather demand, 'leniency', as a calculated economy of the power to punish . . . It is no longer the body, with the ritual play of excessive pains, spectacular brandings in the ritual of the public execution; it is the mind or rather a play of representations and signs circulating discreetly but necessarily and evidently in the minds of all. It is no longer the body, but the soul, said Mably . . . Old 'anatomies' of punishment are abandoned. But have we really entered the age of non-corporal punishment? [28]

In the longer term the dissection as punishment remained to contradict the moves to take the cruelty out of power. By 1832 the only thing to do was to remove the surgeons from the horizon of everyday life.

## Duplication

Hogarth's Surgeon's Hall has the unique atmosphere of a court, an environment in which 'splendour, terror and hope of favour are equally blended'.[29] The elevated chair doubles as the throne; the distance between the king and the condemned man is established vertically. In his account of the transition to modern disciplinary society Foucault highlights a polarity between the king and the condemned man:

---

[27] *Ibid.*

[28] *Ibid.*, 101.

[29] Canetti, 1981, 465.

> In the darkest region of the political field the condemned man represents the symmetrical, inverted figure of the king . . . If the surplus power possessed by the king gives rise to the duplication of his body, has not the surplus power exercised on the subjected body of the condemned man given rise to another type of duplication? That of a 'non corporal', a 'soul' as Mably called it. The history of this 'micro-physics' of the punitive power would then be a genealogy or an element in a genealogy of the modern 'soul'.[30]

I want to outline now how this scheme appears in *Frankenstein*. In the course of Frankenstein's final pursuit of his Creature he encounters 'marks in writing on the barks of trees or cut in stone':

> 'My reign is not yet over,' (these words were legible in one of these inscriptions;) 'you live and my power is complete. Follow me; I seek the everlasting ices of the north, where you will feel the misery of cold and frost, to which I am impassive . . .'[31]

These words invoke what Ernst Kantorowicz (Foucault's source) has called 'the King's Two Bodies' – a relationship between the corporeal frailty of the man and the undying mystique of the Crown. The Creature here is virtually speaking the language of a Shakespearean monarch. 'Tongues in trees' and 'sermons in stones', for example, mark the 'translation' of 'fortune' into 'style' by the deposed monarch in *As You Like It*, Duke Senior, who can only possess the king's double body in the forest of Arden as a projection of pastoral desire, 'feeling not', as he puts it, 'the penalty of Adam' or the harsh winter wind.[32] In an earlier interview between Frankenstein and a magistrate, the public official, hearing the whole story, concludes that Frankenstein's creation is impervious to all environments. He says:

---

30 Foucault, 1979, 29.

31 *Frankenstein*, 171.

32 Shakespeare, *As You Like It*, II. i. 20.

> I would willingly afford you every aid in your pursuit, but the creature of whom you speak appears to have powers which would put all my exertions to defiance. Who can follow an animal which can traverse the sea of ice and inhabit caves and dens where no man would venture to intrude? [33]

As he frames the polarity between the condemned man and the king Foucault comments on the need to analyse 'the least body of the condemned man'.[34] That 'least body' is an effect of power, another body-in-duplication: it is the soul imprisoning the body. Foucault insists that 'the soul' exists and is born in methods of punishment and discipline as the prison of the body, a trace-in-duplication of the king's surplus power exercised over the condemned man. The duplications of the condemned Creature in *Frankenstein* are Justine and Elizabeth, the two young women who are imported into the Frankenstein house from lives spent in poverty. They are the bodies, docile and 'ensouled', which receive training and subjection in their new home. These women, and Elizabeth in particular, play significant roles in the 'gallows wedding' enacted in *Frankenstein*.

## The 'gallows wedding' in *Frankenstein*

There is a drama in *Frankenstein* which recalls the early eighteenth-century public conflict between the surgeons and the poor. It is the drama of the 'gallows wedding', an event performed at the gallows by the labouring poor. The sole spectator to the re-staging of this popular ritual is Frankenstein. The sequence sees the Creature laying claims on Justine and Elizabeth, and contesting the philanthropic initiative which holds them in Frankenstein's household and family. The 'gallows wedding' in Mary Shelley's story culminates on the night when Elizabeth, Frankenstein's bride, is murdered and left on the bed for her husband.

The best available description of the 'gallows wedding' remains

---

33 *Frankenstein*, 167.

34 Foucault, 1979, 29.

Peter Linebaugh's pioneering essay in *Albion's Fatal Tree*, 'The Tyburn Riot Against the Surgeons'. The 'wedding' is a complex of sartorial and rhetorical gestures enacted on and beside the scaffold. Linebaugh comments:

> The full significance of these gallows superstitions cannot be assessed without a greater knowledge than we now possess; nevertheless, the difference between them and surgical dissection is plain: where one honours the powers of the felon's corpse, the other humiliates it. When Mandeville defended the dissection of felons because it allows them to 'make a useful restitution to the Publick', he might with more justice have described these superstitions, for it is in them that the living acknowledged the special powers of those extirpated by the law. It is as though these beliefs were sustained by another: namely, that those killed by the community through its own sanctions should by virtue of their extraordinary death be given an extraordinary opportunity of bestowing some beneficence on the health of the living. The belief seems to appear again at another hanging custom, that of the 'gallows' wedding.[35]

Linebaugh observes that the superstitions in question were rooted in some current dialect meanings in English. For example, the word 'gallows' had multiple meanings, one of which denoted 'smart in appearance': to be 'flash' at one's hanging required a sartorial etiquette befitting a wedding.[36] In other, less frequent, versions of the wedding women dressed in white petitioned for the malefactor's reprieve with a promise of marriage. A host of other practices included the nuptial clothing of the hanged felon amid undercurrents of sexuality in the crowd. Linebaugh points out the intersection of these superstitions with certain symbolic practices observed at funerals of the poor. Of particular significance was the dressing of the corpse in white, which expressed the sense felt by the living that the death of a virgin was the loss of the

---

[35] Linebaugh, 1977, 110–11.
[36] *Ibid.*, 111.

future generation implied by her sexuality.[37] When a virgin or childless woman died, this belief would be indicated at her funeral by dress conventions borrowed from wedding custom. 'At the gallows', Linebaugh comments, 'the history of the poor and the history of English science intersect'.[38]

In recent years some significant attempts have been made to reconstruct imaginatively the unrecorded feelings of people who saw family members go to the gallows. The material I shall use to illustrate the wedding is fictional, but it is an example of how fiction, in alliance with formal history, can focus the cultural limits of our knowledge of the past. Adam Thorpe's 1992 novel *Ulverton*, a historical portrait of Southwest England, features a woman whose son Francis, a typhoid victim, is due to hang at Tyburn in the year 1775. She mends and washes his wedding shirt before sending it on to him in London in time for the execution. Sara Shail is illiterate; her letters to her son are written by intermediaries. Thorpe's linguistic purpose is to render the vernacular culture – and the historical otherness – of a mundane figure. To 'buck' means to wash by bleaching:

> Sonday 17 daye of the instan 1775 sept Surley rew Ulv
>
> Deerst sun francis
> plees replye a meditly els thy mamy shalt die my son off greeve Mr P tak thi to the wagon God speed itt I praye itt bent be cort when bee the day I shll buck thy weddin shirt & soe as itt hev a ter you mus look trim thee mus replye
> thy loving motther
> Sarah Shail[39]

In a letter nearer the event she expresses her view of the 'sur jans' as devils and butchers. The prospect of her son's fate agitates a tumour in her breast:

---

37 *Ibid.*, 113.
38 *Ibid.*, 69.
39 Thorpe, 1993, 102.

Sunday 12th day of this inst Novr 1775 Suleyrowe Ulver

My deer lam francis

wot my son be cutt up inn to ribons wot bee they sur jans jantlemen of the divil to cut upp my ownern sun no hand oll toch thee a hare of thy hed els dam my eies an dam this fifly gurnray of engelin for barin my boddy an thine this woreld hev no massy itt makes my blakk spott biggern afore it maks my eies teart it makkes i blas feeme agin God an al His workes it maks i scroop an skweel like ower doore as thee met bee mendin nowe we shll cum onn a waggern by nite wen bee the daye my lam if so bee as thee ent took afore with thy feverswet an fiflth my lam

thy loveing mother

Sara Shail

use this papper atwen the lines[40]

The 1752 Act, Richardson points out, 'decreed that rescue, or attempted rescue, of a corpse from surgeons' custody would be thenceforth punishable by transportation . . . The surgeons were regarded as agents of the Crown, and protected as such.'[41] Sara Shail's capitalised emphasis in her postscript shows her awareness of this fact:

P.S. mark itt bee TRANS POTASHIN for caryin thy cowpse aff.
I hope ye nkose that john Pounds tailr.[42]

Closer to the day, Sara voices her fear that her son will 'bee slicd upp & throne too the doggs'[43] – which indeed is the criminal's fate in the Hogarth. Francis, however, is reprieved:

My dear Francis,

Mr John Bate our Curate writes this for me . . . I have

40 *Ibid.*, 103–4.
41 Richardson, 1989, 37.
42 Thorpe, 1993, 104.
43 *Ibid.*, 110.

> always been a worthy Church attender. We are all very glad at your Pardon. I believe your Prosecutor was moved by God's merciful example to forgive you I hope he has a fine new hat. Your mother is exceedingly joyous . . . This is the power of Prayer. God be with thee my son . . .
> Your ever loving Mother,
> Sara Shail
> P.S. My black Wen remains very Sore.[44]

'An act of mercy' comments Canetti, 'is a very high and concentrated expression of power, for it presupposes condemnation. There can be no mercy unless there has first been condemnation. Mercy entails *election*: pardons are usually granted only to a limited number of the condemned.'[45] These observations bear on the 'gallows wedding' in *Frankenstein*.

Mary Shelley's story is haunted by the spectre of death in poverty. Caroline Beaufort, Frankenstein's mother, is poverty-stricken and grieving for her father when she meets her future husband. As his wife, she remains aware, and grateful, that her marriage has saved her from destitution. In acknowledgement, she exercises the bourgeois prerogative to grant selective reprieves to deserving people in the social abyss. Mary Shelley sees that this prerogative offers wealthy women an outlet in society; it is on Caroline's initiative that Elizabeth and Justine are admitted into the estate of property. Elizabeth is selected from among 'dark eyed, hardy little vagrants' who endure 'penury in its worst shape';[46] Justine comes from an environment of high child mortality. These two women, however, do not repeat their benefactress's own successful escape. Frankenstein's 'monster' sees to it that both women suffer a death penalty for their aspirations to rise socially. Justine is criminalised and sentenced to death for William's murder; and in due course Elizabeth is murdered on the day which formalises her membership of the family, her wedding-day.

---

[44] *Ibid.*, 110–11.
[45] Canetti, 1981, 348.
[46] *Frankenstein,* 40. See n. 23, ch. 2.

In both cases, the Creature exacts violent death as a symbolic return to the poverty which these women have escaped. As they in the first instance are reprieved, he is condemned at first sight, and henceforth lives as a vagrant. The condemnation shadows the women's lives however, for it is the negative verdict which, as Canetti says, always stands behind the act of mercy. As he revokes their reprieves, the Creature invokes this prior verdict and reimposes it on the women as they die. He uses the womens' deaths to accentuate the key change in the meaning of poverty which is legislatively ratified in 1832: the change in which dissection ceased to be a judicial punishment and became, after 1832, a stigma-haunted social fate. Adam Thorpe's portrait of England in 1775 is instructive here. Sara Shail's fear for what the surgeons will do to her son's body bears witness to Canetti's point that an act of mercy presupposes condemnation. Francis Shail's pardon is a more dramatic version of the philanthropic prerogative which determines the 'election' of Elizabeth and Justine in *Frankenstein*; but Mary Shelley's story constructs the popular perception of the surgeons no less emphatically. The Creature draws the cultural argument about anatomy to a climax on Elizabeth's wedding-night, when her corpse is delivered to the anatomist she has just married.

As noted, Justine is wrongly convicted of William's murder and goes to the gallows. Elizabeth speaks up for her in court, but the contrast between the two women – with Elizabeth the model of domestic virtue – only further impugns the hapless figure in the dock. Even as Elizabeth speaks, however, Justine has since been spoken for by the Creature as a lover and bride:

> I left the spot where I had committed the murder, and seeking a more secluded hiding-place, I entered a barn which had appeared to me to be empty. A woman was sleeping on some straw; she was young, not indeed so beautiful as her whose portrait I held, but of an agreeable aspect and blooming in the liveliness of youth and health. Here, I thought, is one of those whose joy-imparting smiles are bestowed on all but me. And

> then I bent over her and whispered, 'Awake, fairest, thy lover is near – he who would give his life but to obtain one look of affection from thine eyes; my beloved, awake!'
>
> The sleeper stirred; a thrill of terror ran through me . . . I bent over her, and placed the portrait in one of the folds of her dress. She moved again, and I fled.[47]

The placing of the miniature puts Justine into the frame for the murder. Her own reprieve from poverty materialises in court to establish her 'black ingratitude' and her formal condemnation: the portrait of Caroline Beaufort, her benefactress, is the circumstantial evidence which she cannot explain at the trial. Her consignment to legal murder, which Frankenstein witnesses as such, commences here as a separation of lovers: 'the murder I have committed because I am for ever robbed of all she could give me, she shall atone', vows the Creature, refering to William's death.[48] The girl's innocence provokes his knowledge of exclusion, for it signifies an impossible union – and hence, as the sleeper stirs, love at first sight is love at last sight. The trial and the gallows in due course formalise Justine's condemnation, which starts here in this remote spot, the pastoral space of the harvest barn. This drama repeats the story's pervasive first-sight cosmology: as Justine stirs, love at last sight, for the Creature, is love at first sight, as if 'one look' from her would break the cycle and automatism of condemnation. Justine, a figure of Blakean innocence, has a beauty which Elizabeth earlier compares to Angelica: 'one glance'[49] from Justine, she observes, can dissipate anyone's ill humour. The Creature's words of farewell seal the accusation which confronts Justine in court; but, addressed to 'my beloved', they underpin her judicial fate with language evoking *wedding, innocence before God,* and *resurrection,* the ceremonial correlative of which is this secluded barn. As her execution as a murderess is in effect settled, the awakening, 'fairest'

---

47 *Ibid.*, 123–4.
48 *Ibid.*
49 *Ibid.*, 64.

bride is enjoined into the culturally 'other' sexual symbolism of the gallows union and virgin bride.

## The watching ritual

The wedding-day involving Frankenstein and Elizabeth ends with further traces of popular cultural symbolism appearing. The Creature kills the incipient bourgeois bride and denies reproduction to that class; however, he also kills in retribution for his own exclusion from nuptial rites and class progeny. And shortly after Elizabeth's death the world of popular perception delivers a remarkable image. After the Creature departs, a particular ceremony takes place around the corpse in honour of Elizabeth's 'other' identity as an originally destitute child. Frankenstein recalls: 'After an interval, I arose, and, as if by instinct, crawled into the room where my beloved lay. There were women weeping around . . . it.'[50] These are women of unspecified social origin, but the timing of their appearance, as the Creature bars Elizabeth's passage into bourgeois identity, points to what is going on around the body. This is the communal practice of corpse 'watching', the superstitious ceremony in which the poor paid their last respects to their dead.[51] The corpse is watched throughout the sensitive period between death and burial, and the popular conception of the surgeon as a murderer is rooted in the fear of a violation occurring in this period. The ritual exists outside the dominant culture of eighteenth- and early nineteenth-century England. As Richardson notes,[52] the nineteenth century is the prime period of its demise – as 'a healthy basis for the social acceptance of bereavement' – under the pressures of religious opposition. The ritual belongs to a different social culture of death along a class divide, and here in

[50] *Ibid.*, 164.

[51] In *David Copperfield* the superstitious Peggotty 'watches' the corpse of David's mother Clara. See Dickens, 1988, 182.

[52] Richardson, 1989, 23.

*Frankenstein* a gender divide is also apparent. In contrast, the anatomists and spectators in the Hogarth are an all-male assembly.

The 'watching' ritual is the story's final confirmation of Elizabeth's equivocal class identity. The wedding-day sets the symbolic seal on her passage into middle-class life. Not a biological member, she joins Frankenstein's family culturally via the regime of patient self-effacement which trains her for a part in marriage. The nineteenth-century stereotype of the wife beckons: the role of domestic comforter to the husband in his respite from public duty. However, while her fiancé is detained elsewhere – by the Creature – Elizabeth anxiously solicits by letter assurances of Frankenstein's present and future constancy.[53] If the Creature spares her a bourgeois marriage of anxiety, her 'watched' corpse marks an older anniversary belonging to 'the poor' – the long succession of 'gallows weddings' whose historic participants fell victim to the surgeons.

Elizabeth's submerged cultural origins first become apparent in the scene where she makes a strange declaration in the presence of William's corpse. In a letter, Frankenstein's father reports that Elizabeth 'was very earnest to see the corpse',[54] and disregarded his injunction against doing so. This is the only time she is ever disobedient to her superiors. Upon sight of the body she examines the throttle marks and proclaims herself a murderess and a mother: 'Oh God! I have killed my darling child!'[55] – and then she faints. As Frankenstein's father remarks, the self-accusation is unjust; but he remains unaware of the feelings which precipitate the exclamation. Elizabeth is the first to sense the scale of the threat which faces polite society when William's body is discovered. Her irrational confession is her way of taking maternal responsibility. Her words express, and attempt to fill, a void: she assumes – as if someone must – the burden of guilt which lies with Frankenstein, albeit unrealised as he reads the letter. Frankenstein's complicity in William's murder first dawns on him when he is returning

53 *Frankenstein*, 157–8.

54 *Ibid.*, 69.

55 *Ibid.*

home at his father's request. En route, he catches a glimpse of his Creature and attributes the murder to him. Only later, after Justine's execution, does he fully recognise himself, the creator, as the 'true murderer . . . not in deed but in effect'.[56] At the time in question, after seeing the Creature, Frankenstein resolves to withhold his story.

The drama around William's corpse reveals that Elizabeth's adaptation to her new family remains partial from the outset. There is a dimension to her confession which escapes Frankenstein's father. Elizabeth has realised that William's body lies unattended in a room apart. Her first impulse – as her protector moves 'to prevent her'[57] – is a desire to 'see' the corpse. There is a particular meaning carried here by the verb 'to see'. It relates to the ritual of watching and accompanying the corpse, the main example of which, as we have seen, occurs after her own death. What her protector does not understand is that William's murder confronts Elizabeth with her failure, as she sees it, as the surrogate mother in the family, the replacement for Caroline Beaufort. In her confession, notably, she calls herself a murderer first, and then a mother. Richardson points out[58] that in eighteenth-century popular ritual the relationship between the living and the corpse is symmetrical and reciprocal. Elizabeth's first sight of the boy's corpse compounds her crisis, for it reawakens feelings of grief and solicitation which derive from the world she lost when, on Caroline's death-bed request, she became William's 'mother'. This dimension of feeling has remained dormant in her for want of an appropriate outlet.

This symmetry, this *being-with* connection, is at the guilt-ridden root of Elizabeth's utterance over William's body as it awaits burial. The confession speaks her displacement from her origins, from a pre-bourgeois communality of care and regard for the not-yet-departed dead. Her words commence an entreaty to the corpse,

---

56 *Ibid.*, 85.
57 *Ibid.*, 69.
58 Richardson, 1989, 22.

but it is left unfinished as she faints. It is apparent early in the story that Elizabeth possesses remarkable affective qualities. From the moment of her arrival from poverty she exists primarily as a being-for-others. Her powers of benign regard for others stand out in Frankenstein's memory of his childhood; he recalls, for example, that her voice and eyes 'were ever there to bless and animate' those around her.[59] Her power to confer being is concentrated in her face; her being-for-others has an *esse-percipi* dimension which is also integral to the phenomenological structure of the watching ritual. Over William's corpse, however, a less legible emotional repertoire comes to the surface. As she alone knows how, Elizabeth takes responsibility and grieves for William.

Her fainting beside the corpse is the outward sign of an untenable inner crisis. Elizabeth cannot grieve in this way and also confront her failure as the mother figure. In a Laingian scheme, the script of 'parental' but biological non-connection between herself and William is a 'knotted' complexity of conflicting roles.[60] Frankenstein's father reports:

> She told me, that that same evening William had teased her to let him wear a very valuable miniature that she possessed of your mother. The picture is gone, and was doubtless the temptation which urged the murderer to the deed. We have no trace of him at present, though our exertions to discover him are unremitted; but they will not restore my beloved William![61]

The surrogate mother, child-woman, and cultural inferior is 'teased' by her young male charge, and cultural superior, to part with a 'very valuable' emblem of a 'mother' common to both parties. In the exchange, Caroline's son, with playful malice, asserts his prior claim on the mother; it is his way of cruelly reminding Elizabeth of her marginality to the family. The portrait which passes to William symbolises Elizabeth's commitment to fulfil the

---

59 *Frankenstein*, 43.
60 I refer to R. D. Laing's volumes *Self and Others* and *Knots*.
61 *Frankenstein*, 69.

trust placed in her by Caroline to protect the family, and in particular the youngest. As events turn out, the portrait mirrors her failure to protect the two youngest: William dies; and soon afterwards the miniature proves decisive at Justine's trial.

The section of the story which recounts the Frankenstein family bereavement for Caroline is relevant here, for it shows Elizabeth veiling her grief in apparent consideration for her new relations' feelings. The outsider who passively acquires a new kinship orientation also masks herself as she assumes the mother role: 'She indeed veiled her grief, and strove to act the comforter to us all. She looked steadily on life and assumed its duties with courage and zeal. She devoted herself to those she had been taught to call her uncle and cousins.'[62]

'Veiling' is a term which is too charged with associations of complex concealment and mystery for this simply to be unselfish consideration on Elizabeth's part. There is some tact in the gesture: the veil masks her identification with Caroline; but it also separates her as the person who can 'see' Caroline in the miniature in a way that others cannot. The miniature of Caroline Beaufort is a symbolic object which illuminates Elizabeth's culturally determined capacity to grieve. For William, the bourgeois boy, the miniature is only a pictorial representation; for Frankenstein's father, predictably, it is worth a large amount of money. But in the father's letter the phrase 'very valuable' is Elizabeth's word as well. It indicates that she, the newcomer, ascribes a different value to it. The veil which shadows her face is a sign that for her the miniature possesses not 'sentimental' value but value as a sacred or numinous image – it has status in an inverse relationship to its size. Justine's trial sees Elizabeth failing again in a 'maternal' entreaty. When she intervenes and speaks up for Justine, she describes the miniature as a 'bauble'[63] – a jester's trinket, a thing of no value. This description, however, applies to what the object has become in her eyes, for as she speaks Justine's fate looks certain. Via his

---

[62] *Ibid.*, 48.
[63] *Ibid.*, 79.

unknown mediation, the Creature imposes an inversion, a carnivalistic devaluation of the sacred image, and as such it condemns Justine to death. When Caroline dies, the members of the family do not know Elizabeth as she grieves, or how she grieves. Her power to comfort others is the surface vestige of a veiled power to confer being on others – and, in William's case, upon the recent dead. In contrast to Frankenstein's use of science to 'bestow' life, Elizabeth's power is maternal and benign. There is of course no mother involved in Frankenstein's solitary act of creation.

Elizabeth becomes the surrogate mother when, by her protectress's death bed, she and Frankenstein pledge eventual marriage. Left virtually alone in the house by Frankenstein's departure, she is emotionally unassisted in her transition to middle-class identity. Her maternal declaration over William's corpse registers a confused anticipation of real motherhood, but on her wedding-night the Creature denies her this role. In his letter, Frankenstein's father delivers an unwittingly accurate description of Elizabeth's return, after her faint, to bourgeois identity. She is 'restored' with 'great difficulty'[64] and the wording 'when she again lived'[65] suggests an initiation in which Elizabeth dies in a lower social class, to be brought back to life in the higher: death itself divides class from class.[66] Prior to the wedding her culturally antecedent self assumes a vestigial form. After the drama beside William's corpse her life continues to be a round of failing solicitation. She delivers the articulate but futile defence of Justine in the courtroom; and, as noted, she requests assurances of constancy from the long absent Frankenstein. In death, and on her wedding-night, she is cast to her husband, the anatomist, as one of 'the Scum of the People' in Mandeville's phrase.

---

64 *Ibid.*, 69.

65 *Ibid.*

66 Here I am adapting a point made by Canetti (1981, 440) about transformations of status within a class hierarchy.

## *I will be with you on your wedding-night*

Egoist that he is, Frankenstein construes the Creature's words *I will be with you on your wedding night* as a death threat directed at himself. In fact the words address him in his secretly desired, but not yet apparent role as the survivor. The wedding-night ends with 'the monster . . . pointing towards the corpse of my wife'.[67] Murdering Elizabeth the bride, the Creature strikes at the deadliest item in his maker's vocabulary: the possessive pronoun and its variants. The fantasy of possession is heavily marked when Frankenstein and Elizabeth first meet. As he accepts his future mate as 'a pretty present' from his father and mother, Elizabeth sounds much like a fairy-tale answer to his heart's desires. Variants of the pronoun proliferate:

> Everyone loved Elizabeth. The passionate and almost reverential attachment with which all regarded her became, while I shared it, *my* pride and *my* delight. On the evening previous to her being brought to *my* home, *my* mother had said playfully, 'I have a pretty present for *my* Victor – tomorrow he shall have it.' And when, on the morrow, she presented Elizabeth to me as her promised gift, I, with childish seriousness, interpreted her words literally and looked upon Elizabeth as *mine* – *mine* to protect, love, and cherish. All praises bestowed on her I received as made to a possession of *my* own. We called each other familiarly by the name of cousin. No word, no expression could body forth the kind of relation in which she stood to me – *my* more than sister, since till death she was to be *mine* only [italics added].[68]

The 'gift' appears to mark the continuation of a benevolent paternalist relationship to poverty which – in a romance form – is the basis of the parents' own marriage: as noted, Frankenstein's father found Caroline left destitute by her father's death and

---

[67] *Frankenstein*, 164.

[68] *Ibid.*, 35. Added in 1831.

married her. The first meeting between Frankenstein and Elizabeth accords with the fairy-tale convention in which the parent's gift represents heart-felt, if unconscious, desire on the part of the child. Elizabeth's arrival leads to Frankenstein eventually marrying his 'promised gift', and finding her left on the 'bridal-bier' as a potential medical exhibit. On the wedding-night, in other words, the fairy-tale is rewritten by the murderous intellect and answers to the anatomist's amnesia of the heart.

When the Creature 'vows' *I will be with you on your wedding-night* he not only addresses Frankenstein but Elizabeth as well. As directed at 'you' – bride and groom together – the words invoke the execution ritual. Elizabeth's body, as offered to Frankenstein, is no exception to the rule: all the corpses finding their way to surgeons in the pre-1832 era, including murdered bodies, are shadowed by the gallows stigma. The pronoun 'you', however, also directs the vow to Elizabeth exclusively as her death approaches, and, as in the tradition Linebaugh describes, Elizabeth dies a virgin. With equal weight, each of the words invokes the wedding ceremonial which is present in dress convention at the funerals of the poor in the eighteenth century when a virgin, or a childless woman, died. The vow, therefore, is the Creature's promise to Elizabeth that her real identity will be recognised on the night. In particular, the preposition and pronoun *with you* sound the same note of accompanying co-presence which, as the episode with William's corpse shows, is the popular import of Elizabeth's capacity to grieve, to be-with the dead.

The first announcement of the wedding-night assignation follows a significant sequence. I have already commented that the story is prescient where the 'unclaimed' clause in the 1832 legislation is concerned. Most notably, the verb 'to claim' appears just before Frankenstein looks into the Creature's face and destroys the female creation: 'he now came . . . to claim the fulfilment of my promise'.[69] Having witnessed his mate torn 'to pieces',[70] the

69 *Ibid.*, 141.
70 *Ibid.*

Creature withdraws for 'several hours'[71] to grieve. After this interval comes the first announcement of the vow. The haunting words serve notice that the violence done to the mate is the same order of violence which awaits Elizabeth – and her corpse subsequently – in the bodysnatching spirit in which it is offered to the surgeon. In other words, Elizabeth the bride is the double of the mate which Frankenstein promises and then denies to his creation. In Elizabeth the Creature recognises a reflection of his own lost bride – and so the vow acquires, from the first, another addressee: the lost, violated and mourned bride-and-mother-to-be.

*Frankenstein* therefore stages a double wedding. On the night, Elizabeth belongs both to Frankenstein and the Creature: 'the monster' Frankenstein reports, 'pointed towards the corpse of my wife'. The murder just committed is the Creature's demonstration of the schizophrenic, split-in-two identity which Elizabeth has acquired since entering the bourgeois house – as 'mine', Frankenstein's sole possession. For the Creature, the wedding-night is a revenge and a re-claiming drama. To avenge his own loss, he kills Elizabeth on the day which formalises her middle-class status. The body left on the 'bridal-bier' focuses the class hypocrisy which later, in 1832, was set down in law.

By leaving the throttled, stigma-ridden corpse to Frankenstein, the Creature imposes the perception, widespread among the poor in the pre-1832 era, that dissection symbolises not creation, but destruction. Elizabeth's origins in poverty are recognised in the vow. The words invoke a primitive belief in the sentience of the corpse before burial and announce a popular cultural claim on the body. *I will be with you on your wedding-night* is a promise made to Elizabeth by the Creature in his historic identity as a crowd of the corpses of the poor. In a crowd, Canetti argues, the individual unburdens himself of his distance from his fellow beings and is liberated from the commands imposed on him by superiors. Here we rejoin my earlier account of the workings of the sting of command in the pre-1832 anatomy context.

---

71 *Ibid.*

In a discussion that is relevant to Elizabeth, Canetti argues that no one needs the crowd more than the schizophrenic, the person paralysed into isolated torment by the burden of stings. This insight illuminates the unreality which afflicts Elizabeth as her isolation deepens in the Frankenstein house prior to her wedding. The Creature's vow to reclaim Elizabeth – to 'be with you' – first surfaces just after the promise that he too shall have a mate is broken. Canetti comments on the element of illusion which comes into play when the schizophrenic behaves as a member of a crowd would:

> The schizophrenic, overburdened with stings . . . succumbs to the illusion of the opposite state, that of being in a crowd. As long as she remains in it she does not feel her stings. She has, or so she thinks, stepped out of herself and, though the way in which this happened is obscure and questionable, she seems to derive from it at least a temporary relief from the torment of stings; she has a sense of being linked with others again. To be sure, this deliverance is an illusion, for . . . new and stronger compulsions await her . . . [but] no one is more in need of the crowd than the schizophrenic, who is crammed with stings and feels suffocated by them. She cannot find the crowd outside and so she surrenders to one within her.[72]

On the wedding-night the murderous 'monster' relinquishes Elizabeth's body to Frankenstein. With a parting gesture, however, he figures as the angry gallows crowd of the early eighteenth century. Appearing to Frankenstein's sight, he 'jeers', and, in a claiming gesture, points to the corpse as one of his own.

---

[72] Canetti, 1981, 376. I have altered 'he' to 'she' in this quotation.

CHAPTER 6

# Paternalism and poverty: the 1780s and 1790s

## Blake's 'accidental'

In his *Annotations to Laveter* William Blake comments on the word Vice:

> As I understand Vice it is a Negative. It does not signify what the laws of Kings and Priests have call'd Vice . . . Accident is the omission of act in self & the hindering of act in another; this is Vice, but all act is virtue. To hinder another is not an act; it is the contrary, it is a restraint on action both in ourselves and in the person hinder'd, for he who hinders another omits his own *duty* at the same time [italics added].[1]

Blake, in Bakhtin's sense, is accentuating or contesting the sign 'duty'. In this chapter I shall examine some uses of the term 'duty' where Blake's general contention becomes relevant in the anatomy context. Blake gives these examples:

> Murdering is hindering another.
>
> Theft is hindering another.
>
> Backbiting, Undermining, Circumventing & whatever is negative is Vice.[2]

One other term in Blake's moral vocabulary is cognate with 'hindering' – the word 'injury'. The Devil in *The Marriage of Heaven and Hell* says: 'A dead body revenges not injuries.'[3] In

---

1 Blake, 1966, 88.
2 *Ibid.*
3 *Ibid.*, 151.

Blake's scheme Vice is whatever injures or hinders being itself. In medieval thought the 'accidental' equates with the non-essential or the unreal. 'Accident' means non-being, a diminishment or curtailment of being, an ontological demotion.

If we allow it a resonance in the anatomy context, Blake's 'Negative' is an articulation in moral terms which spells out the human devaluation which was imposed by the transference of a criminal stigma on to poverty. The 1832 Anatomy Act has an ontological dimension, of course, for it advanced the cause of life itself. When he gives life to his creation Frankenstein refers to himself 'bestowing'[4] life. The word applies equally well in the case of the beneficiaries of the new law: they enjoyed an improving medical education from which the poor remained excluded for the greater part of the modern era. Frankenstein's dishonouring of his promise of a second creation is the decisive 'hindrance' in Blake's sense: it deprives his Creature of relatives and precipitates him into the 'unclaimed' category of the law as a candidate for dissection. 'Man', says the Creature to Frankenstein at this point, 'you shall repent of the injuries you inflict.'[5] The admonishment repeats the earlier threat that 'I shall revenge my injuries'.[6] In Frankenstein's later self-defence concerning his broken promise the utilitarian accentuation of the term 'duty' can be heard alongside the word 'claim': 'The duties towards the beings of my own species had greater claims to my attention because they included a greater portion of happiness or misery.'[7] Prior to the moment of seeing his Creature live, Frankenstein's main metaphor concerning his great task is paternalistic: he imagines himself as the 'father'[8] of a new race of grateful Creatures. Moreover, he later promises the Creature a mate out of a residual feeling of paternalist obligation. I now examine the late eighteenth-century context of his paternalist ideology.

---

4 *Frankenstein*, 55.
5 *Ibid.*, 142.
6 *Ibid.*, 125.
7 *Ibid.*, 180.
8 *Ibid.*, 55.

## Speenhamland and the market system

The 'Speenhamland system' was established by the Berkshire magistrates, meeting in the Pelican Inn, near Newbury, on 6 May 1795. The substance of the paternalist measure, in Karl Polanyi's words, was that:

> subsidies in aid of wages should be granted in accordance with a scale dependent on the price of bread, so that a minimum income should be assured to the poor *irrespective of their earnings* . . . Very soon it became the law of the land over most of the countryside, and later even a number of manufacturing districts; actually it introduced no less a social and economic innovation than the 'right to live,' and until abolished in 1834, it effectively prevented the establishment of a competitive labour market.[9]

The system in fact was also disastrous for the poor themselves. Polanyi describes the labourer's reduced status and demoralisation under these arrangements. His analysis of the labourer's plight is an example of Blake's category of the 'accidental' – the realm of non-being – in a key phase of the anatomy timetable:

> Unless he was able to make a living by his own labour, [a man] was not a worker but a pauper. To reduce him artificially to such a condition was the supreme abomination of Speenhamland. This act of an ambiguous humanitarianism prevented labourers from constituting themselves as an economic class and thus deprived them of the only means of staving off the fate to which they were doomed in the economic mill.[10]

Polanyi indicates the momentousness of the abolition of the system: 'The abolishment of Speenhamland was the true birthday of the modern working class . . . The hatred of public relief, the distrust of state action, the insistence on respectability and self-reliance, remained for generations characteristic of the British worker.'[11]

---

[9] Polanyi, 1980, 78.
[10] *Ibid.*, 99.
[11] *Ibid.*, 101.

We saw in Chapter 4 how a key figure in the promotion of these attitudes, Francis Place, could by 1832 draw a firm distinction between the labour aristocracy and 'the poor', and on the basis of it successfully divide the world of work from the dissection constituency. Polanyi comments:

> The repeal of Speenhamland was the work of a new class entering on the historical scene, the middle classes of England. Squirearchy could not do the job these classes were destined to perform: the transformation of society into a market economy . . .
>
> Now that we realise the degree to which its paternalist methods were merged with the life of the country, we will understand why even the most radical supporters of reform hesitated to suggest a shorter period than ten or fifteen years for the transition. Actually it took place with an abruptness which makes nonsense of the legend of English gradualism fostered at a later time when arguments against radical reform were sought. The brutal shock of that event haunted for generations the daydreams of the British working class.[12]

It was also the case that after 1834 the abolition of poor relief deprived many in the industrial districts of a vital 'unemployment wage', and this fact undermined the intentions of many who attempted to be self-reliant. It meant, for example, that payments to Friendly Societies to save for funeral expenses were apt to lapse during periods of unemployment. As we shall see in my Conclusion, Mrs Gaskell describes the lapsed payment abyss, and its impact on the burial customs of the poor, in her 1848 novel *Mary Barton*.

The discourse of political economy, as it triumphs in 1832, lends a great weight of legitimation to the Anatomy Act. Political economy introduces a new concept of law into human affairs, that of the laws of nature. As he repeatedly argued for the abolition of poor relief, Bentham counselled the tactic of harnessing needs to motivation. Polanyi notes that the commodification of labour served disciplinary objectives:

---

[12] *Ibid.*

> The solution lay in the abolishment of the Elizabethan legislation without replacing it by any other. No assessment of wages, no relief for the able-bodied unemployed, but no minimum wages either, nor a safeguarding of the right to live. Labour should be dealt with as that which it was, a commodity which must find its price in the market. The laws of commerce were the laws of nature and consequently the laws of God. What else was this than an appeal from the weaker magistrate to the stronger, from the justice of the peace to the all-powerful pangs of hunger? [13]

The Creature in *Frankenstein* is able-bodied, unemployed, and knows the pangs of hunger. The references to extreme privation in *Frankenstein*, in the editions up to 1831, have a historical basis in the fact that 'the scale of bread was actually being whittled down in various counties, and the wretched incomes of the poor were reduced even further'.[14] Polanyi sketches Bentham momentarily caught wrongfooted by his own leading utilitarian premise:

> To the politician and administrator *laissez-faire* was simply a principle of the ensurance of law and order, with the minimum cost and effort. Let the market be given charge of the poor, and things will look after themselves . . . The calculus of pain and pleasure required that no avoidable pain should be inflicted. If hunger would do the job, no other penalty was needed. To the question, 'What can the law do relative to subsistence?' Bentham answered, 'Nothing, directly'. Poverty was Nature surviving in society; its physical sanction was hunger . . . All that was needed was the 'scientific and economical' treatment of the poor . . . Bentham believed that poverty was part of plenty. 'In the highest stages of social prosperity,' he said, 'the great mass of the citizens will probably possess few other resources than their daily labour, and consequently will always be near to indigence . . .' Hence he recommended that 'a regular contribution should be established for the wants of indigence,'

---

[13] *Ibid.*, 116–17.

[14] *Ibid.*, 97.

> though thereby 'in *theory* WANT is decreased and thus industry hit,' as he regretfully added, since from the utilitarian point of view the task of the government was to increase want in order to make the physical sanction of hunger effective.[15]

The food provision which Canetti in *Crowds and Power* locates in the domestication of command is in play here, but with the stipulation that the crust must be worked for in the first place. An uncontrolled system, the market economy, was to create the supply of corpses from the post-1832 workhouse. The hunger-emaciated boys in the workhouse who put Oliver Twist up to asking for more food are a testimony to the power of the laws of nature to break up family life among the poor.[16] Bentham's logic leads to and legitimates pauperism; and it deprives the destitute of the moral world which hitherto formed a part of the body politic: 'Pauperism, political economy, and the discovery of society, were closely interwoven. Pauperism fixed attention on the incomprehensible fact that poverty seemed to go with plenty.'[17]

The argument to abolish poor relief was made by Joseph Townsend in his 1786 *Dissertation on the Poor Laws.* It contained the ringing emphasis that 'Hunger will tame the fiercest animals, it will teach decency and civility, obedience and subjection to the most perverse.'[18] In 1817, a year before *Frankenstein*, Townsend's *Dissertation* was reissued with a preface praising the author's insistence on the complete abandonment of poor relief.

As the early utilitarians saw matters, economic society needed to emerge as distinct from the political State. It did so, and Bentham was a prime mover in the process. Polanyi calls this development 'the discovery of society'.[19] The scandal of the Speenhamland arrangement, as Bentham saw it, was that it impeded the

---

[15] *Ibid.*, 117.
[16] Dickens, 1961, 35–6. The threat to family life posed after 1834 is noted by Richardson, 1989, 267.
[17] Polanyi, 1980, 85.
[18] Quoted by Polanyi, 1980, 117.
[19] *Ibid.*, 85.

construction of the utilitarian utopia; and worse, it in effect sabotaged the very foundations. In his treatise Townsend argued for a ten-year timetable in which to abolish outdoor relief; others, mindful of the suffering the change would entail, counselled a more gradualist transition.[20] In the early 1830s, however, *laissez-faire* imperatives swept aside the gradualist argument. Polanyi observes: 'The laws governing [capitalist society] had asserted themselves, and manifested their radical antagonism to the principle of paternalism'.[21] After the political solution of 1832 the proper foundations of 'society' were swiftly laid: 'The Poor Law Amendment Bill was carried in its most extreme form and rushed into effect without any period of grace.'[22]

## Crabbe's crowd

The anatomy literature of the late 1780s offers a resonant image of failing paternalism. A passage in George Crabbe's poem *The Village* captures a moment of dawning, traumatic disillusionment with paternalistic authority. It surveys the poor as they assemble in a graveyard to bury one of their own. Crabbe's description of the priest's omission of duty illustrates Blake's notion of 'hindering another':

> Up yonder hill, behold how sadly slow
> The bier moves winding from the vale below . . .
> Now to the church behold the mourners come,
> Sedately torpid and devoutly dumb;
> The village children now their games suspend,
> To see the bier that bears their ancient friend . . .
> Him now they follow to his grave and stand,
> Silent and sad, and gazing, hand in hand;
> While bending low, their eager eyes explore
> The mingled relics of the poor,

20 *Ibid.*, 139.
21 *Ibid.*, 85.
22 *Ibid.*, 139.

> The bell tolls late, the moping owl flies round,
> Fear marks the flight and magnifies the sound;
> The busy priest, detained by weightier care,
> Defers his duty till the day of prayer;
> And, waiting long, the crowd retire distrest,
> To think a poor man's bones should lie unblest.[23]

Here in *The Village* the lamenting crowd is a sensitive register of social difference. Crabbe is showing the poor being consigned to Blake's realm of the 'accidental'. In the classifications given in *Crowds and Power*, this is a 'slow' crowd.[24] It gets a long description from an external and higher social standpoint. The form of its movement is an index of its nature. The cortège appears – 'behold how sadly slow' – in the form of a train; it includes all who are going to keep together and move towards its ultimate goal, especially children. The goal, as it were, is postponed to a far distance. There is nothing in Crabbe's ostensible ideology to countenance a 'reversal' crowd, a crowd which forcibly overturns an existing status quo. The reversal crowd enjoys a discharge – a deliverance from the sting of commands – which is denied to the slow crowd.[25] In Crabbe's description such deliverance is contained in the conception of the final state or goal: that is, reversal is deferred to the hereafter. However, this crowd in the graveyard is glimpsed in a moment of stunned reaction to the priest's indifference to the occasion. Canetti's metaphor of the 'sting' is appropriate. The priest's dereliction of his duty stings this crowd into an apprehension that threatens its very character as a dignified social assembly, and on this note Book I of *The Village* ends.

The Blakean terms of 'injury' and 'accident' apply in one further sense to this affronted crowd. As Michael Durey has noted, 'the same fundamentalist religious beliefs which made burial in unconsecrated ground unacceptable applied equally to resurrectionism'.[26]

---

[23] See Barrell and Bull, 1982, 409.
[24] See Canetti, 1981, 44.
[25] *Ibid.*, 66.
[26] Durey, 1979, 174.

Crabbe's image of the 'unblest' bones of the dead implicitly acknowledges the same sensitivities that gave the poor understandable reason to hate resurrectionists.

The priest in *The Village* is more interested in hunting than in ministering to the poor at their funeral. And he has his ideological confederates, as Crabbe's candid irony spells out. The dying man in question, as he lies in the workhouse, is visited by a man on the parish payroll:

> Anon, a figure enters, quaintly neat,
> All pride and business, bustle and conceit;
> With looks unalter'd by these scenes of woe,
> With speed that, entering, speaks his haste to go,
> He bids the gazing throng around him fly,
> And carries fate and physic in his eye:
> A potent quack, long versed in human ills,
> Who first insults the victim whom he kills
> Whose murd'rous hand a drowsy Bench protect,
> And whose most tender mercy is neglect.[27]

Roy Porter has argued that quackery was the entrepreneurial sector of medicine in the eighteenth century.[28] Victor Frankenstein's stated project is to rid the human condition of disease.[29] In my Introduction I linked his ambition to Godwinian utopianism; but behind Frankenstein's idealism, like a shadow, stands the quotidian world of quack medicine. Here in *The Village*, as 'a poor man' dies, medicine is business and time is money. Busy as they are, the medical men in Crabbe's cosmology are still at a loss 'to name the nameless ever-new disease',[30] as indeed, in terms of technical discovery, were their successors right through the inception and early implementation of the anatomy legislation. This is why the quack 'carries fate and physic in his eye' – and why he looks the part. The Bench, as it protected the quack's 'murderous hand',

27 Barrell and Bull, 1982, 407.
28 Porter, 1987, 44.
29 *Frankenstein*, 45.
30 Barrell and Bull, 1982, 406.

continued into the early nineteenth century to fail to supply anything like a sufficient number of corpses to the profession. The resurrectionists and bodysnatchers were informal but logically-minded exponents of *laissez-faire* in the medical field. The 'great inflation' in the cost of 'subjects' escalates in the decade between the first and third editions of *Frankenstein*.[31]

## *Frankenstein* and pauper lunacy

As I noted in Chapter 4, the system of outdoor relief, as the new naturalists in political economy saw it, had the unacceptable effect of eroding a distinction between labourers and paupers. In the decades before the eighteen-thirties there emerges a cultural category of the 'deserving' poor. The 'deserving' existed in contradistinction to a Malthusian category of the 'undeserving'. In *Frankenstein* the spectrum is marked by Elizabeth, Justine and the Creature respectively. In Mary Shelley's story, however, the Creature's constitution as a mass of plebian bodies focuses a further official perception involving the general category of 'the poor' in the pre-1830s period. In his study *Medical Power and Social Knowledge* Bryan Turner comments:

> The problems of lunacy were closely related to the problem of pauperism, since approximately three quarters of the insane came under the Poor Law authorities and the increase in the lunatic population occurred *primarily among the paupers, not among private patients*. In England in 1744 the Vagrancy Act recognised that those suffering from mental disorders required treatment. By the beginning of the nineteenth century there was increasing disquiet concerning the amount of pauper lunacy in the population. The campaign to improve the public management of insanity was directed by Christian evangelicals and Benthamite utilitarians [italics added].[32]

---

[31] See Fido, 1988, Ch. 5.

[32] Turner, 1987, 67–8.

The eighteenth-century history of the private mad-patient universe has recently been told by Roy Porter in *Mind Forg'd Manacles*, in a story in which older 'hard usage' physical regimes were gradually replaced by an assumption that madness was a curable mental disorder. As Porter notes,[33] the 'governable' condition was a frequent metaphor.

Some developments in *Frankenstein* point to Frankenstein himself as an associate of the mad-doctor fraternity. An instance from Porter's story around 1803 is relevant here. Thomas Percival emphasised the importance of keeping a 'regular journal'[34] containing the detailed case-notes of each patient, including 'age, sex, occupation, mode of life, and if possible hereditary constitution'. He advised postmortems: 'When the event proves fatal, the brain, and other organs affected should be carefully examined, and the appearance on dissection minutely inserted in the journal.'[35] The notebooks in *Frankenstein* are discovered by the Creature in the pocket of the garment he takes from Frankenstein's laboratory. They too record minutiae:

> now that I was able to decipher the characters in which they were written, I began to study them with diligence. It was your journal of the four months which preceded my creation. You minutely described in these papers every step you took in the progress of your work; this history was mingled with accounts of domestic occurrences. You doubtless recollect these papers. Here they are. Everything is related in them which bears reference to my accursed origin; the whole detail of that series of disgusting circumstances which produced it is set into view; the minutest description of my odious and loathsome person is given . . .[36]

The emphasis on detailed observation here can be related to Porter's account of the unresolved contemporary debates about

---

[33] Porter, 1990, 212.
[34] *Ibid.*, 211.
[35] *Ibid.*
[36] *Frankenstein*, 113.

the aetiology of madness. In the period between the Restoration and the Regency no hard and fast distinction held between the medico-organic (i.e. the somatic) and the 'mentalist' schools of thought on this question. The persistence of this diagnostic dilemma to some extent furnished a rationale for the emerging 'management' argument,[37] and the gradual eclipse of the hard usage routines. As he evades the postmortem dissection due to the murderer, the pauper-'monster' in *Frankenstein* withholds his brain and the rest of his body from this continuing debate. As the story ends, the Creature indicates that no 'unhallowed wretch' shall obtain his remains. By implication the mad-doctors are included in this repudiation of the medical tribe.

Porter cites an example of late eighteenth-century mad-doctoring discourse which illuminates some of the key social assumptions implicit in the emerging anatomy debate and the actual design of the eventual legislation. It is from Benjamin Faulkner's *Observations on the General and Improper Treatment of Insanity* (1789). Faulkner advises a strategic and empathetic view of a patient's long-term normalisation needs:

> Sudden changes of situation, *and sudden removal from friends and relatives*, may be attended with fatal, rather than happy consequences. Suppose the mind to be deranged for a moment, and in that moment this violent and sudden change takes place, what more can be wanting, on the slightest appearance of recovery, than the soothing attentions and assiduous cares of affection? What can so soon calm the troubled spirit, or enliven the gloomy imagination, just on the point, perhaps, of regaining its powers [italics added].[38]

This statement opens a window into the middle-class world of the late eighteenth-century madhouse. By contrast, Turner's distinction between paupers and private patients indicates a growing constituency in the early nineteenth century of mental disorder

---

[37] Porter, 1990, 212.
[38] *Ibid.*, 213.

where no such empathy obtained. In *Frankenstein* the Creature's first experience is to be at the receiving end of a failure of empathy. The moment precipitates him into solitary vagrancy – and into Blake's realm of the 'accidental'. In his recommendation Faulkner maintains that access to relatives is tantamount to a viable claim upon recovery. It is instructive to apply this argument in the case of workhouse inmates in the post-1832 period who knew about the Anatomy Act's design on unclaimed bodies. By the same rhetoric, the mental state of those in the workhouse *without relatives* outside is constructed in social terms as a lower class of madness, and beyond cure.

In *Frankenstein* one particular moment of mental torment on Frankenstein's own part illustrates Benjamin Faulkner's contention. Upon sight of Clerval's corpse, Frankenstein succumbs to 'strong convulsions', 'ravings', and a fever lasting two months.[39] Held in prison, he stands in the public eye as a murderer. By order of the magistrate, Mr Kirwin, he is accommodated in 'the best room' and provided with 'a physician and a nurse'.[40] One day, 'while I was gradually recovering',[41] he is approached by Mr Kirwin, who brings news of a friend's visitation. As recovery approaches, the timing of Kirwin's tidings puts Frankenstein into the frame of Faulkner's scenario:

> Immediately upon your being taken ill, all the papers that were on your person were brought to me, and I examined them that I might discover some trace by which I could send to your relations an account of your misfortune and illness.[42]

At this point Frankenstein fears, in Faulkner's terms, a 'sudden change of situation'. He is trembling with 'agitation' and expects to be informed of another family fatality. The magistrate in his reply inadvertently blurs the distinction between friend and relative, by withholding the referent:

39 *Frankenstein*, 149.
40 *Ibid.*, 150.
41 *Ibid.*, 151.
42 *Ibid.*

> 'Your family is perfectly well,' said Mr Kirwin with gentleness; *'and some one, a friend, is come to visit you.'*
>
> I know not by what chain of thought the idea presented itself, but it instantly darted into my mind that the murderer had come to mock at my misery and taunt me with the death of Clerval, as a new incitement for me to comply with his hellish desires. I put my hand before my eyes, and cried out in agony, 'Oh! Take him away! I cannot see him; for God's sake, do not let him enter!'
>
> Mr Kirwin regarded me with a troubled countenance. He could not help regarding my exclamation as a presumption of my guilt and said in a rather severe tone, 'I should have thought, young man, that the presence of your father would have been welcome instead of inspiring such violent repugnance.'
>
> 'My father!' cried I, while every feature and every muscle was relaxed from anguish to pleasure. 'Is my father indeed come? How kind, how very kind! But where is he, why does he not hasten to me? . . .'
>
> My change of manner surprised and pleased the magistrate; perhaps he thought that my former exclamation was a momentary return of delirium, and now he instantly resumed his former benevolence. He rose, and quitted the room with my nurse, and in a moment my father entered it.
>
> Nothing, at this moment, could have given me greater pleasure than the arrival of my father [italics added].[43]

The shielding of the eyes by the hand is a reflex defence of the soul. The face which Frankenstein expects bears the marks of the 'hard usage' that was the predominant treatment for insanity in the eighteenth century, and for a moment it throws its shadow across Frankenstein himself. His conviction that the visitor will 'mock' and 'taunt' him recalls the eighteenth-century theatre of madness as an entertainment spectacle. The reversal here enacts an escape from brutalisation and objectification. Kirwin is not refering to Frankenstein's shadow self or double. As the father

---

[43] *Ibid.*, 152.

replaces the Creature, 'every feature and every muscle' in Frankenstein's body registers – or mirrors – the relief. Reality breaks a 'chain of thought'. The episode links the term 'relation' to 'association' and makes play with the Lockeian possibility of a 'mad' misassociation of ideas: the Creature turning up in the mind turns out to be a delusion and, mercifully, not a real relation. This drama shows a relative making a 'claim' on a relative; thus does the story once again prefigure the design of the anatomy legislation. This episode rehearses the bureaucratic ritual which in due course determined the fate of the pauper corpse in the English workhouse. Benjamin Faulkner's normalisation programme for his patients constructs the lower class of madness which in *Frankenstein* remains without name or recognition. It is figured in the Creature, the man without relatives or friends.

# Part IV

# The early nineteenth century

CHAPTER 7

# *Frankenstein* and the resurrectionist culture, 1796–1825

## Southey's *The Surgeon's Warning*

In the mid-1820s the mere possession of a dead body did not in itself constitute a crime. The resurrectionist-man's usual tactic, to avoid a charge of theft, was to leave the shroud behind in the coffin. The grave-robbing cameo shows Frankenstein omitting to do this: 'I thought that I held the corpse of my dead mother in my arms; a shroud enveloped her form, and I saw the graveworms crawling in the folds'.[1] The image cancels the distinction between the surgeon and the resurrectionist, and this, notably, is an emphasis which surfaces in some earlier anatomy literature. Robert Southey's 1796 poem 'The Surgeon's Warning' continued to be pertinent in the early decades of the nineteenth century. It anticipates calls which were to surface in the 1820s for the surgeons to be made to will their own bodies for dissection, alongside those of their relatives. It refers to recent commercial moves, since 1781, to patent metal coffins. As Brian Bailey points out,[2] lead coffins had been used 'by those who could afford them, for a long time, not for protection from grave-robbers so much as from bodily corruption, on the religious grounds that they would be better prepared for resurrection on Judgement Day'. However, in 1818, the year *Frankenstein* appeared, Edward Bridgeman registered his cheaper, wrought-iron Patent Coffin. Bridgeman's was a significant undertaking initiative. The new coffin was designed to appeal to relatively wealthy people, and grim references to the resurrectionist

1 *Frankenstein*, 58.
2 Bailey, 1991, 51.

trade appeared in the product's advertisement promotion. These technological developments give Southey's poem a topical late-eighteen-teens relevance. Southey comments on the way the anatomist's notorious lack of respect for the dead gave offence:

> All kinds of carcases I have cut up,
>   And now my turn will be;
> But brothers, I took care of you,
>   So pray take care of me.
>
> I have made candles of dead men's fat,
>   The Sextons have been my slaves,
> I have bottled babes unborn, and dried
>   Hearts and livers from rifled graves.
>
> And my Prentices now will surely come
>   And carve me bone from bone,
> And I who have rifled the dead man's grave
>   Shall never have rest in my own.
>
> Bury me in lead when I am dead,
>   My brethren, I entreat,
> And see the coffin weigh'd, I beg,
>   Lest the plumber should prove a cheat.
>
> And let it be solder'd closely down,
>   Strong as strong can be, I implore;
> And put it in a patent coffin,
>   That I may rise no more.

Southey's surgeon calls for a defence militia to defend his grave:

> Powder and ball and blunderbuss,
>   To save me if he can,
> And eke five guineas if he shoot
>   A Resurrection Man.
>
> And let them watch me for three weeks,
>   My wretched corpse to save;

For then I think that I may stink
Enough to rest in my grave.[3]

The poem conveys the public perception that the surgeons themselves, whatever they might say about their motives, were to blame for the paid activities of the resurrectionists.[4] Hypocrisy on the surgeons' own part is also Southey's theme, for this surgeon is betrayed by his apprentices and goes to the slab. Dying in 1841, the surgeon Sir Astley Cooper was to have no such mortal fears; his own three-coffined sarcophagus[5] was an exercise in social ostentation long after the charges of hypocrisy had passed.

## William Godwin's *Essay on Sepulchres*, 1809 and Thomas Southwood Smith's *The Use of the Dead to the Living*, 1824

As we now turn to the decade of the first edition of *Frankenstein* the scene, once again, is the graveyard. William St Clair tells us of a favourite book which Mary Shelley 'would take with her to St Pancras Churchyard and read alone as she lay on the grass by her mother's grave'.[6] It was her father's 1809 *Essay on Sepulchres.* In it Godwin comments on the sanctity of the grave:

> The dead body of a man is reserved by the system of the universe to be the great example to us, of the degradation of our nature, and the humility of our origin. *I therefore cast a heap of mould upon the person of my friend, and take the cold earth for its keeper* [italics added].
>
> But my thoughts will not stop here. Where is my friend? As to the thinking principle which animated him, I can follow it, by the close deductions of reasoning, or by the suggestions of faith, through the vast regions of space, and see 'the spirit return to God that gave it.' But this is reasoning and faith; and I am

---

[3] Grigson (ed.), 1970, 53–9.
[4] Noted by Low, 1982, 87.
[5] Noted by Richardson, 1989, 273.
[6] St Clair, 1989, 367.

> to a considerable degree the creature of sense. It is impossible therefore that I should not follow by sense the last remains of my friend; and finding him nowhere above the surface of the earth, should not feel an attachment to the spot where his body has been deposited. *His* heart [Godwin's emphasis] must be 'made of impenetrable stuff' who does not attribute a certain sacredness to the grave of one he loved, and feel peculiar emotions stirring in his soul as he approaches it.
>
> All this consideration of *hic jacet*, it must be granted, is very little. But such is the system of the universe, that is all that we have for it. It is our only reality. The solidity of the rest, the works of my friend, the words, the actions, the conclusions of reasoning and the suggestions of faith, we feel to depend, as far as they are solid to us, upon the operations of our own mind. They stand, and are the sponsors, for my friend; but what the grave incloses is himself.[7]

Godwin's proposal, which went ignored, was to use public subscriptions to erect plain wooden crosses over the graves of the deserving dead, as a proof of human progress and a store of knowledge for future generations. The crosses would be easily renewable and in the permanent honouring of the dead there would be no distinctions of rank. The essay makes no reference to the contemporary graverobbing, but there could hardly be a more direct negation of these sentiments than a deliberate violation of the grave and its contents.

However, Godwin's essay evidently had an appreciative readership amongst the surgeons as the resurrectionist connection was reluctantly maintained. One such reader was Thomas Southwood Smith, the surgeon who was later to dissect Bentham's body in 1832. In 1824 Southwood Smith published an article in the *Westminster Review* in which he expounded the vital importance of anatomy to medicine. Shortly after the Burke and Hare scandal it was reprinted as a pamphlet under the title *The Use of the Dead*

---

[7] Godwin, 1809, 15–19.

*to the Living*; in this form it went through several editions, a copy being presented to members of both Houses of Parliament. Echoing Abernethy's first public call in 1819 (which I discussed in my Introduction), Smith recommended that all unclaimed bodies from workhouses and hospitals should automatically be given over to the surgeons, in line with the Continental system. There is a section in this essay, a discussion of the sanctity of the grave, where it is patently clear that Smith borrows Godwin's idiom of 'my friend' – even to the extent of an unattributed quotation:

> I know that I never more shall see the light of intelligence brighten that countenance, nor benevolence beam in that eye, nor the voice of affection sound from those lips: that which I loved, and which loved me, is not here: but here are still the features of my friend: this is his form, and the very particles of matter which compose this dull mass, a few hours ago were a real part of him, and I cannot separate them, in my imagination, from him. And I approach them with profounder reverence; I gaze upon them with the deeper affection because they are all that remain to me. I would give all that I possess to purchase the art of preserving the wholesome character and rosy hue of this form that it might be my companion still: but this is impossible: I cannot detain it from the tomb: but when I have '*cast a heap of mould upon the person of my friend and take the cold earth for its keeper*,' I visit the spot in which it is deposited with awe: it is sacred to my imagination: it is dear to my heart [italics added].[8]

Smith opens his essay with this large claim for anatomy:

> An enlightened physician and a skilful surgeon, are in the daily habit of administering to their fellow men more real and unquestionable good, than is communicated, or communicable by any other class of human beings to another. Ignorant physicians

[8] Southwood Smith, *Westminster Review*, 1824, vol. 2, 59–79.

> and surgeons are the most deadly enemies of the community: the plague itself is not so destructive.[9]

Southwood Smith here is honing a new rhetoric in support of the surgeons. He is writing in the mid-1820s, but the substance of his point about unskilled surgery would not have been lost on a whole generation of medical students in the eighteen-teens. In his medical apprenticeship the poet John Keats, for example, witnessed incompetent surgery and never forget what he saw:

> in 1799 . . . 'Billy' Lucas . . . began a career of butchery which even his generous colleague Astley Cooper, was to recall with critical horror: 'he was neat-handed, but rash in the extreme, cutting amongst most important parts as though they were only skin, and making us all shudder from the apprehension of his opening arteries or committing some other error.' He put students [e.g. Keats] off surgery not, as has been suggested, because he was dull, but because he was dangerous.[10]

In 1816 Keats left medicine because he feared not being able to use the lancet safely.[11]

Keats' biographer comments that it is 'more than likely'[12] that he personally had dealings with London resurrectionists. A decade later Southwood Smith is much exercised by the continuing resurrectionist trade:

> England [has] almost insuperable obstacles to the cultivation of anatomy. Even at the present the prejudices of the people on this subject are violent and deeply rooted. The measure of that violence may be estimated by the degree of abhorrence with which they regard those persons who are employed to procure the subjects necessary for dissection. In this country there is no other method of obtaining subjects.[13]

---

9 *Ibid.*, 59.
10 Gittings, 1968, 103.
11 *Ibid.*, 132–3.
12 Hewlett, 1970, 39.
13 Southwood Smith, 1824, 83.

As regards the composition of *Frankenstein* it is entirely plausible that the St Pancras graveyard – the location of her mother's grave – furnished Mary Shelley with knowledge of the graverobbing, for which it was well known. A report in *The Times* in 1813 illustrates this possibility. The amused cynicism showed by the resurrection-man is grist to the moralistic tone ten years later in Smith's essay:

> 10 Sept.
> Yesterday a man who said his name was *Joseph Naples*, on a charge of stealing a dead body out of St Pancras new Burying Ground. When the prisoner was put to the bar, he looked with the most daring assurance; the eye of every individual was turned with indignation on him, but particularly when the unfortunate wife and daughter of the deceased, dressed in deep mourning, were introduced into the office.
>
> Lambert the officer stated, that about five o'clock that morning he had met the prisoner with a large bundle on his shoulder near the St Pancras new Burying Ground; witness asked him where he was taking it to, on which the prisoner gave him a card with the address on it of Mr Thompson, cutler, Windmill Street, Haymarket. On examining the bundle, the witness found it to contain the dead body of a man, tied up as close as a trussed fowl, and only covered over with a piece of green baize. He took the prisoner into custody, and went to the Sexton, who, on examining the ground, found the grave open, and the body missing that was buried there the preceding evening.
>
> The prisoner, as he was being taken from the bar, with an air of assurance, asked the magistrate, Mr Capper, was it not a bailable offence? he was answered that it was, on which he made a bow and retired amidst the execrations of all present.[14]

This is an ordinary enough day for Naples. By a stroke of bad luck, he has been arrested by Mr Lambert, a corrupt official in

[14] Cited by Fido, 1988, 50–1.

the pay of another graverobbing gang. He uses a spurious delivery address, a frequent tactic in the trade at the time. This incident occurs only months before Mary meets Percy Shelley by her mother's grave in the famous tryst prior to their elopement in 1814.

As far as the medical profession was concerned, the decade of the eighteen-teens began as it ended, with a perception of problems. In 1810 the surgeon John Bell expressed dissatisfaction on two counts: the poor quality of the anatomy teaching by the Edinburgh establishment and the paucity of subjects. As the decade passed, Bell was to gain professional distinction and at the end of his life he was the Shelley family doctor:[15]

> John Bell (1763–1820), elder brother of Sir Charles Bell, was noted as an excellent classical scholar, as a lover of art, and as a rapid and skilful operator. He observed that the application of anatomy to surgery was neglected in the lectures of Monro *secundus*, and resolved to remedy the defect. He saw that not only demonstration but actual dissection was required.[16]

The Bell brothers belonged to the resurrectionist culture,[17] but still the problem remained the shortage of subjects. Bell commented on the profession's dependency on the hangman in the following terms:

> In his own words: 'In Monro's class, unless there be a fortunate succession of bloody murders, not three subjects are dissected in the year. On the remains of a subject fished up from the bottom of a tub of spirits, are demonstrated those delicate nerves,

15 Bell, an eminent Scottish physician, was unable to prevent the death of William, the Shelley's child, in 1819. His prescriptions for William appear in Mary Shelley's Journal of that year.

16 Cited in Ball, 1989, 97.

17 Noted by Richardson, 1989, 61. In the mid eighteen-teens Percy Shelley's doctor was William Lawrence, who in 1816 raised a controversy in the medical establishment by arguing for the materiality of the mind. See Richardson, 1989, 93–4.

which are to be avoided or divided in our operations; and these are demonstrated once at the distance of one hundred feet'.[18]

This is tantamount to saying, from a medical point of view, that there is not enough murder in society. And as Bell is writing, other developments in the early eighteen-teens confirm once again the long-standing criminal association attached to dissection. As we now see, these concern rising crime figures.

## The hulks

As he reviews the eighteen-teens, Southwood Smith includes prisons in his list of the institutions which potentially could yield unclaimed subjects to the surgeons (this suggestion, however, was not eventually taken up). The increase in crime throughout the decade was precipitous: between 1810 and 1819 the number of adult males committed for trial rose from 66 per 100,000 to 210; and in 1818, as *Frankenstein* appears, the overcrowding in antiquated penal institutions hits unprecedented levels.[19] The Creature's existence at large in Mary Shelley's story enacts the management crisis which Michael Ignatieff identifies as critical to the transition to capitalism: an inexorably rising crime rate and a severe lack of prison provision. The short-term prison provision in the early decades of the nineteenth century was provided in part by the 'hulks', as they were called, the excessively overcrowded ships moored on the water in close proximity to civilisation. The prison hulks are at their most congested in the key phase of the anatomy timetable around 1828, the year of Burke and Hare. In 1815 there existed five hulks holding around 2,500 convicts; by 1828 ten hulks held 4,500.[20] By 1810, Ignatieff notes,[21] the conditions on the hulks were a public scandal. Furthermore,

[18] *Letters on the Education of a Surgeon*, 1810, in Ball, 1989, 97.

[19] The statistics are from Ignatieff, 1978, 154.

[20] The statistics are from Sharpe, 1990, 52. I assume (although Sharpe does not say so) that these are the figures per hulk.

[21] Ignatieff, 1978, 156.

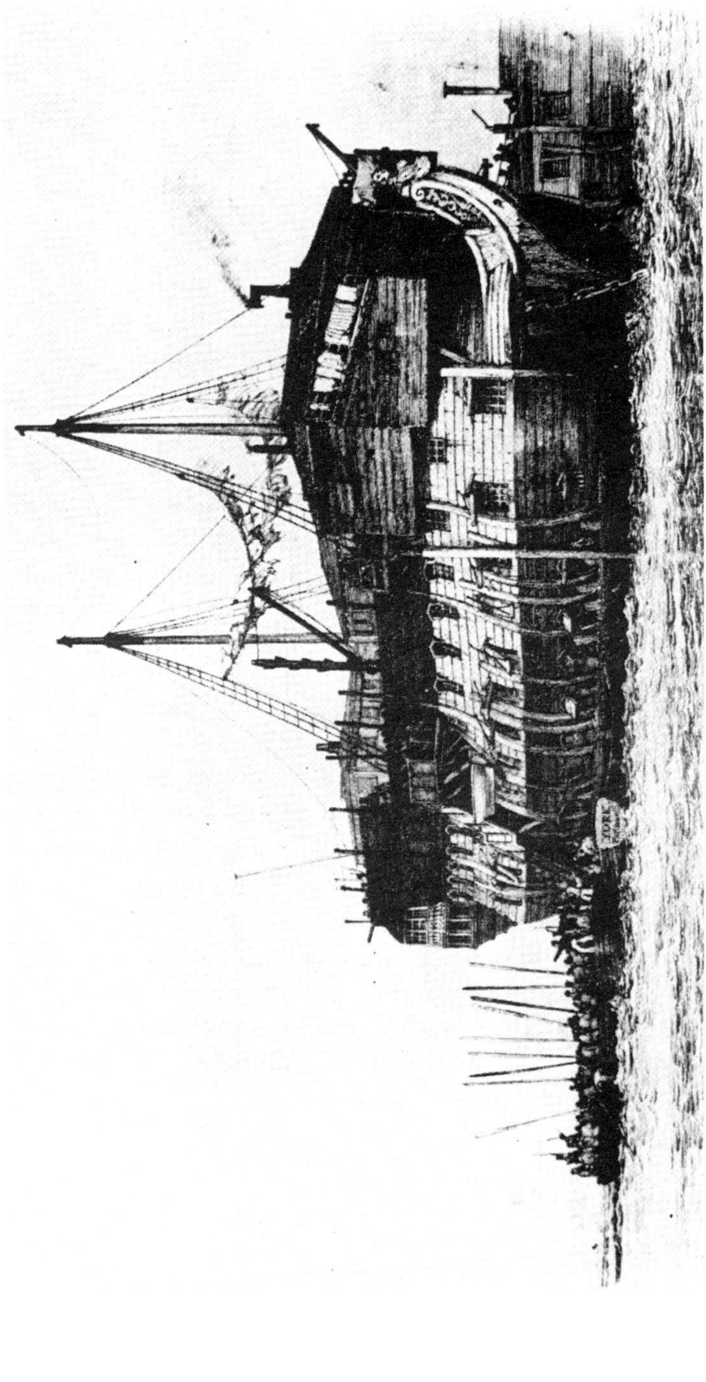

E. W. Cooke, RA, '*H.M.S. York* as a hulk at Portsmouth, 1818'.

while new sentences of imprisonment were inflicted on 'first time offenders convicted of minor larcenies', the 'atrocious and hardened'[22] offenders were sent to the hulks. (Dickens' character Magwitch in *Great Expectations*, a story set in the 1820s, is a convict from the hulks.) J. A. Sharpe comments that:

> conditions on the hulks, and especially in the early days of their use, were appalling. No complete figures for convict mortality have ever been calculated, but it seems that initially something like a third of those incarcerated in the hulks died in them.[23]

The hulks were a convenient source of corpses for the slab. Sharpe indicates the criminal stigma surrounding dissection: 'Their bodies were buried in unconsecrated ground . . . or sent for dissection, a sideline which . . . earned the hulk doctors £5 or £6 a corpse.[24] And the point about unconsecrated burial is relevant to one other social perception in the decades prior to 1832. In the fundamentalist world-view of the poor, resurrectionism was offensive precisely because it deprived the body of a resting place in consecrated ground. In this view, the graverobbing was putting the innocent on a par with the criminal.

The figurative hulk in *Frankenstein* is of course the nameless Creature himself. There is a detailed scheme of imagery in which he is effortlessly amphibious and lively, a large body in water and a figure moving at speed on land. He exhibits on his person the condition of life in the hulks. This 'big person or mass' – this hulk – shadows the growing shortfall in the legal supply of subjects. On the subject of the hulks, Ignatieff records one remarkable rhetorical manoeuvre used in 1810 by the Society for the Diffusion of Information about the Punishment of Death. It was: 'a tract for juveniles that took the form of a letter from Jack Wild, an imaginary convict on board the hulk, to one of his "mates" in

---

22 *Ibid.*, 82.
23 Sharpe, 1990, 53.
24 *Ibid.*

St. Giles warning him against a life of crime.'[25] The Creature of the 1818 edition of *Frankenstein* provides an apt comment on this 'revealing attempt to understand the psyche of the young 'predators' and the milieu that produced them'.[26] On Jack Wild's word – 'the only disgrace that could be incurred was the shame of detection'.[27] The point bears repeating that in *Frankenstein* the surgeon creates a criminal 'hulk' type who escapes both capture and automatic dissection as the killer of William, Clerval and Elizabeth. As he offers his middle-class victims to the surgeon, the Creature withholds his body from the pro-dissection propaganda which begins to emerge in the late eighteen-teens. The 'hulk' man in Mary Shelley's tale exhibits the stigma on dissection as constructed by the law. As he eludes the law's grasp, he provokes the hypocrisy which was to countenance the criminalisation of poverty and the 1832 attempt to conjure away the gallows stigma by a simple act of repeal. He acts out the popular assumption of an unacceptable violation which could not be dissolved by legislative fiat because it remained inscribed in the social memory.

## Joanna Southcott's dissection, 1814

These popular perceptions can be focused in a figure who became famous in the early eighteen-teens, the millennarian prophetess Joanna Southcott. Southcott powerfully represents a specific strand of popular feeling about poverty which begins in the early 1800s; indeed, her impact was such that a residue of 'Southcottism' still survived in the resistance to the New Poor Law in the late 1830s. The prophetess died in 1814 in London. Her subsequent dissection brought the movement she led to a traumatic spiritual climax.

---

25 Ignatieff, 1978, 157.

26 *Ibid.*

27 *Ibid.*

The defeat of British Jacobinism at the end of the 1790s marks the beginning of some fringe religious movements alongside a major development of Methodism in England. Joanna Southcott was a domestic servant in the West Country when in 1792, at the age of 42, she claimed that God had chosen her to proclaim the Second Coming. Joanna first appeared in 1801, with a 'zealous attachment' to the Methodist communion which Southey describes in his *Letters from England*.[28] She was to become, in the modern sense of the word, a phenomenon, a national celebrity with a huge following, particularly among those dependant for guidance on a literal interpretation of the Bible. In 1814 she announced that she was pregnant with a divinely conceived child who was to be called Shiloh, and she was still announcing this right up to her death. Throughout the final drama she could not produce the child. Her disciples kept her body warm, in hope of a resurrection. She had directed in her will that if no signs of 're-animation'[29] had appeared after a lapse of four days, then her body 'might be submitted to skilful operators' – the surgeons.

The events surrounding her death were known to the Godwin and the Shelley circle. William Harwood,[30] a close associate of Godwin's, was present at Southcott's death, dissection and her burial at night away from the large crowds. The drama of her dissection was reported in detail early in 1815 in *The Examiner*, under Leigh Hunt's editorship. The millenarian revivalism of the eighteen-teens, as it climaxes with Southcott's dissection, provides a perspective on the spiritual condition of the poor in the years just prior to the composition and first appearance of *Frankenstein*. I want to suggest that the Creature's part in the story, particularly as it affects Justine, can plausibly be read as a reworking of some key elements of the sensational 'Southcottian' controversy.

E. P. Thompson[31] locates Joanna Southcott within an interpretation of the rapid rise of Methodism during the Napoleonic Wars

---

28 Mentioned by E. P. Thompson, 1980, 421.

29 I am quoting from Southcott's will, as cited in *The Examiner*, 1815, vol. 30.

30 See Hopkins, 1982, 151, 158.

31 E. P. Thompson, 1963, 419.

as 'a component of the psychic processes of counter-revolution'. He presents the Southcott phenomenon under the heading 'the chiliasm of despair', a term which he defines by a quotation from Karl Mannhein: 'Chiliasm has always accompanied revolutionary outbursts and given them their spirit. When this spirit ebbs and deserts these movements, there remains behind in the world a naked mass-frenzy and a despiritualised fury.'[32] In the excitement of the war-time years, Methodism, as Southey observed, made of religion 'a thing of sensation and passion, craving perpetually for sympathy and stimulants'.[33] At her death Southcott had a following of at least 100,000 believers. In Thompson's view of the 1790s onwards, religious revivalism occurs in 'an oscillation between periods of hope and periods of despair and spiritual anguish', taking over 'just at the point where 'political' or temporal aspirations [meet] with defeat'.[34]

By the spring of 1814, no less than seventeen doctors were convinced of Joanna's pregnancy, including Dr Reece, who eventually dissected her.[35] Joanna had refused to allow them to conduct an internal examination, but still they stuck to their conclusions. At her death Joanna's body is a site of conflicting solicitations, popular and medical. *The Examiner* ran the headline 'DEATH and DISSECTION of the PROPHETESS' and reported this scene:

> [Her disciples] . . . proceeded to wrap her body in warm blankets, to place bottles of hot water to her feet, and by keeping the room in a state of warmth, endeavour to preserve the vital spark! After this event, the crowd, daily assembled in Manchester street, opposite the depository of the dead body, was immense; and the inquiries respecting her resuscitation were constant and anxious . . . The prescribed period of four days and nights elapsed . . . [and] preparations were made to dissect her remains . . .

---

32 *Ibid.*
33 Cited in Rule, 1992, 157.
34 E. P. Thompson, 1963, 428.
35 Hopkins, 1982, 200.

> Mr Reece and Mr Want proceeded to perform their disgusting task. The result of this examination were these—first, that there was *no Shiloh;* next, that there was no disease of the *uterine organs,* as imagined by Dr Sims; thirdly, that the *uterus*, instead of being enlarged was remarkably reduced. The intestines were much distended by flatulency, and hence the appearance which led to false conclusions. The *omentum* was loaded with fat, and a very considerable quantity of *calculi* were found in the gall-bladder.[36]

The disciple Colonel Harwood – Godwin's Southcottian associate – witnessed Joanna's last breath.[37] Not ready for despair concerning the fulfilment of her mission, he pinned his hope for her resurrection on the biblical story of Lazarus. Southcott's autopsy is a controversial episode in a gradual cultural development which effectively begins in the second part of the eighteenth century: the medicalisation of death,[38] the taking of death out of the control of the dying and the living. She had stipulated that consideration went first to her disciples, not to the doctors. As Hopkins, her modern biographer, notes, Harwood stood firm:

> [and] refused to allow a medical examination to settle the matter of her pregnancy and determine the cause of her death, if indeed she was dead, until a period of four days elapsed. 'No force' during this time 'should be used to Extricate the child,' she had warned. At the end of that time it would be clear 'to the full Satisfaction of her friends' if 'actual Death' had taken place.[39]

The attending physicians could not establish the cause of her death, and signed a statement to this effect.[40]

Thomas Rowlandson's 1814 cartoon, entitled 'A MEDICAL INSPECTION. Or MIRACLES WILL NEVER CEASE' depicts Joanna

---

36 *The Examiner*, 1815, 30.
37 Hopkins, 1982, 209–10.
38 See D. and R. Porter, 1989, 147–9.
39 Hopkins, 1982, 210.
40 *Ibid.*

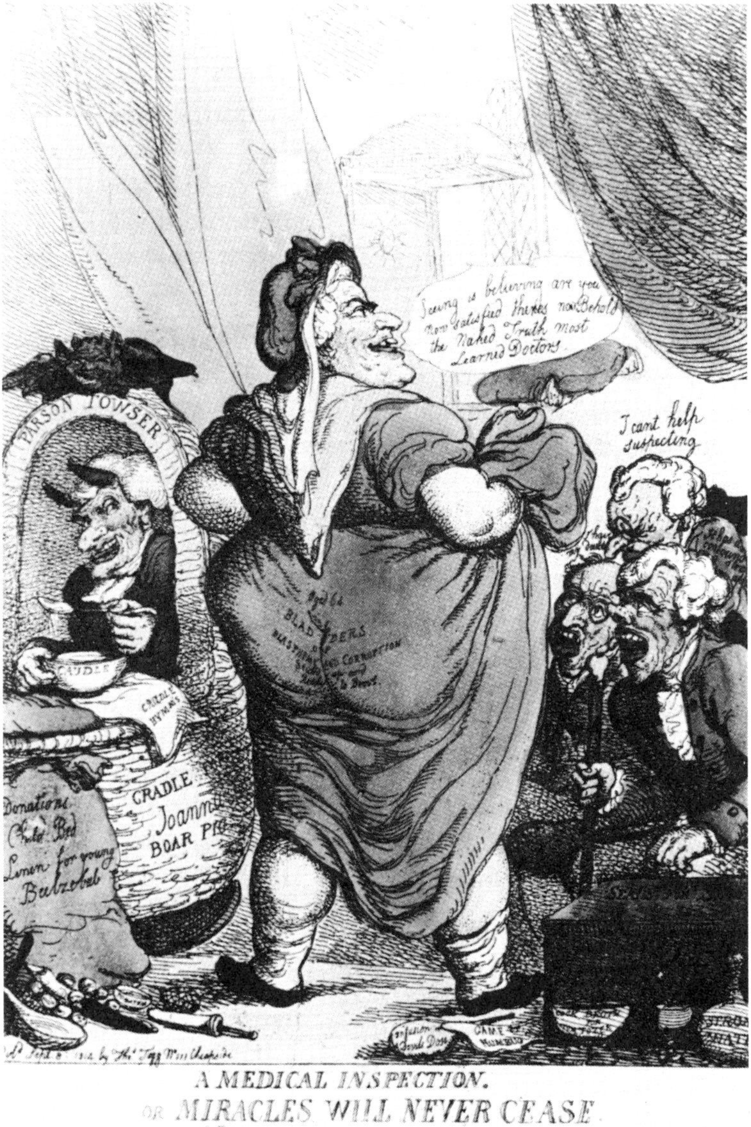
Seeing is believing are you now satisfied thinkes now Behold the Naked Truth most Learned Doctors
I cant help suspecting
PARSON TOWSER
CAUDLE
CRADLE Joanna BOAR PIG
Donations Child Bed Linen for young Belzebub
Aged 64
A MEDICAL INSPECTION.
OR MIRACLES WILL NEVER CEASE

Thomas Rowlandson, 'A Medical Inspection'.

defying the 'most Learned Doctors' while, with a suitably 'plebeian' gesture, exposing 'the Naked Truth'. The cartoon comments on the contending orders of interest and psychic investment in Joanna's body in a number of ways. It shows Joanna simultaneously exposing and withholding her body, as she provokes the surgeons into a show of gaping fascination with her sexuality. 'Seeing is believing', she taunts the doctors, while the trio in front of her confer and opine in unison: 'I can't help suspecting'. During the middle decades of the nineteenth century the medical men were increasingly to assume a right to pronounce upon 'suitable' womanly conduct, particularly where sexuality was concerned; but this pre-Victorian cartoon catches them without the mask of rectitude which accompanied the later professional persona.

*Frankenstein* accommodates an early version of the consensus view of Victorian womanhood which the medical men were to do much to promote. As she awaits her wedding day, Elizabeth uneasily rehearses the role of the 'angel in the house', and her newly assumed maternal role comes to a crisis with William's murder. This view of femininity[41] located the woman's rightful sphere of influence in the home and domesticity; it related to an idea of middle-class as opposed to working-class womanhood. However, as Elizabeth is murdered on her wedding-night, the Creature bars her route into the house and hence into an identification with prescriptive virtues. As we saw in Chapter 5, the Creature insists instead on Elizabeth's other class identity: the corpse he leaves for the surgeon on the 'bridal bier' shares a cultural identity with the plebeian body which the surgeons are ogling in Rowlandson's cartoon. The prescriptive model also asserted another view of the woman as bestial, depraved and possessed of a rampant sexuality. It displaced this sexuality on to the poor and the insane,[42] and the pornographic fantasy in Rowlandson's sketch draws on contemporary perceptions of Joanna as mad.[43] The sexually anarchic

---

41 I am drawing on Owen, 1989, 7.
42 *Ibid.*
43 See Harrison, 1979, 108.

woman proves to be a figment of Frankenstein's mind that is decisive in his move to destroy the promised second creation.

It is appropriate here to review Southcott's own vision of her mission, for some key elements in the *Frankenstein* story become strikingly apparent in the light of it. Harrison comments:

> Joanna's doctrine of the Woman becomes intelligible as a kind of theological feminism. She saw herself as destined to fulfil the promise made to Eve, that her seed [i.e. Joanna] should bruise the serpent's [i.e. Satan's] head. By struggling with Satan, and defeating him, she would redeem woman from the guilt incurred at the Fall, and make woman the 'true helpmate'. As woman tempted man at first, so at the last she is to bring his deliverance. Finally, woman is to be saved through child-bearing, her last and greatest glory. The object of this unorthodox theology was to support Joanna's claim to be the second bride or bride of the Lamb, claims which can be interpreted as part of her fantasizing. She who could never bring herself to have an earthly husband found satisfaction in a spiritual marriage, decked out with all the erotic imagery of the bible. 'My beloved is mine, and I am his', she sighed, echoing the Song of Songs.[44]

The events in *Frankenstein* cancel all chance of this programme ever materialising, but there are signs that lend it implicit support. The Creature never has a mother, of course, only a 'father' who has denied the woman a role in creation – to say nothing of the nurturing role. (In an exit notable for its timing, the benign mother in the story, Caroline Beaufort, is dead before Frankenstein starts work on his project). Furthermore, as the Creature seeks a helpmate he never doubts that the two candidates for this role would fit the 'true helpmate' part. The first candidate, as we have seen, is Justine, the child from the lower orders of society. She is pronounced 'depraved' by Frankenstein's father even before the murder trial confirms she should never have been admitted into the house. To the Creature, however, as he puts the incriminating

44 *Ibid.*, 108.

miniature of the good mother about Justine's person, she becomes 'my beloved', and with these words the gallows-wedding (as discussed in Chapter 5) commences. By making Justine monstrous, the Creature at once disfigures the union he cannot consummate and claims the bride he cannot have. The framing of Justine is the Creature's way of finalising his estrangement from a 'true helpmate' in the temporal world: it is, therefore, the only way he can sufficiently represent his experience of a world of arbitrary injustice to the figure who alone knows that Justine is innocent – Frankenstein. Later, as he demands a mate (and by implication a form of sociopolitical recognition), he offers his maker the 'make me happy and I shall again be virtuous'[45] clause in good faith and expectation. It is only Frankenstein, in the event, who easily persuades himself that the new Eve will bring catastrophe to mankind.

Some historians underplay the 'feminist' strand in Southcott, while others[46] accord her a place alongside Mary Wollstonecraft in the push against restricted opportunities for women. There is a tendency among the former to rank her securely with figures like Hannah More and Mrs Trimmer in 'the onslaught of respectability' of the pre-Victorian decades';[47] but this emphasis really applies only to her earlier 1800–6 phase of exposure. It is arguable that the excitement surrounding Shiloh's 'birth' caused other more directly political ideological currents to inform her broadening appeal among the poor. In Rowlandson's 1814 sketch the 'Condition-of-England' is figured in Joanna's body. The image points to a popular base to Joanna's appeal: the raised skirt gesture has the contemptuous *sans-culottes* dimension which recalls the political role of women in the French Revolutionary crowd. The full title, 'A Medical Inspection, or Miracles Will Never Cease' is partly ironic. Rowlandson does not allow the surgeons to get at the secrets of this gargantuan body. They remain a huddled,

---

[45] *Frankenstein*, 90.
[46] Hopkins, 1982, 216.
[47] Garrett, 1975, 223.

tantalised group, forever pressing towards the body while Joanna plays the pornography queen and lashes them with mockery. The true mystery of her body, and the impropriety of their gaze, is implied by the fact that it remains turned away and veiled from the reader of the cartoon.[48] The image, in other words, denies the historical fact of her actual dissection and its findings. It keeps her in a mythical dimension, with her extraordinary female power on display and her pregnancy intact. With her size, she carries not only Shiloh, but the increasingly politicised hopes and awareness of all her followers. 'Joanna's God', observes Thompson,[49] 'cursed the false "shepherds" of England', the landowners and governors. William Hazlitt even argued that in order to understand 'the people' of England one should first understand the Joanna Southcott phenomenon. As he constructs his counter-category of 'the people' against the 'mob' projections of writers like Edmund Burke, Hazlitt comments:

> Those who prescribe us the study of the miracles and prophecies, themselves laugh to scorn the promised deliverance of Joanna Southcott and the Millennium. Yet they would have us learn patience and resignation from the miraculous interpositions of Providence recorded in the Scriptures. *'When the sky falls'* - the proverb is somewhat musty. The worst compliment ever paid to the Bible was the recommendation of it as a political palliative by the Lay Preachers of the day.[50]

This is a rare sympathetic emphasis, given the context of the intensifying reform debate of the late eighteen-teens. Hazlitt sees in Southcott the lineaments of a coherent world-view held by people who have a legitimate claim to popular sovereignty. He insists they are worthy of recognition as 'the people'. His essay

---

[48] V. A. C. Gatrell's comment on Rowlandson's cartoon 'The Dissection' applies equally to the Southcott cartoon: the anatomists 'ogle a naked female corpse' and Rowlandson's comment 'on the illicit impulses released by anatomisation is clear'. See Gatrell, 1994, 265.

[49] E. P. Thompson, 1963, 424.

[50] Hazlitt, 1991, 19.

*What is the People?* appeared in 1817; it poses the pertinent question just a year before Mary Shelley's story about the nameless Creature who is designated a 'monster'.

In *A Woman to Deliver her People* James Hopkins comments that the 'quietist posture, one of waiting for deliverance from the suffering and injustice of the world, continued to play a significant role in shaping the character of radicalism in the first half of the nineteenth century'.[51] He quotes the political writer Edward Gibbon Wakefield, writing in 1832, giving a name to all those who projected their hopes 'towards some vague, salvific power'. They were, quite simply, 'the rabble',[52] the people completely unknown to the upper classes and the government. The rabble, said Wakefield, were the 'helots of society'.[53] Linking the plebeian hopes of the mid-eighteen-teens to the 1832 context, Hopkins applies this phrase to Southcott herself: 'These "helots of society," however, were not unknown to Joanna, herself once described as one of those whom "society" had "so neglected and despised as scarcely to be considered human beings".[54] In this, her predicament is strikingly similar to the Creature in *Frankenstein*. Shiloh, as Southcott wrote: 'shall spare the poor and needy, and shall save the souls of the needy. He shall redeem their souls from deceit and violence; and precious shall their blood be in his sight.'[55] As he demands a mate the 'monster' promises to abjure violence, but it is Frankenstein who does not keep his side of the bargain. Motherless from the first, the Creature is the crowd without a mother, the unrecognised 'people' in Hazlitt's sense. But the context of the mid-eighteen-teens provides the surrogate mother-to-be figure of Joanna Southcott, whose place, like his, is in the social abyss. Southcottism in fact long survived Joanna herself. There were others who were to claim her mantle in the 1830s and denounce the New Poor Law (and hence the Anatomy Act

51 Hopkins, 1982, 213.
52 *Ibid.*
53 *Ibid.*
54 *Ibid.*, 199.
55 *Ibid.*, 199.

also) as a breach of divine law. As Thompson notes,[56] a final effervescence of Southcottism, 'the last peasants' revolt' as he calls it, was violently quelled in 1838 with a higher death-roll than the notorious Manchester 'Peterloo' massacre of 1819.[57] It is to the era of Peterloo that we now turn.

## The punishment of poverty and *Frankenstein*

In the eighteen-teens philanthropists in England were starting to discern a legitimacy-crisis in the legal system as it was perceived by the poor. In the *Frankenstein* context this fact has a bearing on Justine's trial and provides some clues to the Creature's hand in it. During this decade the philanthropic lobby begins to note a serious erosion in social discipline. In a reference that is relevant to Justine's perceived 'black ingratitude', Ignatieff points to philanthropic anxieties, surfacing in 1816, concerning juvenile crime.[58] This was a development which philanthropists and the wing of political reaction both duly exploited in order to point to – or construct – a larger pathology in society. In the face of it, however, and directly contrary to the voices of political reaction, the senior philanthropists of the mid to late eighteen-teens began to argue for limited political reform. Romilly, Bennet and others believed, as Ignatieff puts it:

> that a strictly constitutional strategy of order should go hand in hand with a program of institutional reform to remove the sources of discontent. They urged the necessity of a moderate parliamentary reform as a stablizing social gesture aimed at conciliating the unenfranchised lower middle classes . . .

---

56 E. P. Thompson, 1963, 881.

57 The 'Peterloo' demonstration took place in Manchester in 1819. A large but peaceful demonstration for political reform was charged by the local cavalry, resulting in the loss of twelve lives, and many injured. After the event the government congratulated the cavalry and imprisoned the leaders of the demonstration.

58 Ignatieff, 1978, 156–7

> Underlying this strategic conception of reform was a pervasive anxiety about the legitimacy of legal institutions. The reformers knew that the severity of the economic depression had forced many of the 'respectable' poor into crime.[59]

Ignatieff distinguishes between two different perceptions of this new development in crime: 'While they themselves [the philanthropists] did not waver on the necessity of imprisoning such people, they did realise that the poor themselves questioned the justice of "punishing poverty"'.[60] This 'punishment of poverty' is a significant formula. Regarded by the poor as unjust, the 'punishment of poverty' is the ideological antecedent of the 'criminalisation of poverty' tactic which promoted the settlement in 1832 and found expression in the Anatomy Act. It is in the context of this repression that the 'monster' in *Frankenstein* increases the political temperature of the late eighteen-teens, the era of Peterloo, as it was to prove. He sees to it that Justine, his 'bride' at the 'gallows wedding', goes to her death innocent of a murder charge.

Ignatieff quotes a revealing statement made in 1818 by the philanthropist MP, T. F. Buxton. It illuminates the deeply negative attitude with which the public receives news of Justine's theft of the miniature:

> Persons may steal for immediate sustenance. I do not contend that they are not criminal. True morality would tell them it is better to starve than to rob; but in truth such a sacrifice of life to principle is an effort of heroic virtue; and perhaps if those amongst yourselves who, free from every temptation, call aloud for rigid and inflexible justice, were placed in the same circumstances, they would have some difficulty in the choice of an alternative, and hunger might make appeals which honesty could hardly reject.[61]

---

59 *Ibid.*, 162–3. Percy Shelley also argued for moderate political reform in his *A Philosophical View of Reform*, 1819.

60 *Ibid.*, 163.

61 *Ibid.*

Justine of course does not steal food. With a murder charge against her, she does something a step worse than Buxton's example. She appears to have despoiled the house in a gesture which abuses the trust – and the memory – of the philanthropic benefactress who first accommodated her, Caroline Beaufort. When she no longer needs food, she has evidently found stealing the very symbol of it irresistible. Her apparent theft of the miniature is regarded as a symbolic vandalism of her new home. In court the portrait of Caroline Beaufort throws a kleptomaniac shadow across Justine; it seems to reveal an unregenerate propensity to steal. In the context of the trial scene in *Frankenstein*, Buxton's appeal for empathy with the poor falls on deaf ears. Only Elizabeth refuses to believe that Justine is guilty, but in her speech on behalf of the accused she fails to get either the court or the indignant public, who attend in their 'thousands', to see beyond the stereotype which the Creature presents to them. The Creature-behind-the-scenes, that is to say, lets the fact of Justine's innocence conflict with the voices of political reaction which pressed a case in the late eighteen-teens to punish poverty by the use of terror in order to deter the soaring rate of crime. Buxton, Ignatieff notes,[62] did not support the deployment of troops at Peterloo, nor the suspension of *habeas corpus* in 1817. As Justine's execution occurs in *Frankenstein* the legal system stands condemned from the viewpoint of the eyes of the poor, that is, in the eyes of the Creature, 'the people'.

---

[62] *Ibid.*, 162. In 1815, a few years prior to these developments, much publicity was given to the case of Eliza Fenning, a domestic servant who was publicly hanged for allegedly trying to poison her master and his family. Fenning's conviction turned on highly dubious circumstantial evidence. She was widely regarded, especially among the poor, as innocent, and her case was taken up by the pamphlet press of the day. The Fenning case, which bears a striking resemblance to Justine's false conviction for murder in *Frankenstein*, is discussed in detail by Gatrell (1994); and by Sales (1994).

## Anti and pro dissection: the pamphlet literature of the 1820s

In *Bodysnatchers*, his history of the resurrectionists, Martin Fido reports the appearance in 1825 of an anonymous pamphlet which intensified the controversy surrounding the surgeons. The pamphlet was indirectly addressed to Sir Astley and Lady Cooper and argued against dissection itself. It was entitled *An Account of the Circumstances Attending the Imprisonment and Death of the late William Millard*, and Fido[63] suspects William Cobbett wrote it. The pamphleteer proposes that the surgeons should be compelled to will their own bodies for dissection as a condition of becoming a licensed surgeon. (This proposal, which Southey's poem moots, was to be restated in 1832 by the radical anti-anatomist Henry Hunt). He develops the argument by suggesting that the surgeons make sure their friends' and relatives' bodies meet the same fate – and this is the sting in the address to the Coopers.

*Frankenstein* rings a version of the formula of the stories in currency during the bodysnatching era, stories in which 'anatomists [suffer] shock and horror when the corpse they are about to dissect turns out to be that of a relative or friend':[64] two of the bodies offered to Frankenstein – Clerval and Elizabeth the bride – answer to the pamphleteer's second suggestion. Elizabeth is the most provocative offering, for reasons which bear on Frankenstein's mode of perception as a doctor. As someone whose public role is to examine bodies, whether dead or living, the early modern doctor has an official and a less than official pair of eyes. In his review of 'moral environmentalism 1830–60' the cultural historian Frank Mort describes a 'cultural distance' standing 'between the male investigator and his female object'.[65] Mort's comments apply to Elizabeth as the Creature keeps the ambiguities of clinical detachment in reserve for Frankenstein's wedding-night. Elizabeth

---

[63] Fido, 1988, 68.
[64] Richardson, 1989, 31.
[65] Mort, 1987, 49.

has endured 'penury in its worst shape' before her arrival and betrothal in Frankenstein's house:

> This process of objectification involved a particular sexualized way of looking which bore close relation to the protocols of official knowledge shaping the public inquiries of these men – the rules of detached observation and classification central to the empirical method. But when applied to working women this discourse eroticized the cultural distance between the observer and the observed. For these professionals, sexual desire was produced at the interface of class and gender oppositions set up by environmentalism. Here was male sexuality constructed through the erotic mechanism of a voyeuristic gaze and the fetishization of cultural difference.[66]

The material advantages of Elizabeth's proposed move into Frankenstein's family are coded as 'Providence'.[67] To use Bourdieu's term (cited in Chapter 3) Elizabeth's change of culture confers 'an ontological promotion akin to a transubstantiation' out of destitution, until the Creature invokes her past working-class identity on the wedding-night. Furthermore, as Londa Schiebinger has shown,[68] investigation of sex differences between men and women was high on the anatomists' agenda in the late eighteenth and early nineteenth centuries. In particular, surgeons sought to delineate and describe the female anatomy. With Clerval and Elizabeth murdered and delivered, Frankenstein is offered the materials for comparative human anatomy.

There are early indications that Frankenstein regards Elizabeth, in sexual terms, as plebeian. In the dream sequence prior to the 'resurrectionist' cameo the anatomist fantasises about his bride-to-be. In the 'wildest dreams' that follow the rejection of his Creature, Frankenstein encounters Elizabeth 'in the bloom of health, walking in the streets of Ingolstadt'.[69] Here in the dream Elizabeth is

---

[66] *Ibid.*
[67] *Frankenstein*, 41.
[68] Schiebinger, 1987, 42–82.
[69] *Frankenstein*, 58.

off-limits: a figure in the street and, equivocally, a figure *of* the street. Mort's scenario of the doctor's sexual arousal is relevant here, for the 'first kiss' sequence which follows hints that the object of male fantasy here is the virgin prostitute figure. Frankenstein's kiss is deadly: 'for as I imprinted the first kiss on her lips, they became livid with the hue of death'.[70] This clinch, this death-at-first-contact, shows the doctor initiating sex and surviving sexually transmitted contagion; it is a fantasy of two desires. Since he moves to embrace her, the image points to the role played by respectable men in the causation of fatally contagious diseases. As with Blake's image of the 'marriage hearse' (in his poem 'London'),[71] the 'bridal bier' in *Frankenstein* condenses a confusion of sanctioned and unsanctioned sexuality. In the dream, the lack of any firm distinction in Frankenstein's mind between extra-marital and pre-marital sex appears sufficient to produce the corpse which duly turns up on the wedding-night. In the time between this dream and the wedding 'the [familiar] name of cousin',[72] with its hint of incest,[73] always stands between Frankenstein and Elizabeth as an equivocal piece of coding. In line with Mort's comments on the doctor's gaze, the long deferred wedding-night – and the convention of first carnal knowledge – is marked by ambiguity. Right up to their final union – and violent separation – the 'cousin' code remains a notional term which covers another order of interest: the corpse on the bed invites both kinds of eye, official and unofficial.

As Fido observes, the anonymous 1825 pamphleteer, puts 'one argument the surgeons really feared, as it was immensely prejudicial to the concept of dissection as necessarily detached and scientific':[74]

Who, we may ask, even among the practitioners of medicine,

---

[70] *Ibid.*

[71] 'The youthful harlot's curse/Blights with plagues the marriage-hearse' is Blake's line.

[72] *Frankenstein*, 42

[73] The suggestion of incest was toned down in the 1831 edition.

[74] Fido, 1988, 68.

> does not shudder at the mere contemplation that the remains of all that was dear to him, *of a beloved parent, wife,* sister or daughter may be exposed to the rude gaze and perhaps to the INDECENT JESTS of unfeeling men . . .
>
> We should observe that this is not mere surmise. It is impossible to be more explicit; we must therefore content ourselves with remarking with reference to such occurrences, that what has happened heretofore may, and in all probability will, happen again [italics added].[75]

As Fido notes, the Coopers 'hated this pamphlet, but wisely made no attempt to answer it'.[76] However, *Frankenstein* assembles the same polemic. In the 'resurrectionist' cameo Frankenstein kisses Elizabeth, his wife-to-be, as she turns into a corpse; and then, as the image changes, he holds his mother in his arms as a corpse from the grave. That is to say, the dream sequence reproduces the same categories as those used in the pamphlet. As the Creature looms into view, the graverobbing cameo fades, as if, like the pamphlet, stopping short of full explicitness.

Explicitness is avoided in the dream cameo, but Elizabeth's death scene contains hints which appear to bear out the anonymous pamphleteer's polemical emphasis. The wedding-night context inevitably supplies a suggestion that the corpse on the bed has been sexually abused:

> She was there, lifeless and inanimate, thrown across the bed, her head hanging down and her pale and distorted features half covered by her hair. Everywhere I turn I see the same figure – her bloodless arms and relaxed form flung by the murderer on its bridal bier . . . I fell senseless on the ground.[77]

As he regains consciousness, Frankenstein recalls Elizabeth's body just after the murder. While he has been unconscious, it has been restored to a dignified posture. But the image which remains with

---

75 *Ibid.*
76 *Ibid.*
77 *Frankenstein,* 163.

him derives from his *first* sight of the violated body upon his return to the bridal chamber just after the attack. Elizabeth's murder, in other words, sees the Creature reversing the terms of first-sight perception against his creator. The rape mirrors the Creature's own original condemnation:

> When I recovered I found myself surrounded by the people of the inn . . . I escaped from them to the room where lay the body of Elizabeth, my love, my wife, so lately living, so dear, so worthy. She had been moved *from the posture in which I first beheld her*, and now, as she lay, her head upon her arm and a handkerchief thrown across her face and neck, I might have supposed her asleep. I rushed towards her and embraced her with ardour, but the deadly languor and coldness of the limbs told me that what I now held in my arms had ceased to be the Elizabeth whom I had loved and cherished. The murderous mark of the fiend's grasp was on her neck, and the breath had ceased to issue from her lips [italics added].[78]

This passage gains in significance from the post-Burke-and-Hare context, but it can also be read alongside Southwood Smith and the anonymous writer, the pro- and anti-dissection lobbies of the 1820s. At the time of the Burke and Hare scandal, as well as before, there were popular perceptions of surgeons committing sexual abuse on the corpse, as the 1825 pamphlet hints. Commenting on these perceptions, Richardson draws the line against the perpetration of actual indecency in Robert Knox's establishment; but she notes the male tone of the proceedings there, and itemises Knox's necrophiliac voyeurism.[79] For the reasons I have given, the contemporary cartoon imagery of the young woman on the Day of Resurrection[80] demanding the return of her virginity is echoed on the wedding-night in *Frankenstein*. Frankenstein's necrophiliac embrace of Elizabeth in the earlier dream sequence

---

[78] *Ibid.*, 164.
[79] Richardson, 1989, 96.
[80] *Ibid.*

culminates in the resurrectionist cameo. As the passage above shows, however, the honeymoon episode obligates him to repeat this embrace at a conscious level – and to confront the now familiar black strangulation marks. Notoriously, Burke and Hare left no signs of violence on the bodies they delivered to Dr Knox. After Edinburgh, however, informed readers of *Frankenstein* could have conjectured that these signs confirm the bodysnatching connection, and imply Knox's collusion.

One other detail on the wedding-night is significant. The handkerchief which covers Elizabeth's face and neck, as it prohibits erotic interest, appears to veil her true identity. It remains ambiguous as to whether the handkerchief is a veil left by the Creature, or a consideration of the people at the inn. As the Creature's gesture, the improvised veil symbolises a traditional attitude to the sanctity of the dead, and is a way of insisting upon it; it assimilates Elizabeth to the popular culture of death where older, superstitious beliefs prevail. In this role, indeed, it is a veil imposed across another 'veil'. Southwood Smith was forging the new rhetoric which emerges in the 1820s to overturn such attitudes:

> The important operations of nature are seldom entirely hidden from the human eye; still less are they obtruded upon it, but over the most curious and wonderful operations of the animal economy so thick a veil is drawn, that they could never have been perceived without the most patient and minute research.[81]

The true man of science – like an artist – penetrates the veil, as Smith himself did when he anatomised Bentham.

## Utilitarianism: morality and secrecy

Jeremy Bentham, the architect of the Anatomy Act, sought to ground moral duties in the principle of 'the greatest happiness of the greatest number'. He held a particular view of man's natural state. It surfaces as a condemnation of indulgence:

---

[81] Southwood Smith, 1824, 61.

> To enjoy quickly – to enjoy without punishment, this is the universal desire of man; this is the desire which is terrible, since it arms all those who possess nothing against those who possess anything. But the law, which restrains this desire, is the most splendid triumph of humanity over itself.[82]

Taking this as Bentham's basic assumption, I want to identity the aspects of utilitarian moral psychology which lend support to the disciplinary dimension of the anatomy legislation, and consider how Mary Shelley in *Frankenstein* appears to comment critically on the secrecy dimension of the utilitarian system.

At the basis of Bentham's way of thinking is the conviction that indulgence was in principle a curable evil. The aim of the utilitarian psychological science was to induce activities done not for their own sake, but for the sake of getting some pleasure or avoiding some pain. The law, in Bentham's view, enables humanity to triumph over itself. Anthony Skillen comments that, as the British Utilitarians sought 'to ground moral duties in the substantial, empirical end of "the greatest happiness of the greatest number"', their own thinking 'was obsessed with abstinence, with restraint, with control, through a law-and-ordered mind, of the dangerously seductive forces of impulse'.[83] In *Ruling Illusions* Skillen comments that:

> For the utilitarians . . . pleasure was not a distracting lure but, along with pain, the 'sovereign master' to whose 'governance' all mankind is wholly subject . . . The monarchical irony of Bentham's expression has a real point: in his vision inertness is man's natural state. Activity is undertaken, not for its own sake, but for the sake of obtaining some pleasure or avoiding some 'pain', these being conceived of as sensations produced as more or less direct consequences of activity [i.e. labour] . . . Naturally, then, in the interest of minimum effort, since effort is itself

---

[82] *Principles of the Civil Code*, Ch. 9, *Bentham's Work's*, ed. Bowring, vol. 1, 309. Quoted in Skillen, 1977, 139.

[83] Skillen, 1977, 138–9.

> painful, mankind's first tendency is to seek the most immediate, effortless, and readily available pleasures. And to follow that tendency is, as the utilitarian tracts of the nineteenth century repeat, to follow the road to ruin, since, unlike the gratifications produced by arduous forbearance, its fleeting pleasures bring untold pains in tow. Hence the role of morality as one of the road blocks. Pleasure, for the utilitarians, was indeed a strict master.[84]

This analysis applies to the figure I discussed in Chapter 4, Simon Tappertit in *Barnaby Rudge*. It points to Tappertit's workshy attitude, his hatred of his apprenticeship and his inclination to take the royal road to ruin. Bentham and his followers, Skillen continues,

> consistently present morality in terms of their utilitarian psychology, and in particular in terms of social sanctions operating through the 'association of ideas' so as to produce pain at the thought of certain acts . . . Moral action, therefore, was action motivated by 'obligation', that is by a sense of fitness or repugnance associated with an action through its being attended in experience with certain socially administered pleasures and pains.[85]

One such sanction was dissection, or the threat of it. Exemption from such a fate was a reward for acceptable conduct, as well as a privilege that could be withdrawn. Likewise, the gallows ritual served the utilitarian psychology in the moves to inculcate 'obligation' in the 'susceptible classes'. Its insufficient provision of felons to the surgeons moved Bentham, in the meanwhile, to initiate a secret discussion of a solution to the ever-pressing problem, as we can now see in the context of *Frankenstein*.

The utilitarian scheme is based on a dualistic conception of the higher and the lower, of conscience and natural inclination in man. As Skillen memorably phrases it,[86] it is a scheme which splits

---

84 *Ibid.*, 139.

85 *Ibid.*, 139–40.

86 *Ibid.*, 138.

man 'into a celestial bureaucrat administering to a bestial psychopath'. The split validates a role for morality:

> Morality, then, according to this bourgeois picture, is 'self-control'; but between the self who controls and the self who is controlled there is a gulf, a gulf as wide as that between a bestial state-of-nature and an ordered society, and a gulf as narrow, since the forces of anarchy ever threaten to overwhelm their internal ruler. Morality is the political 'problem of order' as it is solved in the head, and the long process of moral education is the authoritarian struggle to achieve that solution. Morality's target, then, is the baseness that is at the core of man's natural, unimproved state.[87]

Justine's moral education in the Frankenstein family effectively ends the moment Frankenstein's father pronounces on her 'depravity',[88] in a prejudgment prior to the trial which convicts her.

The dualism, Skillen notes, is a characteristic structure. The Utilitarians tended to divide society into two distinct groups or mentalities. There were the administrators of sanctions 'acting consciously in terms of the Principle of Utility', and then 'the stratum of administered'. The latter act 'on one hand' in response to sanctions and rewards, and 'on the other hand to the inner prohibitions and commands received from parents and mentors'.[89] Skillen focuses one problem in particular, however, which Bentham acknowledged and faced up to within his own system. *Ruling Illusions* pinpoints this uneasy consideration:

> But since utilitarian calculation is itself far from a mere reflex, and since, if adhered to among the masses, reflex morality is so 'utilitarian', the utilitarians were concerned that the popularisation of their doctrine *might* be counter-productive: in the wrong hands, the Utilitarian Calculus could cause a lot of

---

87 *Ibid.*, 134.
88 *Frankenstein*, 75.
89 Skillen, 1977, 141.

> mischief. Bentham urged heads of state under pressure to avoid stimulating unmanageable reflection among the masses.[90]

He did so with one specific counsel:

> Every favour, everything which bears the character of benevolence, ought to be represented as the work of the father of his people. All rigour, all acts of severity, need to be attributed to no one. *The hand which acts must be artfully hidden.* They may be thrown upon some creature of imagination, some animated abstraction – such as justice, the daughter of necessity and the mother of peace whom men ought always to fear, but never to hate, and who always deserves their first homage. [italics added][91]

Secrecy, it would appear, is an option which the creed itself can happily sanction and accommodate when necessary. In their early private correspondence concerning possible anatomy legislation, Bentham and Robert Peel played the secrecy card: 'Recognising Peel's "personal apprehension" of incurring "odium", Bentham promised to observe his desire for secrecy.'[92] The ambit of secrecy that surrounded the late-night Parliamentary timetabling of the anatomy legislation was to earn the first unsuccessful phase of its utilitarian advocacy the nickname the 'Midnight Bill'. Richardson comments [93] on the nickname that it came from the Bill's opponents, who perceived an attempt to limit discussion of the social implications of the proposal: by being scheduled for debate at midnight the Bill was conveniently buried in Parliament – under the same cover of darkness as the activities of the graverobbers. As he contemplates his task of creation in secretive isolation, Frankenstein uses a paternalist metaphor identical to Bentham's:

> No one can conceive the variety of feelings which bore me onwards, like a hurricane, in the first enthusiasm of success. Life and death appeared to me ideal bounds, which I should

90 *Ibid.*, 141–2.
91 *Ibid.*, 142.
92 Richardson, 1989, 111.
93 *Ibid.*, 157.

> first break through, and pour a torrent of light into our dark world. A new species would bless me as its creator and source; many happy and excellent natures would owe their being to me. No father could claim the gratitude of his child so completely as I should deserve theirs.[94]

To draw out the penchant for secrecy and the opportunism implied by Bentham's candour, Skillen quotes Henry Sidgwick, a later utilitarian theorist:

> Thus, the Utilitarian conclusion, flatly stated, would seem to be this; that the opinion that secrecy may render an action right which would not otherwise be so should itself be kept comparatively secret; and similarly it seems expedient that the doctrine that esoteric morality is expedient should itself be kept esoteric. Or if this concealment be difficult to maintain, it may be desirable that Common Sense should repudiate the doctrines which it is expedient to confine to an enlightened few. And thus a Utilitarian may reasonably desire, on Utilitarian principles, that some of his conclusions should be rejected by mankind generally; or even that *the vulgar* should be kept aloof from his system as a whole, in so far as the inevitable indefiniteness and complexity of its calculations render it likely to lead to bad results in their hands [italics added][95]

The ruling illusion, as Skillen puts it, is 'act-utilitarianism for some; rule-utilitarianism for the others'.[96] It is possible to read a good part of the irony in *Frankenstein* as a reply to the enlightened minority, particularly where the opportunist inclination to secrecy is concerned. The same category of 'the vulgar', with an emphasis identical to Sidgwick's, turns up in Frankenstein's falsely confident and judiciously phrased decision to remain silent throughout Justine's trial for William's murder:

---

94 *Frankenstein*, 55.
95 Skillen, 1977, 142.
96 *Ibid.*

> I was firmly convinced in my own mind that Justine, and indeed every human being, was guiltless of this murder. I had no fear, therefore, that any circumstantial evidence could be brought forward strong enough to convict her. My tale was not one to announce publicly; its outstanding horror would be looked upon as madness by the vulgar.[97]

Frankenstein's promise to the Creature, in the event, is to provide no let-out clause, for his own projection of an anarchic lower-order bestiality – 'a race of devils' – delivers him a terrible scenario of its likely consequences. The logic of the private nightmare which encloses Frankenstein from the creation onwards derives, in other words, from utilitarian premises. Moreover, in Bentham's phrase, the hand that acts – as Frankenstein alone well knows – is a murderous hand of his own making. The fact that he resolves after William's murder to remain tight-lipped on the point – in effect, to wear a mask and hide – is the seal on his isolation throughout the social nightmare. In this respect, then, the hand that acts in *Frankenstein* draws explosive attention to the power and danger of secrecy, to what Canetti [98] defines as the concentration of a secret: 'the ratio between the number of those it concerns and the number of those who possess it'. Always *en route* to a corpse, Frankenstein finds his secret turning up again and again. While he remains silent he is always on the way to another family bereavement: it is a version of the middle-class nightmare which made Bentham's anatomy reform an acceptable option.

## Pain and grief in *Frankenstein*

As he grieves for his son William after Justine's execution, Frankenstein's father offers his distraught eldest son these observations:

> 'Do you not think, Victor,' said he, 'that I do not suffer also? No one could love a child more than I loved your brother' –

---

97 *Frankenstein*, 75.
98 Canetti, 1981, 345.

> tears came into his eyes as he spoke – 'but is it not a duty to the survivors that we should refrain from augmenting their unhappiness by an appearance of immoderate grief? It is also a duty owed to yourself, for excessive sorrow prevents improvement or enjoyment, or even the discharge of daily usefulness, *without which no man is fit for society*' [italics added].[99]

Frankenstein acknowledges that the counsel is good advice, even as it causes him to shrink from his father's company and contemplate suicide. He rejects this step, however, in consideration of the feelings – and the security – of those in his family who would survive him. His father's words are worth focusing on for a moment. They touch upon something crucial: the condition in which the intimate life of the individual shapes itself, or not, as fit for society – that is to say, fit for public appearance. The father's words bear upon an element in Bentham's own scheme, a Cartesian component. Hannah Arendt comments:

> Bentham's invention of the 'pain and pleasure calculus' combined the advantage of seemingly introducing the mathematical method into the moral sciences with the even greater attraction of having found a principle which resided entirely on introspection.[100]

And:

> His 'happiness,' the sum total of pleasures minus pains, is as much an inner sense which senses sensations and remains unrelated to worldly objects as the Cartesian consciousness that is conscious of its own activity. Moreover, Bentham's basic assumption that what all men have in common is not the world but the sameness of their own nature, which manifests itself in the sameness of calculation and the sameness of being affected by pain and pleasure, is directly derived from earlier philosophers

99 *Frankenstein*, 83.
100 Arendt, 1958, 309.

> of the modern age. For this philosophy . . . 'hedonism' is . . . a misnomer.[101]

It is a misnomer because:

> The principle of all hedonism . . . is not pleasure but avoidance of pain, and Hume, who in contradistinction to Bentham was still a philosopher, knew quite well that he who wants to make pleasure the ultimate end of all human action is driven to admit that not pleasure but pain, not desire but fear, are his true guides.[102]

Before his father's rebuke Frankenstein compares his own mind to a hellish torture chamber, and adds that such a state of mind 'preyed upon my health'.[103] He adds that 'my father's health was deeply shaken by the horror of the recent events.'[104] These developments, then, are grist to Hume's point:

> If you . . . inquire, why [somebody] desires health, he will readily reply, because sickness is painful. If you push your inquiries further and desire a reason why he hates pain, it is impossible he can ever give any. This is an ultimate end, and is never referred to by any other object.[105]

Arendt explains Hume's point:

> The reason for this impossibility is that only pain is completely independent of any object, that only one who is in pain really senses nothing but himself; pleasure does not enjoy itself but something besides itself. Pain is the only inner sense found by introspection which can rival in independence from experienced objects the self-evident certainty of logical and arithmetical thinking.[106]

---

101 *Ibid.*
102 *Ibid.*
103 *Frankenstein*, 83.
104 *Ibid.*, 84.
105 Arendt, 1958, 309.
106 *Ibid.*, 309–10.

In Bentham's case, Arendt maintains, the foundation of hedonism in the experience of pain was

> inspired by a deep distrust of man as such . . . by doubt of the adequacy of the human senses to receive reality, the adequacy of human reason to receive truth, and hence by the conviction of the deficiency and even depravity of human nature . . . [and] it was of course interpreted in terms of original sin.[107]

In *Frankenstein* this distrust and the conviction informing it is exemplified in the death sentence passed on the hapless Justine. By an apt irony, the public illusion of her guilt seals Frankenstein into his corrupt silence.

William, Clerval, Elizabeth and his father all die before Frankenstein breaks this silence to the magistrate, and still the Creature proves altogether elusive. Instead of his own body – that is, the innumerable bodies which comprise it – the Creature tauntingly delivers the surgeon victims from his own family and social class. This escalating state of affairs makes sense as a direct intervention against one of Southwood Smith's main thrusts of argument when he pressed for the appropriation of unclaimed pauper bodies. As Smith puts down the following claim, he uses the same key term – the word 'injury' – which the Creature uses in rebuke to Frankenstein after the dishonoured promise.[108] The appropriation, Smith contends,

> would inflict no injury on the poor; it is the rejection of it that would really be unjust and cruel. The question is, whether the surgeon shall be allowed to gain knowledge by operating on the bodies of the dead, or driven to obtain it by practising on the bodies of the living. If the dead bodies of the poor are not appropriated to this use, their living bodies will and must be. The rich will always have it in their power to select, for the

107 *Ibid.*, 310.
108 See *Frankenstein*, 142.

> performance of an operation, a surgeon who has already signalized himself by success.[109]

Frankenstein has freely used the dead bodies of the poor in the making of his creation in the first instance. Now, however, he confronts a living Creature who refuses all further surgical violation, and who instead puts forward another class of corpse. The accusation carried by this gesture concerns the social hypocrisy informing attitudes towards dissection. Indeed, the point in principle was to weigh even with Smith himself eventually, as he came to reconsider (and to boldly voice) the social bias emerging in the legislative text;[110] but there is no hint of this later stance in the 1824 article.

The medical context of his argument concerning experimentation on live patients is the pre-anaesthetic era. It is the sentient Creature himself who figures the primacy of pain. Unrecognised, he is also unrecognisable, a man in pain. Great bodily pain, Arendt observes,[111] 'is perhaps the only experience which we are unable to transform into a shape fit for public appearance'. In *Frankenstein* the Creature's face bears the marks of terrible, unacceptable pain. In *Uses of the Dead to the Living* Southwood Smith spells out the prospect of surgery being practised on the living. He accepts that the wealthy can purchase surgical competence whereas the poor have no choice: money has the power to convert public hospitals

---

109 Southwood Smith, 1824, 94.

110 Noted by Richardson, 1989, 161. As the 1820s proceeded, Southwood Smith came to see more clearly the hypocrisy which was involved in the proposed legislation's design to requisition the bodies of the poor. In an altogether laudable intervention Smith used the occasion of his dissection of Bentham to speak candidly about the need to encourage bequests of bodies: this, he argued, was a fairer system. He pointed out that the social bias in the Anatomy Act would only deepen the popular hostility to dissection. The select audience which heard him speak contained a number of people who had closely associated themselves with the anatomy reform, and there is no record of their reaction to Smith's principled advocacy of a fairer solution. I shall discuss Southwood Smith's criticism of the legislation more fully in Chapter 8.

111 Arendt, 1958, 51.

into 'so many schools where the surgeon by practising on the poor would learn to operate on the rich with safety and dexterity'.[112] In 1824, then, Smith used the spectre of the living suffering pain beyond all recognition to urge for the dissection of dead, unclaimed paupers; and Bentham incorporated this proposal into law in 1832. As the 1820s proceeded, the question of 'recognising' the poor inevitably involved the legislative solutions of 1832, and on both counts – the Reform Act and the Anatomy Act – the working-class remained excluded.

In the story the Creature learns language from its rudiments and uses it successfully to rehearse with Frankenstein a claim to a worldly self – but his hopes are dashed. As the Creature tells his story, however, he reveals another dimension of his 'invisible hand',[113] as he calls it. He describes chopping firewood at night for the de Lacey family and leaving it for their use. This is a pure act of goodness, done in a completely non-phenomenal capacity; its informing motive is to test the water of the family's possible reaction to his appearance among them. The bid fails. Afterwards, as he rescues a young girl from drowning, his appearance causes a passing rustic to fire his gun at him. It is again his appearance which frightens William in the encounter that follows, confounding the Creature's benign intent and precipitating the first killing. The search for the bridge to society is marked by acts of genuine benevolence, as Frankenstein belatedly learns. With this information the story is making a case for the Creature in the late eighteen-teens context as potentially a politically acceptable consideration. In the realm of the political, Arendt observes, appearance is reality:

> appearance – something that is being seen and heard by others as well as by ourselves – constitutes reality. Compared with the reality which comes from being seen and heard, even the greatest forces of intimate life – the passions of the heart, the thoughts

---

[112] Southwood Smith, 1824, 37.
[113] *Frankenstein*, 100.

> of the mind, the delights of the senses – lead an uncertain, shadowy kind of existence unless and until they are transformed, deprivatized and deindividualized, as it were, into a shape to fit them for public appearance.[114]

What the Creature lacks is the possibility of a shaping or a transformation of himself *without which,* as the grieving father says, *no man is fit for society.* As the invisible figure dramatises the social dimension of the anatomy question, these are apt words. The murders – and the hand which acts – are the unacceptable public face of the whole problem. In 1824 Smith is writing well before Burke and Hare of course, but he intimates the possibility of murderous developments:

> there is something in the violation of the grave, which tends . . . to degrade the character and harden the heart. This offence is connived at; nay, it is rewarded; these men . . . are paid by men of reputation and influence in society. The transition is but too easy to the commission of other offences in the hope of a similar connivance, if not similar reward.[115]

And in 1826 Bentham raises the possibility of murderous developments in private correspondence with the Home Secretary, Robert Peel, who was initially reluctant to countenance legislation.[116] The murders in *Frankenstein* lend urgency to the case for the law to intervene, as the Burke and Hare scandal was to do in 1828–29. The scandal, and a philosophically sanctioned form of secrecy, was to carry the anatomy question to its legislative apotheosis in 1832. By the time of the 1831 edition of *Frankenstein* reality had started to imitate fiction and history was busy promoting a pertinent rereading of the story.

---

114 Arendt, 1958, 50.
115 Southwood Smith, 1824, 90.
116 Richardson, 1989, 132.

CHAPTER 8

# Burkophobia, choleraphobia and the law: *Frankenstein* in 1831

## Edinburgh

Approximately midway through the story, Frankenstein agrees to his Creature's demand for a mate. Not long afterwards he is pressed by his father on his commitment to marry Elizabeth, but decides he must keep the promise to his Creature first. There are specialists in England whose knowledge and discoveries can help him to construct the female body. Seeking their advice, he sets out with Henry Clerval on what Chris Baldick aptly describes as 'ostensibly a pre-marital vacation'[1] first to London, and then, via the Lake District, to Scotland. On the way north the two men visit Edinburgh. Here is Burke and Hare's adopted city:

> I visited Edinburgh with languid eyes and mind; and yet that city might have interested the most unfortunate being. Clerval did not like it so well as Oxford, for the antiquity of the latter city was more pleasing to him. But the beauty and regularity of the new town of Edinburgh, its romantic castle and its environs, the most delightful in the world, Arthur's seat, St Bernard's Well, and the Pentland Hills compensated him for the change and filled him with *cheerfulness* and admiration [italics added][2]

For readers of the 1831 edition Edinburgh would not have been such an unqualified tourist delight. The events of 1828–29 constituted an enduring crisis of public awareness and this passage would have acquired a quite different accentuation. The inference

---

[1] Baldick, 1987, 203.
[2] *Frankenstein*, 138.

drawn from the commercial traffic in murdered bodies was that anybody anywhere could be killed and sold to the surgeons.

Frankenstein is *en route* to Edinburgh when he realises that he, his threatened family and his associates can never assemble in safety:

> I had now neglected my promise for some time, and I feared the effects of the daemon's disappointment. He might remain in Switzerland and wreak his vengeance on my relatives. This idea pursued me and tormented me at every moment from which I might otherwise have snatched repose and peace. I waited for my letters with feverish impatience; if they were delayed I was miserable and overcome by a thousand fears; and when they arrived and I saw the superscription of Elizabeth or my father, I hardly dared to read and ascertain *my fate*. Sometimes I thought that the fiend followed me and might expedite my remissness by murdering my companion. When these thoughts possessed me, I would not quit Henry for a moment, but followed him as his shadow, to protect him from the fancied rage of his destroyer [italics added].[3]

Frankenstein himself here is suffering burkophobic anxiety, which erupted nationwide after 1828. The passage evokes a terrorised, egoistic sensibility. It shows Frankenstein, as a doctor, using a language of individual survival. One effect of the rapid pronoun alternations here is that a concern for his family appears to vie with a desire to survive them: 'to ascertain *my* fate'. This is the language of incipient panic. After Edinburgh – that is to say, after Burke and Hare – *Frankenstein* becomes the portrait of a whole society on an escalating panic footing.

In the passage just quoted, Clerval, the middle-class man, is the Creature's next impending victim. In the frame of Frankenstein's uneasy reflections, Clerval exemplifies the post-Edinburgh projection of middle-class apprehensions which lent momentum to the efforts to secure a legislative solution to the bodysnatching problem. Moreover, the Edinburgh sequence gains another historical

---

3 *Ibid.*, 137–8.

accentuation in the third edition context. Alongside the continuing burkophobia, 1831 saw the arrival of a huge cholera epidemic in England. In *Aids and Its Metaphors* Susan Sontag discusses the moralistic responses to this disease. She cites the advice issued in 1832 by the Central Board of Health in the absence of specific treatments for the disease. The Board prescribed fresh air and cleanliness. It asserted: 'The true preventatives are a healthy body and a cheerful, unruffled mind.'[4] This describes Henry Clerval, who is 'filled' with 'cheerfulness' by the prospect of Edinburgh. Clerval's excellent bill of health in mind and body exemplifies the ideological subtext which supports the voice of medical officialdom: the adoption of middle-class habits and values. The same implicit directive is no less true of the social meanings carried by the Anatomy Act.

In the year of the cholera, the burkophobia was described in the press, in a predictable metaphor, as an 'epidemic'.[5] At the same time the graverobbing trade continued. In *Death, Dissection and the Destitute* Richardson describes the historic origins of popular feelings against the surgeons in the early nineteenth century. The dissection was perceived as a deliberate destruction of identity:

> Popular hostility to dissection derived from sources older and deeper than its use in public execution – it would not have been introduced in the Tutor era as a punishment for 'the most heinous kind of criminal homicide' had government not recognised its power in infringing popular taboos. It continuing success as a punishment is evidenced both by its bitter unpopularity and its regular use right up until 1832. This success resulted from its flagrant trespass upon popular belief and the insolence of its denial of customary observances. Dissection represented a gross assault upon the integrity and identity of the body *and* upon the repose of the soul, each of which – in other circumstances – would have been carefully fostered.[6]

---

[4] Sontag, 1990, 55.
[5] Richardson, 1989, 197.
[6] *Ibid.*, 76.

As I commented in my Introduction, the resurrectionist dream-cameo in *Frankenstein* shows the surgeon stealing his mother's corpse from the grave, at which point he wakes up to confront the 'monster'. The Creature's appearance here veils the mother's subsequent fate by censoring the continuation of the dream; but the timing involved suggests this is a protective intervention on his part, based on identification. His sudden appearance demonstrates a recognition of Caroline Beaufort, who has extreme poverty in her background as a formative and never-forgotten experience. Before she became Frankenstein's mother, Caroline lived in the culture of popular beliefs which Richardson describes; and had she not been rescued by her marriage she would have remained in poverty.

By 1831 the 'unclaimed' clause had been put into the draft of the impending anatomy legislation, and in this context the figure of Caroline Beaufort acquires a particular accentuation. Caroline meets her future husband, Alphonse Frankenstein, when he enters the world of poverty in a vain attempt to rescue her ruined, spendthrift father, his friend Beaufort. Alphonse Frankenstein's first sight of his future wife is when she is kneeling beside Beaufort's coffin, 'an orphan and beggar'.[7] This posture is preserved in the portrait of her which has a special place in the Frankenstein house. Recalled home after William's murder, Frankenstein enters the library:

> I gazed on the picture of my mother which stood over the mantelpiece. It was a historical subject, painted at my father's desire, and represented Caroline Beaufort in an agony of despair, kneeling by the coffin of her dead father. Her garb was rustic, her cheek pale; but there was an air of dignity and beauty that hardly permitted the sentiment of pity.[8]

In a less sentimental light, however, the painting is a visual equivalent of the 'unclaimed' clause in the legislation, for it captures

---

7 *Frankenstein*, 39.
8 *Ibid.*, 74.

the moment in Caroline's life when she is truly fallen into destitution and helplessness. The word 'relation' in the relevant passage is ambiguous:

> [Caroline] knelt by Beaufort's coffin, weeping bitterly, when my father entered the chamber. He came like a protecting spirit to the poor girl, who committed herself to his care; and after the interment of his friend, he conducted her to Geneva, and placed her under the protection of a relation. Two years after this event Caroline became his wife.[9]

This does not say whose relation it is; it could be either his or hers. There is therefore no confirmation that Caroline has any surviving relations when her father dies. This ambiguity aside, however, the language here spells out the human face of the 1832 legislative clause: the need for relatives. Her suitor-to-be arrives 'like a protecting spirit' and, lacking other options, Caroline straight away 'commits' herself to him. Contrary to the portrait's idealised version, a telling comment by Frankenstein focuses Caroline's real predicament when her father is dead. With her father, Caroline lives 'unknown and in wretchedness'.[10] With or without relations, therefore, her obscurity before she marries Alphonse Frankenstein marks her as a potential candidate for dissection.

The murders in the story, in 1831, would have hinted loudly at burking as the logical extension of resurrectionism. This was the inference drawn in many quarters after William Burke's execution and dissection in 1829, as Hazlitt's commentary on Burke and Hare,[11] 'The Late Murders', confirms. Hazlitt is quite clear that the utility principle murders to dissect:

> We may see by this example (in spite of what the *Utilitarians* tell us) how impossible it is to sanctify the means by the end;

---

9 *Ibid.*, 39.

10 *Ibid.*, 38.

11 See 'The Late Murders', *New Writings* by William Hazlitt, 100–5. The essay shows Hazlitt well abreast of the utilitarian arguments promoting dissection, but not, however, the legislative design on the poor.

> or to direct bad instruments and passions merely to the salutary objects we may have in view. We cannot say to vice, *Thus far shalt thou come and no farther!* It may appear proper to have dead bodies to dissect, and necessary to get men to steal them; but from stealing them they shall proceed to *making* them as the shorter cut. Harden the feelings, debase the imagination – and you strike at the root of all morality and at the whole social system. There is no answering for the consequences. From the resurrection-man with his yellow fingers and torpid load, the transition is obvious to the assassin with blood-stained hands and his struggling victim.[12]

Frankenstein's artificial man – the man he 'makes' to use Hazlitt's apt word – turns out to be an assassin of the kind described here. Hazlitt comments on the way informal *laissez-faire* initiatives can harden the sensibility. In a similar way to the resurrection cameo in *Frankenstein*, Hazlitt blurs the distinction between the grave-robber and the anatomist:

> By familiarity (unredeemed by any other views but of his own sordid interest) he loses the repugnance due to death, and by degrees the reverence due to life. He looks at human bodies as containing so many bones and muscles, as so many moving anatomical preparations, and thinks that every pound of flesh, if it were *dead*, would be worth so much gold. This is a fearful train of ideas.[13]

Indeed, 'The Late Murders' reads almost as a commentary on *Frankenstein*. In the following remarks Hazlitt could well be commenting on Frankenstein's silence. Behind the reference to Jack Ketch the executioner stands the surgeons' pre-1832 supply of corpses:

> The abstract utility does not purify these men's motives, as long as their imagination is a charnel-house, and they are accustomed

---

[12] *Ibid.*, 101.
[13] *Ibid.*

> to *stop the mouth* of all their own natural scruples by main force – they will find no difficulty after that in stopping any other mouth in the same way. Nobody would be, or would sit in company with, *Jack Ketch*: yet his is an indispensable calling. There is then something besides Utility.[14]

This prediction was correct. 1831 saw the onset of copy-cat crimes following in the wake of Edinburgh; and Bishop and Williams, the London burkers, were graverobbers as well as murderers. The third edition of *Frankenstein* is an imitation – and clarification – of reality. In the popular perception, Dr Robert Knox, the recipient of Burke and Hare's victims, was as guilty as the killers themselves. When Edinburgh appears in the story it is remarkable to find the fictional surgeon equivocating on his criminal guilt: 'I felt as if I had committed some great crime, the consciousness of which haunted me. I was guiltless, but I had indeed drawn down a horrible curse upon my head, as mortal as that of crime.'[15] By remaining socially invisible, the Creature plays to Frankenstein's rationalisation that nobody would believe him if he were to disclose the murderer. He therefore holds the surgeon to a guilty public silence which uncannily resembles Robert Knox's own controversial stance. As Frankenstein remains silent, his Creature's killings mirror the widely publicised copycat developments.

There is another way to describe the new burking script in the third edition. In this edition least of all, Frankenstein cannot present a favourable, or, in Bakhtin's terms, a uniaccented spectacle of surgery in society. As the Edinburgh scandal rewrites *Frankenstein*, the 1831 edition of the book prefigures the Bishop and Williams copycat murders, as fact and fictional invention enter into a dynamic symmetry. Frankenstein galvanises into life a 'resurrected' body which acts out the spirit of the age in its decisive turn towards the utilitarian culture. As he evades capture, the Creature easily scorns the utilitarian injunction that the dead can prove themselves useful to the living through dissection. As he attacks

---

14 *Ibid.*

15 *Frankenstein*, 138.

the wealthy, however, the case builds to put the injunction into law.

In the pre-1832 context the Creature embodies a particular kind of coveted anatomical subject which was to be excluded, and even tabooed, by the legislation. Richardson cites a private admission by Somerville, the official Inspector of Anatomy for England and Wales, to the effect that 'the Bodies from the Hulks' were considered more 'interesting'. These 'are most prized at the Schools on account of their being for the most part young subjects and better adapted for the display of human structure than the aged inmates of the workhouses.'[16] This official admission comes in 1841, but it confirms a long-standing attitude. As I have commented, Frankenstein creates a great 'hulk' he cannot subsequently control. As a mass of many bodies reborn in a single figure, his Creature is a repository of anatomically young subjects; with an athleticism denied to ordinary mortals, he repeatedly demonstrates supreme physical fitness. Notoriously, Dr Knox is reputed to have marked his approval of the bodies delivered to his School by Burke and Hare with the word 'fresh'. In his own language therefore – if not in his mind – there was an equivocation between young bodies and/or recently murdered bodies.

The social bias written into the anatomy legislation attracted criticism in due course from within the medical profession itself. As Richardson notes,[17] the London surgeon William Roberts, a campaigner against the Act, even argued that bodysnatching had been a fairer system since it brooked no social distinctions. Campaigning against the law's post-1832 implementation, Roberts, writing in the 1840s, drew attention to the fact that 'advantage had been taken of burkophobia to gain the Bill's passage'. The Bill 'had been accomplished . . . with consummate art. One of its main objectives was to victimise a certain class, and it accomplishes this purpose without naming this class.'[18]

---

[16] Richardson, 1989, 248.
[17] *Ibid.*, 246–52.
[18] *Ibid.*

The moves to use the burkophobia to assist the passage of the law are prefigured in the 1827 instalment of De Quincey's *On Murder considered as one of the Fine Arts* in a strange conjunction of fiction and reality. De Quincey's speaker offers his private audience some 'principles of murder . . . to regulate . . . your judgement'.[19] As he does so, he observes that London is a good source of subjects – and indeed four years later the spate of copycat killings took place in the capital. In what is an uncanny coincidence, reality in 1831 was to imitate De Quincey's words of four years earlier:

> the subject chosen ought to be in good health: for it is absolutely barbarous to murder a sick person, who is usually quite unable to bear it. On this principle no Cockney[20] ought to be chosen who is above twenty-five, for after that age he is sure to be dyspeptic. Or at least, if a man will hunt in that warren, he ought to murder a couple at a time . . . The world in general, gentlemen, are very bloody minded; and all they want in a murder is a copious effusion of blood; gaudy display in this point is enough for *them*. But the enlightened connoisseur is more refined in his taste.[21]

This spells out the desirable condition and age-group of subjects. The corpses in *Frankenstein* meet these requirements. Here, for example, is Clerval: 'It appeared to be a handsome young man, about five and twenty years of age. He had apparently been strangled, for there was no sign of any violence except the black marks of fingers on his neck.'[22]

As I have noted, Knox's collusion with Burke and Hare was assisted by the killers' art of suffocation which left no signs of violence. Where Clerval and Elizabeth are concerned, Frankenstein's eye is always drawn first to the black finger marks on the body, as they conspicuously spell out the popular belief that Burke

---

19 De Quincey, 1918, 332.

20 A 'Cockney' is a Londoner born within the sound of Bow Bells.

21 De Quincey, 1918, 334.

22 *Frankenstein*, 148.

and Hare's victims were throttled. Furthermore, before the journey north via Edinburgh, and Clerval's death, Frankenstein and his friend spend some months in London, the territory of Bishop and Williams. By 1831 the objective, as Roberts puts it, 'to victimise a certain class' was in the draft version of the Anatomy Act. In the third edition of *Frankenstein* the Creature's three victims all qualify as highly prized subjects on account of their age and health; and by selecting victims of their social class, the Creature spells out the hypocrisy at the root of the social argument.

As Richardson observes, the injustice written into the law in 1832 has this pre-1832 face:

> It could truthfully be said that high hospital mortality was the price paid by the poor both for the advancement of scientific surgery, and the advancing social status of surgeons . . . That Astley Cooper ran a free clinic for the poor to trawl for 'interesting' cases is recorded by his biographer Brock.[23]

The last victim of the 'trawl' in *Frankenstein* is Elizabeth. The bridal corpse left for the anatomist in the wedding chamber draws into focus the deathly nuptials of a marriage of heaven and hell. Blake's famous contraries of 'Heaven' and 'Hell' are the apposite social categories where the political allegory in the story is concerned. Elizabeth has known 'Hell' in the time she spent as a child, alongside other children, amid 'penury in its worst shape'.[24] When Caroline Beaufort first sees her, Elizabeth stands 'far above all the rest . . . of a different stock . . . a being heaven-sent'.[25] There is a hint here of 'natural' aristocracy, but this role – when it is finally assumed – is reserved for Elizabeth on her 'heavenly' wedding-day: the day which puts the symbolic stamp on her husband's advancing professional and social status. Elizabeth's latent upper-class status is only disclosed on the eve of her marriage, when part of her parents' aristocratic fortune is released to her.

---

23 Richardson, 1989, 49.
24 *Frankenstein*, 40–1
25 *Ibid.*, 41. See n. 23, ch. 2.

This development belongs to the final frame of the story's metaphor of 1832, the political marriage of the upper and the middle classes, who are figured by the bride and groom respectively, Elizabeth and Frankenstein. Her special-day elevation in status makes Elizabeth the Creature's target in a timely and pointed reversal: the aristocratic bride is murdered in Como, the location of her original penury.

As I showed in Chapter 5, the Creature's words *I will be with you on your wedding-night* are in part a promise to Elizabeth, as he perceives her. On the night in question the Creature demonstrates the class contradiction Elizabeth embodies: the bride is attacked for her class betrayal *and* claimed by the mass of bodies comprising the Creature's body. As he departs after her death, the figure confronting Frankenstein silently points to the antecedent identity Elizabeth retains from the abyss of poverty – that is, he lets her corpse speak the difference between poverty and power. Throughout the story Frankenstein's fiancée, who is brought into the family by benevolent philanthropy, remains an ambiguous body: she stands on both sides of an incipient social divide. As she awaits marriage, Elizabeth begins to qualify as a political beneficiary of the Anatomy Act. The dutiful, patient bride-to-be is a docile or 'ensouled' body of the kind famously described by Foucault in *Discipline and Punish*. As he affirms the soul's reality, however, Foucault inverts the traditional Christian paradox: the soul exists – and constitutes individuality – but it is the prison of the body. The soul holds the body, divesting it of its power as a signifying force.[26] On the 'bridal bier', however, Elizabeth's corpse is reinvested with a power to signify: it is drawn across – and back across – the social class demarcation which after 1832 was to sanction exemption from dissection as a mark of the rights and freedom of the individual.

---

[26] See Foucault, 1979, Pt III.

## The political allegory

*Frankenstein* enacts an allegory of civil society in an early nineteenth-century time frame. The story charts the changes in England's ideological climate which culminate in the political settlement of 1832. Before he creates the Creature, Frankenstein fixates on the success of his project with a paternalist metaphor: 'No father could claim the gratitude of his child so completely as I should deserve theirs.'[27] These words invoke a bond of gratitude which, where his Creature is concerned, he will revoke as the story proceeds. His pre-creation paternalist rhetoric is mirrored in Caroline Beaufort's attitude towards Justine as reported by Elizabeth in her first letter to Frankenstein:

> My aunt conceived a great attachment for her, by which she was induced to give her an education superior to that which she had at first intended. This benefit was fully re-paid; Justine was the most grateful little creature in the world . . . [She] paid the greatest attention to every gesture of my aunt. She thought her the model of all excellence, and endeavoured to imitate her phraseology and manners, so that even now she often reminds me of her.[28]

Further into the story, however, it becomes apparent that a climate of benevolent paternalism is failing to guarantee social order: this is the public perception following Justine's conviction. Frankenstein's family, as we have seen, shows a hybrid class complexion. With Elizabeth and Justine as members, it is constituted by Caroline's philanthropy. On her deathbed, Caroline obtains Frankenstein's and Elizabeth's pledge of eventual marriage. That is to say, within the story's allegory, she secures a romance version of the bond – or constancy – between benevolent philanthropy and the poor which sees Elizabeth admitted to the house. In this respect the family belongs – as does *Frankenstein* in its first three

---

[27] *Frankenstein*, 55.
[28] *Ibid.*, 64.

editions – to a pre-1832 ideological climate in which poverty was bonded to forms of humanitarianism in ways that, post-1832, it ceased to be.[29] Justine, as Elizabeth says, is philanthropy – and gratitude – incarnate: she acquires Caroline Beaufort's body by imitation. In court Justine's social condemnation is marked by the unfavourable evidence represented by the miniature portrait of her benign aunt. But something else is suggested when Justine goes to the gallows: her remarkable resemblance to her aunt sees the Creature staging a mock execution of Caroline Beaufort and the philanthropy she represents. In the home, by contrast, the young servant's docile body is the appropriate and fitting reminder of her aunt. In what Elizabeth intends as a compliment, Justine is a body schooled in grief: 'she was much altered since the death of my aunt: grief had given softness and a winning mildness to her manners which had before been remarkable for vivacity.'[30]

As she grieves, Justine learns to keep her place in her new home. Bereavement is an appropriate metaphor for a subjection coming from ideology, but accepted as 'from within', from within the individual subject. For Justine, grief is her *rite de passage*, her initiation into the social contract. In court, her 'winning mildness' – which contrasts so strongly with the assumption of her guilt – is her damnation. Foucault's gloss on the social contract applies to Justine in *Frankenstein*:

> a formidable right to punish is established, since the offender becomes the common enemy. Indeed, he is worse than an enemy, for it is from within society that he delivers his blows – he is nothing less than a traitor, a 'monster'.[31]

The 'he' in this sentence is apt. Justine's wrongful conviction is set up by the common enemy of civil society, the 'monster'.

The 1832 Anatomy Act, as it passed into law in the shadow of the Reform Bill, spelt the end of benevolent philanthropy: this

---

29 Richardson, 1989, 266.
30 *Frankenstein*, 64.
31 Foucault, 1979, 90.

much is the Creature's own perception when Frankenstein confronts him pointing at Elizabeth's corpse on the wedding-night. By the end of the 1820s, comments F. M. L. Thompson:

> Viewed through the ruling class end of the telescope, all workers, irrespective of their precise status . . . being propertyless were either potentially dangerous as liable to subvert property and the social order, or at best not worthy of political recognition as being incapable of taking a balanced and responsible view of the public interest.[32]

The first murder in the story, which claims William, reinforces this perception. Frankenstein's return home, upon the news of this killing, is marked by his glimpse of the miniature portrait of William which stands alongside the mantelpiece image of Caroline Beaufort, the benign but now deceased mother. The 'monster's subsequent violence lends ideological ammunition to those who sought to harden class lines and persecute the poor in the immediate pre- and post-1832 era. (Under the new regime a number of recorded cases[33] involved open accusations of 'murderousness' in the implementation of the New Poor Law). It is decisive that the murderous developments intensify *after* Frankenstein breaks his promise to assemble a female mate for his creation. The Creature demands a mate 'as a right'.[34] It is a dutiful, if profoundly uneasy, paternalism which leads Frankenstein to give his word.

On the Creature's provocation, the hardening class attitude becomes more marked in Frankenstein's tone of voice and feeling after Henry Clerval's murder. After the death of his friend – and in renewed bereavement – he can talk only the language of harsh antagonism and reprisal against his creation. The abandoned promise reads as a remarkable anticipation – or prolepsis – of 1832, the political bad faith of which has caused some historians to employ

---

32 F. M. L. Thompson, 1988, 15–16.

33 Richardson, 1989, 268

34 *Frankenstein*, 124.

a vocabulary of betrayals and dishonoured bargains. Richardson comments:

> after the 1832 election . . . it became clear that the main beneficiaries of the immense mobilization for reform had been the very people who had dishonoured their bargain with the working class – who had created the Anatomy Act, and who promised yet worse . . . The *coup de grâce* would come in the New Poor Law.[35]

By the time of the 1839 instalment of *On Murder considered as a Fine Art* the fear of the abyss felt by the respectable paled somewhat beside the fear felt in the abyss itself in respect of the orders above. Rule by social division in the 1830s, as Richardson observes,[36] was born in the political convenience of alliances forged between elites and rising middle-class aspirations. In Chapter 4 I examined the reverberations of this divide-and-rule tactic in *Barnaby Rudge*. We shall observe it again in my Conclusion, where I shall show the common people's fear of dissection surfacing in Mrs Gaskell's *Mary Barton*.

Where these historic alliances are concerned, the event which prefigures them in *Frankenstein* is Frankenstein's and Elizabeth's wedding-day. On its eve, as I have noted, the bride comes into repossession of part of her parents' aristocratic fortune. On the day itself Elizabeth's life reaches its climax in a crisis of competing claims on her. The showdown argument between Frankenstein and his 'monster' over who Elizabeth is begins in earnest soon after the second creation is destroyed. The female mate is coveted by the Creature as the *bona fide* relative, the only kind of relation recognised by the impending anatomy law in its notorious claiming clause. Having witnessed the violent destruction of his mate, the Creature serves notice that he will be present on the wedding-night. As I commented in Chapter 5, Elizabeth doubles as Frankenstein's bride and the bride denied to the Creature. The

---

35 Richardson, 1989, 265–6.

36 *Ibid.*

multi-accentuation in play on the wedding-day focuses the ambiguities which lie at the political core of the 1832 legislative package. Lord Grey, who took the Reform Bill into law, spelt out the tactic that carried the day at the climax of the national drama. The aim was: 'To associate the middle with the higher orders of society in the love and support of the institutions and government of the country.'[37]

The situation in 1830–32, as Whig ministers saw it, is summarised by F. M. L. Thompson: 'The vital thing . . . was to break the radical alliance by driving a wedge between the middle and the working classes, buying off the one with votes and representation and leaving the other, isolated and weak, outside the pale.'[38] Being outside the pale meant being inside the newly created dissection constituency. Prior to her wedding-day, Elizabeth is a submerged repository of the social spectrum whose division-and-rule manipulation begins in 1832. Hers is a story, however, of upward class aspiration, and the political configuration which she embodies on her wedding-day is a sentimental sham. On the day in question she accommodates the entire class macrocosm which Grey was aiming to reconstitute by division: Elizabeth the bride is a newly reinstated aristocrat whose middle-class groom is a surgeon, a man aspiring to professional and social legitimacy – but she remains originally a child reprieved from destitution. The wedding-day in *Frankenstein*, that is to say, is a charade rehearsal of the political marriage of 1832. As she marries, Elizabeth plays to the part and the idea of an inclusive 'nation' – and this the Creature cannot accept. Since the breaking of the promise made to him he has repeatedly indicated his dissent, and, as he vows, he intends to have his word. For him, after the loss of his own mate, the parading of Elizabeth is a provocation.

The Creature swiftly demonstrates the punitive nature of the impending political settlement. Elizabeth's body is left on the 'bridal bier' on the night of first intimacy. The corpse is Elizabeth

---

37 Cited in F. M. L. Thompson, 1988, 16.

38 *Ibid.*

as the Creature alone recognises her – the less than familiar face of the destitute woman before she was singled out for bourgeois identity. As the bride denied to the Creature, Elizabeth is the pauper body with no relative at hand to claim her. In his eyes, she belongs in death to the communities which were targeted by the impending law's clause concerning the 'unclaimed' dead – and so her body is left to the surgeon on the ceremonial day of his professional legitimation. By the same token, the Creature's estrangement from his mate is a portent of the notorious sexual segregation which, on Malthusian logic, was imposed on the inmates of the post-1832 workhouse to limit their numbers. On the eve of her true caste's historic persecution, Elizabeth becomes the law's first victim: the Creature offers her to the new political leviathan in a timely clarification of its premeditated designs on the poor. She is of course also Frankenstein's bride, and hence the offering of the bourgeois corpse to the surgeon is a final provocation to the hegemonic group in society to secure an anatomy legislation.

One image in particular draws Elizabeth into focus on the most important, and the last, day of her life, On her wedding-day Elizabeth's body announces her elevation to the aristocracy. As the day approaches:

> The sweet girl welcomed me with warm affection, yet tears were in her eyes as she beheld my emaciated frame and feverish cheeks. I saw a change in her also. She was *thinner* and had lost much of that heavenly vivacity that had before charmed me; but her gentleness and soft looks of compassion made her a more fit companion for one blasted and miserable as I was [italics added].[39]

Frankenstein's own feverish emaciation I shall comment on in due course. The immediate image here is Elizabeth's weight-loss and her appearance as it coincides with the part-restoration of her aristocratic inheritance. In *Illness As Metaphor* Sontag makes a

[39] *Frankenstein*, 159.

number of comments which bear pertinently on the political 'marriage' settlement of 1832 and its dress-rehearsal here in *Frankenstein*. Identifying illness as 'a trope for new attitudes to the self', Sontag observes: 'Consumption was understood as a manner of appearing, and that appearance became a staple of nineteenth-century manners.'[40] And:

> The TB-influenced idea of the body was a new model for aristocratic looks – *at a moment when aristocracy stops being a matter of power, and starts being mainly a matter of image.* ('One can never be too rich. One can never be too thin,' the Duchess of Windsor once said.) Indeed, the romanticising of TB is the first widespread example of that distinctly modern activity, promoting the self as an image. The tubercular look had to be considered attractive once it came to be considered a mark of distinction, of breeding [italics added].[41]

Elizabeth does not, of course, have tuberculosis, but, with her middle-class fiancé, she is starting to look the part for the honeymoon. She is shrinking to fit the image. In a preposterous piece of semiotic bodysnatching the wealthy and the image-conscious steal a sign, and a self-promotion, from a deadly disease. In contrast, when Caroline Beaufort first sees Elizabeth she is 'thin' for reasons which have to do with poverty, but even here her appearance – her natural aristocracy – distinguishes her from the crowd,[42] and she is chosen for the Frankenstein home. As the passive figure she is, Elizabeth, likewise, does not choose her wedding-day body-image; on the contrary, its powerful, mythic attributes choose her. The lowered vitality that 'becomes' her on her wedding-day is a sign of a romantic and 'interesting' individuality: Elizabeth, as Frankenstein says, is a model form of companion.

Everything Frankenstein ever says about Elizabeth's keen and

---

40 Sontag, 1983, 33.

41 *Ibid.* Apropos of Sontag's aside, the Duchess of Windsor, when she honeymooned in Como in 1936, was not setting a trend – she was following the one set in *Frankenstein.*

42 *Frankenstein*, 40–1.

sad sensitivity has its iconic focus in her ceremonial attribute, her wedding-day thinness. Sontag instances Italy[43] as the place which was considered in the nineteenth century to be especially good for tuberculars; the disease which was socially appropriated as the 'special person's disease' started to furnish models for fashionable kinds of life style. As we see from Frankenstein's honeymoon in Como, travel is a part of this. The story at this juncture indirectly invokes the Shelleys' own Continental elopement, and perhaps also the drug diversions of the Diodati villa. Frankenstein has for some time, since his return from Ireland, been taking a double nightcap of laudanum. The newly-weds' journey south quickly dissolves the bourgeois reality-principle. Frankenstein's wedding-night encounter with Elizabeth on her bridal bier occurs in a space which is temporarily free of constraints. As Sontag observes: 'The Romantics invented invalidism as a pretext for leisure, and for dismissing bourgeois obligations in order to live only for one's art. It was a way of retiring from the world without having to take responsibility for the decision.'[44] The honeymoon in Como resembles a banishment to an idyllic lake; however, it is also a disenchantment, a beautiful place which cannot be enjoyed.[45] Nevertheless, the ego-world of aestheticism invites the Creature, as he enters the villa, to take the line of least resistance.

Elizabeth's bridal-bier is a sexually charged representation of the surgeon's energies of interest in the bodies of the poor, on the day of all days which symbolises his access to them. The TB-body is a social totem and the wedding day is inevitably the occasion for its grandest exhibition. This above all makes Elizabeth the object of the Creature's attack in Como, the place where she originally existed in 'penury': in his eyes she is a class traitor. When Frankenstein first sees her on his final return home Elizabeth stands on the threshold of formalising an alien identity. Marriage, status and family life beckon – and she is losing weight. In the

---

43 Sontag, 1983, 37.

44 *Ibid.*

45 I am adapting a remark made by R. L. Stevenson which Sontag quotes. *Ibid.*, 37.

event, on the ceremonial day of union, the bride's 'manner of appearance', in Sontag's sense, is accepted by the Creature as the final provocation – and a licence to produce the corpse. The third edition of *Frankenstein* appeared just months before England finally put an end to its *ancien régime.* The body on the bridal bier – as aristocrat and pauper – is divided between the winners and the losers.

## From crowd to social class

Before Frankenstein's wedding, the Creature seeks to negotiate a place for himself in society. Franco Moretti highlights Frankenstein's fear of his Creature in their exchange:

> The creature's explicit demands cannot in fact produce fear. They are not a gesture of challenge; they are 'reformist'/'Chartist' demands. The creature wishes only to have right of citizenship among men: 'I will not be tempted to set myself in opposition to thee. I am thy creature, and I will be ever mild and docile to my natural lord and king . . . I was benevolent and good; misery made me a fiend. Make me happy and I shall again be virtuous'. Furthermore, when all friendly relations with humans have failed, the creature humbly accepts his marginalization, begging only to have another creature who is 'as deformed and horrible as myself'. But even this is denied to him. The creature's sheer *existence* is frightening enough for Frankenstein, let alone the prospect of his producing children and multiplying.[46]

'The creature is disfigured,' Moretti observes,[47] 'because this is actually how things were in the first decades of the industrial revolution'. However, these observations only apply accurately to the 1831 edition of *Frankenstein* as it appears on the eve of 1832. They cannot apply to the editions of 1818 and 1823 which long

[46] Moretti, 1983, 86.
[47] *Ibid.*, 87.

precede the beginnings of Chartism. As E. P. Thompson argues,[48] there is a sense in which Chartism 'commenced at the moment when the Reform Bill received Royal Assent' – and, we may add, not least as the Bill overshadows the passage of the Anatomy Act into law.

The historical research on the legislative phase of the anatomy reforms was not available when Moretti gave his pioneering reading in which the Creature figures as the industrial proletariat. I do not entirely agree with him when he emphasises the Creature's sheer existence – rather than his demands – as the source of fear. Frankenstein's ambivalence concerning his promise is sanctioned even as the Creature binds the demand for a mate to his pledge to be virtuous. The appeal for citizenship has a threatening dimension. The words quoted by Moretti above hold a particular fear for Frankenstein even in their sincerity, for a virtuous Creature is nevertheless still a Creature who desires to increase in numbers. In *Crowds and Power* Canetti[49] uses the term 'increase pack' to describe social groups whose propelling energies centre in a desire to *be more* in numbers. It is the prospect of growing numbers of the proletariat which threatens Frankenstein:

> The *hubris* of production goes back to the *increase* pack . . . It is worth pointing out that the strict and exclusive combination of proletarian and production, which has acquired such prestige during the last hundred years, re-establishes in a particularly pure form the old conception which was the core of the increase pack. The proletariat are those who increase fastest, and they do so in two ways. First, they have more children than other people and thus, through their progeny, come to resemble a crowd, and secondly their numbers are increased by the influx of people from the country to the centres of production.[50]

As Mark Harrison comments, 'it is this notion of crowds of people

---

[48] E. P. Thompson, 1963, 909.
[49] Canetti, 1981, 125–32.
[50] *Ibid.*, 224–5.

permanently representing the possibility of an organised crowd which concerns most historians when they refer to nineteenth-century anxieties about "the crowd"'.[51]

Frankenstein's fear of crowds determines his decision to break his promise. It is his reservations about a propagation of children, or, as he calls it, 'a race of devils',[52] which lead him to dishonour his side of the bargain. His anxiety surfaces as he works on the female anatomy. The 'devils' are figured as children, 'who might make the very existence of the species a condition precarious and full of terror':

> now, for the first time, the wickedness of my promise burst upon me; I shuddered to think that future ages might curse me as their pest, whose selfishness had not hesitated to buy its own peace at the price, perhaps, of the existence of the whole human race.[53]

Imagining posterity, Frankenstein conjures a large crowd indeed and a vast billingsgate of curses. Since the creation, he admits, only Clerval has been able to call 'forth the better feelings of my heart':[54] Clerval 'again taught me to love . . . the cheerful faces of children'.[55] And likewise, only his friend's presence sustains Frankenstein's pleasurable communion with romantic nature when they travel together through the pastoral haunts of England. As he rationalises abandoning his promise, Frankenstein is on the verge of losing his benign sympathies, for the broken promise seals Clerval's fate. Henceforth, after his friend's murder, an uncompromising rejection of the Creature informs the story's political allegory.

---

51 M. Harrison, 1988, 36
52 *Frankenstein*, 140
53 *Ibid.*, 141
54 *Ibid.*, 68
55 *Ibid.*

## Microscopic vision and the plague

As I will now show, there are various kinds of crowd conception which conspire to intensify Frankenstein's fear of the Creature. These crowds are always associated with the Creature, but assume a number of forms. For example, his imagination of posterity necessarily involves an invisible crowd – a hostile and limitless mass of children – which reverses his earlier pre-creation fantasy of a grateful new species full of 'happy and excellent natures'.[56] The anxiety about 'a race of devils' is typical of the apprehensions and ambitions which haunt the preventative efforts of early modern social medicine. The specific threat here was the high incidence of epidemics. Before he makes the Creature, Frankenstein is inspired by Waldman's vivid cameo of the eyes of the 'modern masters' poring 'over the microscope' and 'acquiring new and almost unlimited powers'.[57] Frankenstein belongs to a small minority which, by means of the microscope, has observed one particular phenomenon. His vocabulary of a 'race of devils', however, suggests the extent to which his own experience as a microscopist has left a remnant of potential nervousness[58] in him. In *Crowds and Power* Canetti describes the invisible, hostile crowd which was becoming apparent in the nineteenth century:

> If we consider the *fate* of the invisible crowds we have spoken of [i.e. the Christian Middle Ages conception of the devils], we shall conclude that some of them have disappeared completely, and others in large part. Among the latter are the devils. In spite of their former numbers, they are no longer to be found anywhere in their familiar shape. But they have left their traces. The fact that they were small is proved by the striking instances

---

[56] *Ibid.*, 55.

[57] *Ibid.*, 51.

[58] In *The Human Province* (the notebooks to *Crowds and Power*), Canetti discusses the disquiet which a person who is obsessed with order can feel after looking through a microscope. Such a person retains 'a remnant of potential nervousness'. See Canetti, 1985, 160.

> adduced by Caesarius von Heisterbach, who was contemporary with the time of their flowering. Since then they have given up all the traits which might remind us of a human figure and become much smaller still. It is greatly changed, and in even larger numbers, that they turn up again in the nineteenth century as *bacilli.* Instead of the souls, they now attack the bodies of men; and to these they can be very dangerous. Only a tiny minority of people have looked into a microscope and really seen them there. But everyone has heard of them and is continually aware of their presence and makes every effort not to come into contact with them – though this, considering their invisibility, is a somewhat vague endeavour. Their power to harm and their concentration in enormous numbers in very small spaces is undoubtedly taken over from the devils.[59]

In 1831, at the height of the burkophobia, the cholera epidemic engulfed England and Scotland with mortality estimated at around 23,000. Special services were organised to plead for divine mercy, and in his Parliamentary speech of that year the King indicated that 'precautions against the introduction of so dangerous a malady'[60] should be taken. No cure existed, and no cause was known, for the bacillus was not identified until 1884, after two more epidemics in 1849 and 1854. As Frank Mort observes, amid the lack of agreement about causation one firm understanding nevertheless prevailed:

> medics, clerics and other local officials were all agreed that the *urban poor* were the human agents responsible for spreading the contagion . . . the hastily constituted Board of Health confirmed that the environment and the physical and moral habits of the poor actively stimulated the disease.[61]

Frankenstein's 'race of devils' projection carries an apprehension of hosts of bacterial life – it is a pre-eugenicist vision of the

---

59 Canetti, 1981, 53
60 Quoted by Mort, 1987, 14
61 *Ibid.*

working class as rampantly procreating bacilli. As he constructs the female anatomy, his thoughts turn to his Creatures' breeding proclivities – and then to his promise. Frankenstein, whose original project was to rid humanity of disease, now stands in trepidation of initiating a terminal global plague. The scenario is a Malthusian apocalyse, a crowd scene to end all crowd scenes. He is emphatic on the point of a menace in mass form. The logic of the demonising metaphor, Mort points out,[62] twins poverty and immorality with contagion; it facilitates intentions of a greater surveillance and regulation of the poor.

Helman[63] has described how, in the nineteenth century, 'diseases of uncertain origin could become metaphors, carriers of social and moral meaning'. The developments in *Frankenstein* which are the work of the Creature's hand can be cast into a 'germ-ism' scenario of the invisible enemy.[64] The infection is a social event which announces itself suddenly with William's murder; it quickly reveals Justine's 'criminal' origins in poverty as the source of contagion; as a scapegoat is sought, thousands of people attend the young girl's trial and subsequent punishment. The Creature, the unseen host, places society on a war-footing in an uneven struggle. In the escalating crisis he kills Henry Clerval in a parody of a sacrificial offering. Eventually, the invader brings about a state of total helplessness. As he withdraws from view and remains unpredictable, the Creature provokes, but foils, society's xenophobic projections. And with the wedding-night assignation the 'monster' haunts Frankenstein with the certainty of his germ-like power to enter – and hence in Como he enters the property unseen.

Waldman's description of medicine's microscopic vision applies to the eighteenth-century context of pathology and John Hunter's early emphasis on observing diseased organs. It also accommodates Bichat's directive to concentrate attention not on whole organs but on their constituent tissues as the sites of disease. (Although

---

62 *Ibid.*

63 Helman, 1991, 31; Sontag, 1983, 65.

64 My comments here owe to Cecil Helman's essay 'The Rise of Germism' in *Body Myths*, 1991, 29–47.

not a microscopist himself, Bichat led others to study disease with the microscope and anticipated the major discoveries of the nineteenth century in this area.)[65] Waldman's image also recalls Antoni van Leeuwenhoek spotting the germs through his crude microscope. Simply listening to Waldman holding forth on medical power causes Frankenstein to feel 'as if my soul were grappling with a palpable enemy';[66] and this moment in the lecture, he declares, is unforgettable. Canetti focuses the contrast:

> Man's power and the conception he had of himself had already expanded enormously when he stumbled upon the bacillus. This discovery made the contrast immeasurably greater . . . [he] easily persuaded himself to see as vermin everything which opposed him; as such he regarded and treated all animals which he could not use. And the despot who reduces men to animals and only manages to rule them by regarding them as belonging to a lower species, reduces to vermin all who do not qualify to be ruled and ends by destroying them by the million.[67]

Some of the specific ideological developments of 1832 were legitimated within the larger scheme of this panoptic regime.

As regards 1832, Bentham and the anatomy legislation, Canetti's general proposition is implicit in these observations by Ignatieff:

> Bentham's two personae – the advocate of parliamentary reform, and the publicist for the Panoptican – were not contradictory but complementary. The extension of rights within civil society had to be compensated for by the abolition of the tacit liberties enjoyed by prisoners and criminals under the *ancien régime*. In an unequal and increasingly divided society, this was the only

[65] In *The Birth of the Clinic* (1986, 146) Foucault argues that Bichat's famous recommendation to 'open up a few corpses' saw the birth of anatomo-clinical medicine. In George Eliot's *Middlemarch*, a story which refers to Burke and Hare, the surgeon Tertius Lydgate is a follower of Bichat.

[66] *Frankenstein*, 51.

[67] Canetti, 1981, 420. Evidence of the poor being treated as if they were herds of animals in the post-1832 era is noted by Richardson (1989, 268).

> way to extend liberty and fortify consent without compromising security.[68]

The process facilitated, and was facilitated by, a transposition to metaphor:

> Like the hospital, the penitentiary was created to enforce a quarantine both moral and medical. Behind its walls, the contagion of criminality would be isolated from the healthy, moral population outside. Within the prison itself the separate confinement of each offender in a cell would prevent *the bacillus of vice* from spreading from the hardened to the uninitiate [italics added].[69]

On his death-bed, and close to the end of his story, Frankenstein presents his decision to abrogate his promise as the recovery of his reason. He uses the philosophical principle of Utilitarianism to support a firm renunciation of paternalism:

> In a fit of enthusiastic madness, I created a rational creature and was bound towards him to assure, as far as was within my power, his happiness and well-being. This was my duty; but there was another still paramount to that. My duties towards the beings of my own species had greater claims to my attention *because they included a greater portion of happiness or misery*. Urged by this view, I refused, and I did right in refusing, to create a companion for the first creature. He showed unparalleled malignity and selfishness in evil; he destroyed my friends; he devoted to destruction beings who possessed exquisite sensations, happiness and wisdom; nor do I know where this thirst for vengeance may end [italics added].[70]

This in effect is a rehearsal of the criminalisation of poverty, the ideological lever of the legitimation accorded to the anatomy legislation. The race of devils projection is an instance of the way

---

[68] M. Ignatieff, 1978, 212.
[69] *Ibid.*, 61–2.
[70] *Frankenstein*, 180.

political and medical discourses intersect in the vocabulary of official anxieties. Confronting the Creature, Frankenstein directly associates the devils with vermin: '"Devil," I exclaimed, "do you dare approach me? . . . Begone, vile insect!"'[71]

Canetti observes that the discovery of the bacillus provides an illustration of 'the exact model of the dynamics of power':[72] 'Man, with his enhanced opinion of himself, increasingly seeing himself as an individual detached from his fellow creatures, was suddenly confronted with entities much smaller even than vermin, multiplying even more rapidly and invisible to the naked eye.'[73] This concept is first identified in *Crowds and Power* in another context. Canetti argues that opportunities to study crowds 'as they appear in the minds of individuals'[74] are provided by the visual hallucinations and the crowd-sensation experiences of persons in certain drug-induced states of delirium, in which this same basic situation obtains. Where *Frankenstein* is concerned, there is warrant to take this suggestion seriously. Frankenstein notes 'the nervous fever with which I had been seized just at the time that I dated my creation'.[75] Virtually all the people who are privy to his 'nervous fever', his 'ravings' and his outbursts of guilt, assume he is affected by delirium. They include Clerval;[76] Frankenstein's father, who construes such outbursts to be 'the offspring of delirium';[77] the magistrate;[78] and Walton, the interlocutor[79] who mediates Frankenstein's narrative. As I have noted, there is also a drug factor. After his trip to Ireland, while recovering from fever, Frankenstein becomes a regular night-time laudanum user[80] – and, as a result, a fitful sleeper prone to nightmares.

---

71 *Ibid.*, 90.
72 Canetti, 1981, 419–20.
73 *Ibid.*, 418.
74 *Ibid.*, 414.
75 *Frankenstein*, 73.
76 *Ibid.*, 61.
77 *Ibid.*, 156.
78 *Ibid.*, 168.
79 *Ibid.*, 175.
80 *Ibid.*, 155.

John Barrell has recently described the connection between Thomas De Quincey's opium-influenced vision of the working class and his attraction to extreme reactionary politics.[81] Frankenstein's own opium-assisted delirium places him in a similar pathology and persuasion, for it underlies his death-bed defence of his decision to retract his promise to his Creature. The basic situation of the delirium states documented in *Crowds and Power* involves an original relation to vermin. Canetti calls it the 'Lilliput effect':

> the Lilliput effect . . . is a single large individual seeing himself in opposition to a numberless host of tiny aggressors . . . It begins with the peculiar feeling about vermin, by which all mammals (to speak only of them) are plagued. Whether these are mosquitoes or lice, locust or ants, they have always occupied men's imaginations. Their threat lies in the fact that they appear in great crowds and very suddenly. They have often stood as symbols for crowds.[82]

What matters decisively – the physiological explanation aside – is that the sufferer thinks of verminous creatures, such as insects, and imagines himself assailed by them in large numbers.

This scheme figures in Mary Shelley's story when Frankenstein the microscopist contemplates the global threat represented by the 'devils'. Where this pivotal moment is concerned, it is notable that the developments in lens technology in the medical culture of the 1820s illustrate Waldman's emphasis on the microscopists acquiring new powers. Poynter and Keele comment:

> The first compound microscopes were of very limited value. The failure was due to chromatic aberration blurring the visual images. This defect received intense study by lens-makers in London and Paris, as a result of which 'modern' microscopes appeared about 1820. Almost at once there were great discoveries . . . the complex anatomy of the cell came into sight.[83]

---

81 See J. Barrell, 1992.
82 Canetti, 1981, 419–20
83 Poynter and Keele, 1961, 62.

As a student Frankenstein discovers ways of improving scientific instruments, and this achievement wins him recognition in Ingolstadt's specialist academic circles;[84] later, as he works on the female anatomy, he has his instruments with him. Canetti's description of the Lilliput-effect can help us to see the way the new access of perception turns Frankenstein himself into a kind of giant:

> Everything is multiplied and everything is reduced in size. But the sufferer himself keeps his normal size and, even in delirium, knows who and what he is. He himself remains the same while his surroundings undergo a radical change. The monstrous flux they are suddenly caught up in is one of masses of tiny things, most of which he sees as alive. In every possible way there is *more life* around him, but it affects him as though he were a giant . . . These changed proportions are not as astonishing as they may appear at first sight: one should remember how numerous and how small are the cells of which the human body is composed. These cells are of very different kinds and act on each other continuously. They are attacked by hosts of bacteria and other minute creatures which settle among them and which, being alive, are always active in their own way.[85]

Frankenstein of course retains a sense of his own identity, as his own name in the eyes of posterity unhappily reminds him. A reference to vermin is implicit when he thinks of the unborn of the future, the children who will curse him as 'their pest'.[86] Behind the meaning of 'to plague' attached to the verb 'to pester' stand two older meanings: 'to entangle' and 'to crowd'. In this context another observation by Sontag is relevant. She comments that epidemic diseases ('pestilence', she notes, is the older term) are usually conceived of as a moral disorder in the social fabric.[87] In this scheme, as the community appears to be under mass attack by unseen powers, scapegoats are looked for. In *Frankenstein* Justine

---

84 *Frankenstein*, 53.
85 Canetti, 1981, 418–19.
86 *Frankenstein*, 141.
87 Sontag, 1983, 63; Helman, 1991, 44.

serves the purpose. And in England in 1832 the Anatomy Act scapegoated the poor.

As Canetti observes, within the Lilliput-effect 'the constant trend . . . towards the concrete and the small . . . has some resemblance to a dissociation of the body into its component cells'.[88] And in the giant's eye, the hallucinations have a content. The person suffering the delirium sees

> the relationships and processes of his own body, and principally the crowd-phenomena of all its minute component parts, transposed into concepts with which he is already familiar. This is, of course, only a guess, but it is worth remembering that there are moments when the whole life of the 'giant' man, all his qualities and all his inheritance, are concentrated in minute individual cells, massed together and moving as a crowd: the animalcules of the sperm.[89]

For Frankenstein, sex is a deadly business. The reader of the story is well entitled to ponder his avoidance of sex, his projections concerning it, and his fantasies about it. The most revealing example of the latter occurs just after the first encounter with the Creature. In a 'wild' dream, Frankenstein meets Elizabeth in an Ingolstadt street. There and then, he initiates, and survives, a deathly sexual encounter with her – and this with a woman who was once a pauper.[90] In reality, of course, he is never amorous with Elizabeth – on the contrary, their long engagement sees him forever preoccupied elsewhere. As he breaks his promise to his Creature, Frankenstein contemplates the Creatures' sexual energies and all their offspring. In his history of the devils Canetti comments: 'It is clear that the importunity of these devils was as monstrous as their numbers.'[91] The microscope reveals for the first time the crowd of the normally invisible spermatozoa.[92] The

---

[88] Canetti, 1981, 419.
[89] *Ibid.*
[90] *Frankenstein,* 58.
[91] Canetti, 1981, 51.
[92] *Ibid.*, 53.

'race of devils' scenario hints at an impending miscegenation threat, a global anarchy of the spermatozoa. As he procrastinates on marriage, Frankenstein is already withdrawing from intimate physical contact. The wedding-night provides an illustration of Frankenstein's earlier description of a dead body as 'food for the worm', for on this night he is left with a corpse instead of a bride. With this gesture the Creature forces his maker to comprehend bereavement and, as an anatomist, his own emotional disfigurement. The Creature's intervention here is prompted by the loss of his own promised mate, and it carries a further comment on Frankenstein's suspicion-ridden image of women generally. It is notable, for example, that when Frankenstein breaks his word a male assumption comes into play to support an official surveillance subtext. The medical man easily persuades himself to imagine a concupiscent female Creature, disdainful of the Creature, and quick to turn to 'the superior beauty of man'.[93]

Frankenstein's fantasy of sexually active monsterdom has a place in the double cosmology of the plague, as Foucault describes it:

> A whole literary fiction of the festival grew up around the plague: suspended laws, lifted prohibitions, the frenzy of passing time, bodies mingling together without respect, individuals unmasked, abandoning their statutory identity and the figure under which they had been recognised, allowing a quite different truth to appear. But there was also a political dream of the plague, which was exactly its reverse: . . . not masks that were put on and taken off, but the assignment to each individual of his 'true' name, his 'true' place, his 'true body', his true disease. The plague as a form, at once real and imaginary, had as its medical and political correlative discipline.[94]

The modern penal system, Foucault maintains, came into being when a large number of individual criminal acts began to assume a political meaning. From around the time of the French Revolution:

---

[93] *Frankenstein*, 140.

[94] Foucault, 1979, 197

'A whole series of illegalities was inscribed in struggles in which those struggling knew that they were confronting the law and the class that had imposed it.'[95] The double legislative package passed in England in 1832 was a rampart which successfully averted revolution. The relatively quiet passage of the Anatomy Act into law behind the public drama of the Reform Bill marks the presence of an implicit agenda, a mastering of the body in Foucault's sense. The theatrical metaphor of the mask in Alan Sheridan's reading of *Discipline and Punish* is appropriate:

> two processes are interdependent: economic expansion provided the means of sustaining and using the increase in population, while the disciplinary techniques accelerated the accumulation of capital. The process by which the bourgeoise became the politically dominant class . . . was masked by the establishment of a coded, formally egalitarian constitution, supported by a system of representative government. But this 'Enlightenment' politics had its dark underside in the ever-proliferating network of disciplinary mechanisms. While the first was based on the notion of the freely negotiated contrast, the second ensured the submission of forces and bodies.[96]

In the English context, Frankenstein's elusive Creature refuses to assume the discipline which enables human beings to be accumulated, organised and set to work; indeed, he embodies the able-bodied unemployment 'problem' which, for the early utilitarians, was a scandal sustained by the Old Poor Law.

## Clerval

In *Frankenstein* each new victim marks a widening of the political and cultural points of reference carried by the plot. The attack on Clerval is another tilt at the toppling edifice of benevolent

[95] *Ibid.*, 247. See also Harland, 1987, 164.
[96] Sheridan, 1980, 157.

paternalism. It is logical that Frankenstein's benevolent friend should be next in line after the broken promise. The letter from Clerval, urging their mutual and speedy return to London, is Frankenstein's cue to leave the Orkneys, but on the sea passage he is blown off course towards Ireland. Clerval indicates his plans to embark soon on a voyage to India, which was a major British colony in 1831:

> He said he was wearing away his time fruitlessly where he was; that letters from the friends he had formed in London desired his return to complete the negotiation they had entered into for his Indian enterprise. He could no longer delay his departure but as his journey to London might be followed, even sooner than he now conjectured, by his longer voyage, he entreated me to bestow as much of my society on him as I could spare.[97]

The Creature's perception of Clerval is inevitably bound up with his own recent failure to wrest political recognition from Frankenstein – so he is not likely to regard Clerval's colonial venture favourably. Clerval is the idealised representative of the new hegemonic class in England. He is murdered just at the moment when England, with its own threat of revolution averted, is poised to assume major imperial status. Clerval, Frankenstein comments:

> was also pursuing an object he had long had in view. His design was to visit India, in the belief that he had in his knowledge of its many languages, and in the views he had taken of its society, the means of materially assisting the progress of European colonisation and trade.[98]

Clerval is accorded the character-references of humanist man. Henry Clerval, a being 'formed in the very poetry of nature',[99] is *par excellence* the expressive soul. 'In Clerval I saw the image of my former self',[100] remarks Frankenstein. Clerval doubles with

---

[97] *Frankenstein,* 144.
[98] *Ibid.*, 135. Added in 1831.
[99] *Ibid.*, 133.
[100] *Ibid.*, 135.

Frankenstein: he is a portrait of Frankenstein as he might have been, *minus* the Creature. Equally, therefore, Clerval is the bourgeoisie in 1832 idealised, minus the Anatomy Act. The Creature attacks this ideal on the eve of its imperial journey abroad to follow the flag. His attack on Clerval is not arbitrary: it is an attack on the British Empire. By the same token, however, the Creature's violence hands a propaganda victory to those in England in 1831 who were pressing the case for the tougher domestic politics of democratic liberalism.

## The surgeon's alibi

Clerval's death draws forth officialdom's darker side as Frankenstein helplessly proclaims his murderous guilt in connection with all the victims, including Justine; but he does so behind the acoustic mask of his native language. Clerval's murder is an episode which presses further questions concerning the surgeon's guilty silence and, in particular, his criminal association. In the Irish episode, however, the story constructs Frankenstein's alibi in the face of these questions. From the moment he receives Clerval's letter in the Orkneys, up to the arrival of his father in Ireland and the clearing of his name, a revealing sequence of events takes place. Frankenstein departs the island with the half-formed female body on board, which he dumps in the sea. He is later assumed by the Irish crowd to have murdered Clerval and to have dumped the body on the spot where it is found. The crowd's assumption of his guilt is false, but the overall sequence represents Frankenstein as someone with, and then without, a corpse: that is to say, at first in possession of a body, but then innocent in respect of the body which turns up later. Indeed, the wind blows the boat back towards Henry Clerval's corpse – as if he, Frankenstein, cannot deny his relation to it – and thus does the criminal connection lodge in the public mind.

The Irish episode exemplifies the surgeon-bodysnatcher complicity. The 'monster' – Frankenstein's other double – kills Clerval, while the surgeon turns out to be innocent; but Frankenstein still cannot disburden himself of the association which shadows him.

His ravings in his dungeon sickbay lend support to the widespread public assumption of his guilt. This belief is then contradicted by the alibi, and the charges are dropped. The authorities are satisfied that Frankenstein was on the Orkneys when Clerval's body was found.[101] The surgeons likewise, in their relations with the resurrectionists, were always, as it were, somewhere else at the time. Here it is worth examining the nature of an alibi. As Canetti observes,[102] the suspect establishes an alibi, if he can, by 'setting place against place, identity against identity'. Thus:

> The first question concerns identity, the second is about place. Since both presuppose speech, one is led to ask whether there was an original situation which preceded this verbal questioning and corresponded to it. If there was, place and identity must have coincided in it, for one without the other would be meaningless. Such a question existed, and still exists; it is the hesitant examination of prey. 'Who are you? Are you good to eat?' An animal, which is continually in search of food, touches and sniffs at everything it finds, and sticks its nose in everything. 'What is this? Is it something to eat? What does it taste like?' The answer is a smell and either a movement or a lifeless rigidity. The strange body is simultaneously also a place; by smelling and touching it the animal makes itself at home with it and in it; translated into our terms, it names it.[103]

It is relevant here to recall one other fact in the story. Justine's conviction turns decisively on the production in court of the miniature portrait of her step-mother which is found about her person after William's murder. Elizabeth places the portrait around the boy's neck in the first instance, as she confirms to the court,[104] but it is the nameless and displaced Creature who transfers it. Inexplicable to the accused, this evidence affirms Justine's inability to establish a credible alibi concerning the time in question – that

101 *Ibid.*, 153.
102 Canetti, 1981, 337.
103 *Ibid.*, 334.
104 *Frankenstein*, 77.

is to say, to set place against place, identity against identity. The miniature compounds her plight, for under the public gaze it throws the shadow of 'ingratitude' across her identity and place in the Frankenstein home. Where dangerous, or potentially dangerous, persons are concerned, the name and the address are the first two questions.[105] The Irish episode shows this procedure at work where the stranger Frankenstein is concerned. The letters about Frankenstein's person provide Mr Kirwin, the magistrate, with the name and address of Alphonse Frankenstein. A letter is dispatched, and in due course Frankenstein's identity is established.

The 'original situation', as Canetti describes it, is relevant to the claiming-by-relatives clause in the legislation. In 1832 dissection became the fate of those who died inside the workhouse with no one to vouch for their having a name and address – an identity and a place – in the world outside the workhouse. The claiming ritual here in Ireland, as the father claims the son, holds social meanings which ramify in the Victorian context. The first and second questions point to an invidious implication which is implicit in the ideological move to criminalise poverty. On the same logic under review here, a successful workhouse claim is tantamount to nothing less than the formal judicial process of establishing innocence: the production of an alibi, and a real identity somewhere other than the scene of the crime.

By the time of the 1831 edition of *Frankenstein* Ireland was the known place of origin of Burke and Hare. The Irish episode inevitably comments on the anatomists' desire for legitimacy and is a cameo of their worst nightmare: the slide of the resurrectionist trade into murder scandal. Clerval is Frankenstein's closest associate – and close is the operative word. As Clerval's body is offered to the surgeon, his murder strikes at the bourgeois fears aroused by the bodysnatching culture in the 1820s. But in 1831 the class Clerval represents was close-to-home where the legislative solition was concerned. The murder of Clerval – of so perfect a man – is the provocation which draws the Anatomy Act into existence

---

[105] Canetti, 1981, 336.

with its implicit agenda of discipline and class reprisal. The genuine benevolence which informs Frankenstein's initial paternalist idealism is an appropriate preliminary mood in the story's allegory of the legislation; after Clerval's killing, however, Frankenstein's attitude towards his creation is nothing if not punitive. Richardson[106] describes the Anatomy Act, in its synchronicity with the Reform Bill, as the measure which completed 'the rout of benevolent paternalism'. And when the bride Elizabeth is murdered, the political betrayal of the working classes is answered by reprisal. The 'Condition-of-England' is worsening as the story proceeds.

## Choleraphobia

'Condition' is a medical metaphor. In *The Great Transformation* Polanyi points to the critical 'Condition-of-England' which remains the great might-have-been of English nineteenth-century history:

> It is a fair guess that had [Edmund] Burke lived, the Parliamentary Reform Bill of 1832, which put an end to the *ancien régime*, would have been passed only at the cost of an avoidable bloody revolution. And yet, Burke might have countered, once the masses were fated by the laws of political economy to toil in misery, what else was the idea of equality but a cruel bait to goad mankind into self-destruction?[107]

One early source for the 'Condition-of-England' metaphor, a good time before Carlyle's coinage of the term, are the three words in Frankenstein's great creation fantasy which evoke epidemics and the fear of them: he speaks of pouring 'a torrent of light' into 'our dark world'.[108] In 1831, as the cholera arrives, the burkophobia hysteria continues. The wedding-night corpse is the last body-snatcher 'commission' in the story; the bride's murder completes

[106] Richardson, 1989, 267.
[107] Polanyi, 1980, 118–19.
[108] *Frankenstein*, 55.

the sequence in which systematic murder makes the case for the legislation. In the context of the year in question, the appearance of each corpse parallels the stages of a plague. With William's killing, the burkophobia 'epidemic' strikes suddenly in the first instance, but involves a cumulative destruction of unknown duration. It brings visible death in ever larger numbers, with the greater number foreshadowed by the first few cases. In *Frankenstein* the first few are the most precious: the family and its closest friend. The Creature reproduces the conditions of a battle in which he alone is active, the hidden enemy who strikes at will at the postures of rank and power.[109] In his chapter on 'Panopticism' in *Discipline and Punish* Foucault comments that the plague, 'envisaged as a possibility at least, is the trial in the course of which one may define ideally the exercise of disciplinary power.'[110] The plague and the panopticon are the two main stage-sets in Foucault's account of modernity and in *Frankenstein*, likewise, the omniscient Creature leads the cast as the centralised eye of power. The jewel in the design of Bentham's panopticon is the principle that power should be visible and unverifiable:

> Visible: the inmate will constantly have before his eyes the tall outline of the central tower from which he is spied upon. Unverifiable: the inmate must never know whether he is being looked at at any one moment; but he must be sure that he may always be so.[111]

This ambiguity is reproduced in the story but now, however, with the 'knower' himself – Frankenstein – under surveillance. In one of his parts the Creature is a spy, the concealed enemy. He sees to it, as Frankenstein affirms, that those eyes 'as I first beheld them'[112] haunt the man who made him.

As a metaphor for moral collapse, an epidemic also illustrates what disrespect for the sanctity of the grave, in the resurrectionist

---

109 Canetti, 1981, 319.
110 Foucault, 1979, 199.
111 *Ibid.*, 201.
112 *Frankenstein* 153.

sense, means: the abandonment of all restraints and pieties. Instead of single burial and formalised ceremonial, large scale epidemics produce heaps of corpses in public places; they impose a more or less total breakdown of all respectful burial procedures across the social scale. In these circumstances all ordinary relationships are abrogated.[113] When he breaks his promise, Frankenstein unconsciously links the likely mischief of the female Creature and her offspring with an intensifying bodysnatching culture. She 'might . . . delight, for its own sake, in murder and wretchedness',[114] and her children likewise. Throughout the 1820s, Richardson reports,[115] the voices of self-interest which pondered aloud the alternatives to the resurrectionist monopoly were not above suggesting the sites of open pit burial as feasible official sources of supply. By the time of the third edition, these sites are the 'charnel houses' which Frankenstein visits as he prepares his creation.

It is relevant here to read the following statement from *The Poor Man's Advocate* of July 1832 which R. J. Morris cites in *Cholera 1832*. As a voice from the radical platform, it expresses sceptical working-class reactions to the cholera measures proposed by officialdom in 1832 as well as a census carried out in 1831. The statement rebuts the plague announcements as nothing more than a conspiracy of the medical profession. It is a forthright expression of the conflict of popular and administrative values where the sensitive issue of the burial of the dead was concerned. Its tone is heavy with the political radicalism occasioned by the Reform Bill debate:

> The people, they assert, have been numbered and classified for the purposes of selecting the most populous districts wherein this new disorder might be introduced with the greatest success. The poor are made the victims of it, they contend, for no other reason than that they are found to be too troublesome to their richer neighbours. The parliament have passed acts empowering

113 Canetti, 1981, 320.
114 *Frankenstein,* 140.
115 Richardson, 1989, 163.

> the local authorities to erect hospitals in the infected districts, to which hospitals all patients are obliged to be removed; and these measures are pronounced to be nothing more than bare-faced jobs in the first instance, and the means of removing the poor sick from the sight of their friends so that they may more conveniently be butchered and anatomised by the doctors whose gratuitous services are adduced in confirmation of this view.[116]

'In order to see perfect disciplines functioning,' comments Foucault, 'rulers dreamt of the state of plague.'[117] The cholera, however, was real and the rulers did not need to dream. The facts notwithstanding, this perception of the medical profession is valid as it stands. As Morris observes,[118] Malthus was 'part of the demonology of radical discourse' in the plague year.

Well back in the anatomy timetable, the Reverend Malthus preached and moralised that poverty was part of plenty. Thomas Hood included his 'Ode to Malthus' in the *Comic Annual* for the 1832 Christmas gift season:

> Too many girls, men, widows, wives and maids,-
> There is a dreadful surplus to demolish;
> And yet some Wrongheads,
> With thick not long heads,
> Poor metaphysicians!
> Sign petitions
> Capital punishment to abolish;
> And in the face of censuses such vast ones
> New hospitals contrive,
> For keeping alive,
> Laying first stones, the dolts! instead of last ones![119]

Hood's irony, Morris comments, indicates the welcome which Malthus would have given to the cholera. 'Such irony was not

116 Morris, 1976, 99.
117 Foucault, 1979, 199.
118 Morris, 1976, 99.
119 Hood, 1906, 275.

funny for those who suspected the medical profession and believed that the census taken in the summer of 1831 had been a government enquiry into surplus population.'[120] Malthusianism informs the statement carried by the Creature's mass-ive body, particularly when, late in the story, Frankenstein determines to hunt and destroy his creation. The middle-class poor law reformers were to accommodate Malthus in the decades flanking 1832. The Creature in *Frankenstein* is the 'surplus'. If this was not in the event to mean extermination in the post-1832 era, it certainly did mean the withdrawal of relief and an intensified workhouse culture.

## Disease, deformity and dissection

In 1831 the medical authorities entertained two hypotheses of the cause of cholera. The disease was either contagious and spread by contact or it was caused by local miasma (effusions from something unclean). As Simon During notes,[121] the miasma theory was favoured because a sensationalist language of putrefaction and unclean places and people easily accommodated a case for surveillance – but years later it was shown to be the wrong hypothesis of the two. During comments that the contagion hypothesis, on the other hand, 'could not provide the impetus to re-order the material basis of proletarian lives' because the bearer of contagion 'spread invisibly . . . in a deadly inversion of the power of sympathy'.[122] And this, as he craves sympathy and longs 'to be known and loved',[123] is how the Creature moves in *Frankenstein*.

The impediment which stands in the Creature's way is his appearance, his 'monstrosity' or 'deformity' as he calls it. His difficulties really begin when he looks at himself in a pool of water and accepts the socially imposed 'monster' label:

> I had admired the perfect forms of my cottagers – their grace,

---

120 Morris, 1976, 99.
121 During, 1992, 55.
122 *Ibid.*
123 *Frankenstein*, 115.

> beauty, and delicate complexions: but how I was terrified, when I viewed myself in a transparent pool! At first I started back, unable to believe that it was indeed I who was reflected in the mirror; and when I became fully convinced that I was in reality the monster that I am, I was filled with the bitterest sensations of despondence and mortification, Alas! I did not yet entirely know the fatal effects of this deformity.[124]

The 'monster' label first surfaces in Frankenstein's immediate, horrified reaction to his Creature's 'hideous countenance'.[125] In the cholera outbreak of 1831–32 the poor were in many cases obliged by emergency regulations to bury their dead quickly in isolated mass graves which were often preyed upon by resurrectionists. When Frankenstein speaks of his 'loathsome'[126] employment and 'filthy creation'[127] the reference to the dissection-room also characterises the graveyards he raids as sources of disease-carrying atmosphere. After the first encounter, however, the Creature keeps himself out of sight from society and offers no hostage to sensationalist miasma rhetoric.

There were nevertheless many other similar reactions to deformity when the cholera arrived in England. In *Aids and Its Metaphors* Sontag comments that 'while cholera killed fewer people in Western Europe in the nineteenth century than the smallpox did, it was more feared, because of the suddenness with which it struck and the indignity of its symptoms . . . [which] anticipated the horror of postmortem decomposition.'[128] There is, Sontag argues, a scale of dread where debilitating disease is concerned, depending on the degree to which 'the privilege of the face'[129] is threatened.

The Anatomy Act was part of the surveillance and reordering

---

124 *Ibid.*, 101.
125 *Ibid.*, 59.
126 *Ibid.*, 56.
127 *Ibid.*
128 Sontag, 1990, 39.
129 *Ibid.*, 40.

of working-class life to which During refers above; and so too were the burial regulations which were imposed on districts housing the poor in the pre-legislative 1831–32 period. As I now want to suggest, it is not inappropriate that many of the anxieties aroused by the burkophobia-choleraphobia era should have had their psychological correlative in the miasma hypothesis, the view that sickness and its disfigurements spring from contaminated atmospheres. In the late 1820s the fear of disease and physical deformity – and facial deformity in particular – is a revealing index of peoples' feelings about monstrosity generally and ultimate forms of disfigurement such as dissection. To argue this suggestion, I will now show how Mary Shelley herself, when she was disfigured by disease in 1828, and Thomas Southwood Smith, the man who dissected Bentham in 1832, are two figures of the age who strikingly illustrate feelings about disfigurement where the human face is concerned.

An illustration of Sontag's argument about the face can be found in a letter which Mary Shelley wrote in 1828. It contains a description of Mary's own face when it was temporarily marked by smallpox. Her account of herself without 'the privilege' of the face bears comparison with Frankenstein's reaction to his 'monster' in her novel. In the year the Burke and Hare scandal took place, Mary Shelley spent part of the summer in self-imposed quarantine recovering from her illness. Her June letter from Dover to Mrs Isabel Booth records a journey from Paris to London broken at the south coast to take the cure. It shows her availing herself of the growing middle-class health resort culture:

> Dover, June 15 [1828]
>
> MY DEAR GIRL,– You will have heard from Mr Godwin of my hateful illness and its odious results. Instead of returning to town as I most exceedingly desired – to join my friends there, and to see again dear Isabel – I am fain to hide myself in the country, and as I am told sea-bathing will assist materially the disappearance of the marks, I remain on the coast . . .
>
> I was sickening of my illness when I left town – my journey was so painful that I shudder at the recollection, and I arrived only to go to bed. What will you say to my philosophy when

at the end of three weeks in brilliant health *but as ugly as the — I went into society* – I was well repaid for my fortitude, for I am delighted with the people I saw – and some I love and they merit my attention. What will you say also to the imagination of one of the cleverest men in France, young and a poet, who could be interested in me in spite of the mark I wore – it was rather droll to play the part of an ugly person for the first time in my life, yet it was very amusing to be told – or rather not to be told but to find, that my face was not all my fortune.

I have excellent news of my darling boy, whom I long to see again – I hope you are well . . . Mrs G. mentioned in her last letter that your children had called there and that all seemed well with you. When I last saw you, dear friend, I very little anticipated this long separation . . . – Patience! my malady has made me lose a year of my life – but in spite of the marks that still remain (I am in no danger of permanent disfigurement) I am in good health – and so different from my dreary state all last winter – and looking younger than when you saw me last [italics added].

Affectionately, MS[130]

This is someone for whom the ready facility of a health culture is a welcome part of life – as the shaming facial disfigurement is not. The murders at Edinburgh must not be seen in isolation; they were, metaphorically, the unacceptable face of a lucrative and fast developing everyday medical culture which was edging closer to the big breakthrough discoveries of the modern era. Shelley's letter from Dover belongs to the archive of this culture and offers a glimpse of its seaside leisure dimension. According to her *Journal* in the 1830s, the author of *Frankenstein* often recuperated her health on the English south coast, and at Brighton in particular. Her 1828 letter gives us direct access to her as a denizen of this world.

---

130 Quoted in Ingpen, 1917, 601–2.

In my third chapter I introduced Michel De Certeau's argument that the incarnation of the law and the intextuation of the body becomes graphically visible during moments of transgression: the Burke and Hare case is an example of this. The same process, however, is at work in ordinary everyday situations, as Mary's letter shows. A comment by John Fiske is relevant here:

> the relationship between the body beautiful and the body ugly, between the healthy and the unhealthy . . . are social relationships of norms and deviations, and therefore political relationships aimed at naturalizing in the body the norms of those with most power in the social formation.[131]

In this connection it is revealing that Godwin, Mary's father, referred to Mary's condition at this time in a way that virtually demotes her in social class – 'Poor Mary is terribly disfigured & *squalid* at present, as to the surface of her face' [italics added].[132]

In her letter, Mary does not spell out that she has smallpox; the actual word she leaves to the grapevine. The most remarkable deletion (which I have italicised) is the suppressed reference to the devil: 'as ugly as the –'. However, the elision is supplemented in her *Journal* of this time. Having moved to a resort in Hastings, she recalls being 'a monster to look at'[133] in Paris. In Mary Shelley's letter, the English widow, the famous author of *Frankenstein*, draws and enjoys compliments from the Frenchman. The mask of ugliness stands between them unmentioned and the reality of her disfigurement is suspended. As her letter sketches her subjectivity, Mary Shelley is the inverse double of her fictional Creature of lower status. With the mask in place, she 'finds' that 'my face was not all my fortune'. This is admiration, from a stranger,[134] that

---

131 Fiske, 1989, 92.

132 Quoted in Feldman and Scott-Kilvert, 1987, vol. 2, p. 508. (Alongside the general meaning of 'squalid' as 'repulsive' or 'loathsome to look at' the *OED* notes a 1773 usage which associates poverty with vermin life: '*State Poor* 34: Rags and vermin, squalidity and disease'.)

133 *Ibid.*

134 The man was Stepan Mérimée, the poet.

passes beyond appearances and first impressions; it is recognition and acknowledgement of a kind that Frankenstein's Creature can never hope to command. Mary's face shames her, but her power in male company 'to play the part' transfigures her. Sontag's commentary on the face applies here:

> Underlying some of the moral judgements attached to disease are aesthetic judgements about the beautiful and the ugly, the clean and the unclean, the familiar and the alien or uncanny. (More accurately, these are judgements which originate before the stage at which aesthetics and moral categories split apart and, eventually, come to seem opposed.) What counts more than the amount of disfigurement is that it reflects underlying, ongoing changes, the dissolution of the person.[135]

Mary, however, is not literally faced – as the victims of cholera a few years later were – with the signs of an ineluctable organic decomposition. On the contrary, her marks, in Sontag's terms, 'are precisely the stigmata of a survivor.'[136] In Mary's story, Frankenstein sets a high premium on physical beauty: there is recurring emphasis on the facial beauty of the people who end up burked by the 'monster'. The Creature strikes at Frankenstein's judgements of the beautiful, the clean and the familiar, not least because he confronts their negative face when he looks at his reflection in the water.

'There can be no real argument against the aristocracy of the face', comments Sontag: 'our very notion of the person, of dignity, depends on the separation of face from body, on the possibility that the face may be exempt, or exempt itself, from what is happening to the body'.[137] There were others in the 'face culture' of early nineteenth-century England whose actions illustrate this conviction. Thomas Southwood Smith, the surgeon who dissected Bentham, is a case in point, as his friend's auto-icon demonstrates.

---

135 Sontag, 1990, 41.
136 *Ibid.*
137 *Ibid.*, 40.

As he sits reassembled and fully clothed, having donated his body to medical science, Bentham practises the utilitarianism he preached. In a paper about his auto-icon written shortly before his death he had projected a future world in which, following his example, the dissected bodies of famous or wealthy people would enjoy secular resurrection[138] as auto-icons and serve as subjects for phrenological demonstration. The self-image artefacts would dispense with the need for conventional burial, expensive statues and imperfect representation. Bentham planned to represent himself. In his paper he posed the question: 'Is not identity preferable to similitude?' But in a development after the dissection Bentham's head was exempted from the utility principle. Dr Southwood Smith was to comment years afterwards:

> I endeavoured to preserve the head untouched, merely by drawing away the fluids by placing it under an air pump over sulphuric acid. By these means the head was rendered as hard as the skulls of the New Zealanders; but all expression was of course gone. Seeing this would not do for exhibition, I had a model made in wax . . . The artist succeeded in producing one of the most admirable likenesses ever seen.[139]

Southwood Smith's move to replace Bentham's head with a model strikingly resembles the most famous scene in *Frankenstein*, the encounter scene. When the Creature is first sighted the fictional anatomist generalises that 'no mortal could support the horror of that countenance'[140] – and it seems a similar conclusion was drawn by Southwood Smith when it came to his revered friend's countenance. It is apparent – although Southwood Smith does not use the word – that Bentham with his own head is a kind of monster. The dissector himself can bear the spectacle, but he judges that

---

138 'Secular resurrection' is the phrase Richardson and Hurwitz use to describe Bentham's fantasy of corporeal immortality. My observations in the next three paragraphs owe much to their illuminating article on Bentham's auto-icon in *British Medical History*, 298, July 1987.

139 Quoted in Marmoy, 1958, 81–2.

140 *Frankenstein*, 59.

Bentham cannot appear in the eyes of eternity in a disfigured state. By erasing Bentham's monstrosity he perpetuates an illusion of wholeness where the reassembled corpse is concerned. This looks like a hypocritical manoeuvre to exempt Bentham from the physical obliteration which his own Anatomy Act was to impose on paupers

The historical record shows, however, that Southwood Smith in 1832 was the last man in England who could be called a hypocrite where the anatomy of bodies was concerned. His manipulation of the auto-icon must be seen in the context of the principled stand he took against the Anatomy Act when Bentham died. It is true that in his influential 1824 article *Use of the Dead to the Living* he had proposed the wholesale appropriation of unclaimed pauper bodies – and Bentham indeed drafted this idea into the 1832 Act. But, as few others did in the late 1820s, Southwood Smith underwent a sea-change in his attitude to the corpse-supply problem. He came to regard the social bias in his original proposal as the unacceptable face of the Anatomy Act, and was prepared to say so publicly. Bravely, he used the occasion of his dissection of Bentham to express his opposition to the new law and to propose a fairer bequest system. He spelt out to the Parliamentarians in his audience – many of whom had lent their support to the passage of Anatomy Act – the hypocrisy of a requisition system:

> How is it to be expected that the uninstructed and ignorant . . . will sacrifice their own feelings for the public good, when the best regulated shrink from the obligation? . . . It is our duty, not by legislative enactments to force others to submit to that which we are unwilling should be done to ourselves, but to set the example of making a voluntary sacrifice for the sake of a good which we profess to understand and appreciate.[141]

Requisition, Smith pointed out, would maintain public opposition

[141] Southwood Smith, quoted by Richardson and Hurwitz, 1987, 196.

to dissection and make it more difficult to gain widespread acceptance for a voluntary bequest system.

Bentham bequeathed his body to Southwood Smith in a gesture which was intended to promote bequests for anatomy – yet he also designed the coercive Anatomy Act. The old man's hypocrisy would not have been lost on Southwood Smith, even as he admired Bentham's willingness to set an example and submit to a fate normally reserved for murderers. When he commissioned the wax head Southwood Smith showed consideration for the audiences of the future who would see Bentham as an exemplary opponent of the prejudice against dissection. But with this gesture Southwood Smith colluded in one other dimension of his master's hypocrisy and egocentricity. Bentham cannot have been unaware that any medical museum would have welcomed the chance to obtain his remains and, given his intellectual stature, his cranium in particular.[142] By bequeathing his body to his friend, he made certain he would not fall victim to the bodysnatchers after his death.[143] He feared the routine anatomical fate under these circumstances, the journey into non-identity. His corpse would not be put together again and preserved in the manner he required – but the bequest arrangement enabled him to avert this possibility. Southwood Smith conscientiously carried out every instruction Bentham left in his will concerning his own reassembly. The replacement of the head with the model was the finishing touch on a process in which the great philosopher of utility was endowed with a posthumous whole physical identity. It was an act of collusion with Bentham's desire to avoid the victim's fate of dismemberment to the point of anonymity. Even Southwood Smith, the most admirable advocate of anatomy reform in 1832, was prepared to accommodate Bentham's wish to be – and not to be – dissected.

The auto-icon's shadow falls across one other scene in *Frankenstein*. In an episode after his father's death, and following a spell

---

142 Noted by Richardson and Hurwitz, 1987, 197.

143 Richardson and Hurwitz (1987, 197) write: 'Even had [Bentham] been buried in multiple coffins his corpse may not have remained underground for long'.

as a confined 'madman', Frankenstein seeks an interview with a criminal judge. In the presence of this figure he divulges what has been going on. Frankenstein ends his disclosures with a demand that the magistrate 'exert his whole authority for the apprehension of the murderer':

> he may be hunted like the chamois and destroyed as a beast of prey. But I perceive your thoughts: you do not credit my narrative, and do not intend to pursue my enemy with the punishment which is his desert.'
>
> As I spoke, rage sparkled in my eyes; the magistrate was intimidated:- 'You are mistaken,' said he, 'I will exert myself; and if it is in my power to seize the monster, be assured that he shall suffer *punishment proportionate to his crimes*. But I fear, from what you yourself have described to be his properties, that this will prove impractical [italics added].[144]

When the 1831 edition of *Frankenstein* appeared – on the eve of the anatomy reform – the resurrectionist market continued unchecked by the government. And for just a few more months, dissection remained the proportionate extra punishment for murder. This is the punishment which was inflicted on William Burke, and which Frankenstein demands here for his Creature.

The magistrate replies to Frankenstein here with the utilitarian proposition that justice, instead of taking revenge, should simply punish. Bentham's own major alterations to the penal code during his long life were a comprehensive attempt to make punishment, as this magistrate says, proportionate to the crime. Ignatieff's summary of Bentham's conception of punishment, namely that it 'should not be scattered by a monarch's wrathful hand, but apportioned to each crime as precisely as the market allocated prices to commodities',[145] is a telling gloss on Frankenstein's royal 'rage' in this scene. Bentham knew, however, that dissection could not be assimilated to this calculation; the stigma which Frankenstein

---

144 *Frankenstein*, 167.

145 Ignatieff, 1978, 76.

invokes as fit punishment for his Creature stood in the way. The long term utilitarian agenda could only be served by a legislative intervention to decriminalise dissection – and the surgeons themselves. As Bentham authorised this agenda the Edinburgh scandal delivered a crude public parody of his metaphor of an exact price for a crime: a burking for an exact price. Burke and Hare received £7 10*s*. for their first corpse, a victim (who was not murdered) who died in debt to Mrs Hare. Sold to recoup the money, the price paid for this body provided an incentive to their own crime of serial burking – and to the further copy-cat killing which Bentham's colleagues in Parliament used to hasten the anatomy reform into law. With the Anatomy Act passed in 1832, it was the stigma which exacted the price: dissection became the punishment for the crime of being poor.

## The graveyard

The episode which follows the interview with the magistrate finds Frankenstein in the graveyard as night is falling. Simon During has commented on the way the utilitarians in Victorian England sought to displace the graveyard in England's cultural tradition:

> [To loosen old traditions] a technology of 'reculturation' was required – a secular and bureaucratic apparatus to acculturate British subjects in ways which reduce the presence both of old religious beliefs (which made of graves sacred places) and of values tied to the local memories (to which graveyards were central), and replace such beliefs and memories with a sense of belonging to, and working for, an abstract Humanity.[146]

The changes During identifies here are a feature of the 1870s and the arrival of mechanical cremation played a major role in them. However, the cultural moment of *Frankenstein* predates these developments, as an episode in Mary Shelley's life as a widow reveals.

---

[146] During, 1992, 57–8.

In 1824, the same year that Southwood Smith published his *Use of the Dead to the Living* article, Mary Shelley wrote an entry in her *Journal* which indicates the extent to which she herself gave emotional assent to the values traditionally memorialised by graveyards. It concerns an anniversary visit on 8 June of that year to the spot where ten years previously she and Shelley first declared their love for each other in a tryst before their elopement. The scene is St Pancras churchyard in London, a resurrectionist haunt. Mary stands by her mother's grave: 'The lamp of thought is again illuminated in my heart – & the fire descends from heaven that kindles it – Such, my loved Shelley now ten years ago – at this season – did we first meet – & these were the very scenes.' In Sontag's metaphor, Mary's rhetoric summons 'the privilege' of her husband's face:

> That churchyard with it[s] sacred tomb was the spot where first love shone in you[r] dear eyes – My own love – we shall meet again – the stars of heaven are now your country & your spirit drinks beauty and wisdom in those spheres – & I, beloved, shall one day join you – Nature speaks to me of you – in towns & society I do not feel your presence – but there you are with me, my own, my unalienable.
>
> I feel my powers again – & this is of itself happiness – the eclipse of winter is passing from my mind – I shall again feel the enthusiastic glow of composition – again as I pour forth my soul upon paper.[147]

Percy Shelley's atheism made Mary into a self-conscious if intermittent churchgoer;[148] here, however, she writes as a widow of nearly two years. It is worth observing the sublimation of grief that is in play here. The reunion with Shelley by her mother's grave restores her – the author of *Frankenstein* and publicly known as such since 1823 – to her compositional 'powers' and her 'soul'. Her creative energies are sanctioned by a recognition of herself

---

147 Feldman and Scott-Kilvert, 1987, vol. 2, p. 479.
148 *Ibid.*, vol. 1, p. 386.

by Shelley – and indeed by her dead mother – which she feels is real here beside the grave. This is the same order of recognition – of kind recognition – which her fictional Creature craves and yet cannot command in face-to-face encounters. And this comparison can be taken further. In the journal entry the phrase 'My own love' magically cancels any distinction between Mary and her lover. The equivalent moment of desire in *Frankenstein* occurs at the commencement of the gallows-wedding which I described in Chapter 5. It sees the Creature addressing Justine as 'my beloved' as she stirs from her sleep in the barn, just before he moves to frame her for William's murder. Here, however, unlike Mary's 'first love' recognition, the address to the beloved summons the Creature's knowledge that he is forever excluded from the recognition which he so greatly desires. And by framing and losing Justine he enacts – for the eyes of God – his exclusion from human recognition and love.

In *Frankenstein* the graveyard inevitably is the place where Frankenstein declares outright class war on his creation. The language he uses as he kisses the earth is revealing. Gone is the earlier rationalist rhetoric in which 'a churchyard to me was merely the receptacle of bodies deprived of life'.[149] He now intones an impassioned invocation of 'the spirits of the dead' and the 'ministers of vengeance'.[150] As Frankenstein kneels deep in grief on 'the sacred earth' the same rage which surfaced in his earlier interview with the magistrate reappears: 'I had begun my adjuration with solemnity, and an awe which almost persuaded me that the shades of my murdered friends heard and approved my devotion; but the furies possessed me as I concluded, and rage choked my utterance.'[151]

The Creature, however, hears Frankenstein and answers with loud derisive laughter. It is as if he is laughing at the way the word 'almost' in the sentence above just holds the line against a

149 *Frankenstein*, 53.
150 *Ibid.*, 169.
151 *Ibid.*, 169.

complete abandonment of the rationalist posture on Frankenstein's part. And actually this posture is abandoned, as the passive verb constructions in Frankenstein's subsequent pursuit of the Creature indicate. They reveal a psychically transformed Frankenstein who – as the occasion now demands – is responsive to superstition and ancestral communication. For example, he speaks of himself being 'instigated to toil and revenge' by 'the [hovering] spirits of the dead'.[152] In effect, what Frankenstein does when he vows his revenge in the graveyard is rehearse a bellicose rhetoric and summon a belligerent crowd. His family are among this host and in the subsequent hunt for the Creature Frankenstein conjures the 'ecstasy' of reunion in the grave with his family as 'a reward' for his vengeance.[153] On the eve of the great decade of emerging class division, Frankenstein's adjuration beside the family tomb, as the night falls, is theatrically apt and forward-looking. A decade or so after the legislation the graveyard exhibition of class difference in the Victorian era was to furnish his rhetoric with a fitting apotheosis and monument. The mortal remains of the Duke of Wellington were buried in a four-coffined sarcophagus.[154] In 1829 Wellington's own government bowed to mass opposition to the first proposed Anatomy Bill.

What is decisive in Frankenstein's evocation is that the dead, an invisible crowd, are imagined and summoned as an expeditionary and fighting host. In *Crowds and Power* there is a statement about war, the import of which clarifies the Anatomy Act as a tactic, or weapon, of class war. War is a double crowd phenomenon:

> The aim is to transform a dangerous crowd of live adversaries into a heap of dead. The victor is the one who kills the largest number . . . Each side wants to constitute the larger crowd of living fighters and it wants the opposing side to constitute the larger heap of dead.[155]

---

152 *Ibid.*, 172.
153 *Ibid.*, 171.
154 Richardson, 1989, 273.
155 Canetti, 1981, 78.

The 'respectable' crowd which forms during the anatomy era comprises all the beneficiaries of the legislation; its apotheosis is in 1832, as the burkophobia ends. In his 1827 instalment of *On Murder considered as one of the Fine Arts* De Quincey characterises this crowd's vicarious engagement with violence by referring to it as 'the mob of newspaper readers'.[156] After 1832, however, this crowd survived intact in a changed form:

> The baiting crowd is preserved in the newspaper reading public, in a milder form it is true, but, because of its distance from events, a more irresponsible one . . . it is the most despicable and, and the same time, most stable form of such a crowd. Since it does not even have to assemble, it escapes disintegration.[157]

The signs of this 'respectable' crowd appear in *Frankenstein*, as we can now see.

## Panic

In the honeymoon villa the word 'panic' enters Frankenstein's vocabulary. Elizabeth has been murdered and Frankenstein feels 'a kind of panic'[158] as the 'monster' appears at the moonlit window, pointing at the corpse. As he awaits the wedding-night assignation Frankenstein is armed. He comments: 'suddenly I reflected how fearful the combat which I momentarily expected would be to my wife'.[159] Canetti describes the respectable crowd's panic when its everyday cohesion is threatened:

> the crowd, a moment ago at its apex, must disintegrate violently; and the transmutation shows itself in violent individual action: everyone shoves, hits and kicks in all directions. The more fiercely each man 'fights for his life', the clearer it is that he is fighting *against* all the others who hem him in. They stand there

156 De Quincey, 1918, 332.
157 Canetti, 1981, 59–60.
158 *Frankenstein*, 164.
159 *Ibid.*, 163.

> like chairs, balustrades, closed doors, but different from these in that they are alive and hostile. They push him in this or that direction, as it suits them or, rather, as they are pushed themselves. Neither women, children nor old people are spared: they are not distinguished from men. Whilst the individual no longer feels himself as 'crowd', he is still completely surrounded by it. Panic is a disintegration of the crowd *within* the crowd. The individual breaks away and wants to escape from it because the crowd, as a whole, is endangered. But, because he is physically still stuck in it, he must attack it . . . in such a moment a man cannot insist too strongly on his separateness.[160]

The coexistence of the cholera and the burkophobia[161] in 1831 underlines the survival imperative which asserts itself in epidemics: the need to distance oneself from the sick and the seized. Frankenstein, who does put distance between himself and others, is accorded the experience of survival. As noted, even while his relatives and friends live, his constant desire – as on the road to Edinburgh – is to 'ascertain *my* fate'; and he takes the Creature's wedding-night assignation as a threat directed solely against himself. When he panics, the story – or the Creature – is making the point that a survivor is not necessarily someone strong in moral resources.

The infectious panic of the burkophobia era is foreseen in the first instalment of *On Murder considered as one of the Fine Arts*. On the eve of the disclosures from Edinburgh, De Quincey's speaker delivers an ironic commentary on the social uses of fear:

> There remain many excellent works of art in a pure style, such as nobody would be ashamed to own, as every candid connoisseur will admit. *Candid*, observe, I say; for great allowances must be made in these cases; no artist can ever be sure of carrying through his own fine preconception. Awkward disturbances will arise; people will not submit to have their throats

[160] Canetti, 1981, 29.
[161] Richardson, 1989, 223.

> cut quietly; they will run; they will kick; they will bite; and, while the portrait painter often has to complain of too much torpor in his subject, the artist, in our line, is generally embarrassed by too much animation. At the same time, however disagreeable to the artist, this tendency in murder to excite and irritate the subject, is certainly one of its advantages to the world in general, which we ought not to overlook, since it favours the development of latent talent. Jeremy Taylor notices with admiration, the extraordinary leaps which people will take under the influence of fear . . . Talents of the most brilliant description have sometimes been developed by the panic which accompanied our artists.[162]

These remarks about 'advantages to the world' and 'latent talents' are double-edged: the successful avoiding action is a stimulus to the artists 'in our line' to develop and refine *their* talents. The imitators of Burke and Hare turned up in London in 1831. Bishop and Williams, who were bodysnatchers as well as burkers, were rumoured to have disposed of about sixty people and to have perfected a form of killing which left no signs of violence on the body. Richardson recovers officialdom's vocabulary in 1831:

> Somerville [the future official Inspector of Anatomy] plausibly argued that there were 'many others' in addition to Burke and Bishop, 'whose greater caution in the selection of their subjects, greater skill in the various arts of destroying life, and more circumspection in their dealings, have screened from the hand of justice.'[163]

With this sort of language the bureaucrats in England's officialdom were talking like De Quinceyian connoisseurs. In the meanwhile, their utilitarian confederates in Parliament, behind a language of 'advantages to the world', were acting as such: in 1832, after 'too much animation', the art of murder was perfected in the legislative solution.

---

162 De Quincey, 1918, 326.
163 Richardson, 1989, 197.

Frankenstein's emergent panic vocabulary is a revealing index of the terror spread by his Creature. Frankenstein often comments on his inclination to avoid crowds, but after the Edinburgh and the Ireland episodes (after Burke and Hare, as it were) the mounting threat leads him to seek safety in numbers with the greatest urgency. His avowed aversion to crowds is not borne out by what he says when the pressure is on. It is significant, as a statement to his father shows, that his most desperate rhetoric invokes a crowd in flight from acute danger. In the wake of Clerval's death, Frankenstein asserts:

> I am the assassin of those most innocent victims; they died by my machinations. A thousand times I would have shed my own blood, drop by drop, to have saved their lives; but I could not, my father, indeed I could not *sacrifice* the whole human race [italics added].[164]

In *Crowds and Power* Canetti traces the origin of sacrifice to a moment of cartharsis:

> The collective fear of a herd in flight is the oldest and perhaps the most common example of a crowd state. It seems very likely that *sacrifice* originated in this state of crowd fear. A lion pursuing a herd of gazelles, all fleeing together in fear of him, desists from pursuit as soon as he succeeds in seizing one of them. This animal, his victim, is a kind of sacrifice which procures a respite for its companions in the herd. As soon as the other gazelles see that the lion has got what it wants their fear abates. From mass flight they revert to the normal state of a herd, each animal grazing on its own and doing as it pleases. If the gazelles had a religion and the lion was their god, they could, in order to appease his appetite, voluntarily surrender one of their numbers to him. This is exactly what happens among men: religious sacrifice springs from a state of crowd fear.[165]

---

164 *Frankenstein*, 156.
165 Canetti, 1981, 358–9.

The word 'sacrifice' shows Frankenstein retaining a religious vocabulary for the entailment of real emergency. An identical image of the lion seizing its prey is used by the Creature when he reports his personal catastrophe in the de Lacey cottage. Kneeling, the Creature clings in desperate supplication to the blind man. Felix, arriving suddenly on the scene, 'tore me from his father', and 'I could have torn him limb from limb, as the lion rends the antelope. But my heart sank within me with bitter sickness, and I refrained.'[166] In a cameo of his cherished childhood Frankenstein recalls that he and Clerval played masquerade enactments of the Crusades, 'the train who shed their blood to redeem the holy sepulchre from the hands of the infidels'.[167] Here, however, as he speaks to his father, Frankenstein is not talking make-believe. In dire need of halting the leonine pursuit, his rhetoric turns to the sacrifice of the one for the many in a bid to appease his Creature. It is most appropriate that the lion image occurs at the precipitate moment of the Creature's worst calamity, for soon afterwards he commences his 'reign'[168] of terror.

The following morning, with the cottage deserted, the Creature recalls the women 'flying' at the sight of him. He overhears Felix in conversation with his landlord recounting 'the horror' and indicating his desire 'to fly from this place'[169] forthwith. Here at the start of the terror is a reaction to the Creature in which fear and panic combine to cause flight, and this reaction, as we have seen, has occured once before in the story. The momentum into flight reproduces the original character of the command – the compulsion to flee – which characterises Frankenstein's own first reaction to his Creature. The cottage scene reassembles the configuration of the 'arche command' which, as I argued in Chapter 4, is the basis of the dissection threat during the anatomy era. As the women's escape shows, the threat announces death

---

166 *Frankenstein,* 117. An antelope is a gazelle – therefore Canetti's and Mary Shelley's images are identical.
167 *Ibid.*, 42–3.
168 *Ibid.*, 171.
169 *Ibid.*, 119.

and flight simultaneously. This matches Canetti's emphasis: 'flight is the final and only appeal against a death sentence. For the roar of a lion *is* a death sentence . . . The oldest command – and it is far older than man – is a death sentence, and it compels the victim to flee.'[170] From the lion image onwards in the story's time-sequence, society itself is in effect compelled into flight.

Frankenstein's rhetoric of the sacrifice occurs as the terror escalates. But his language here is a verbalisation of an earlier dream in which he himself figures as the sacrificial victim. The journey from Ireland to Geneva sees Frankenstein in an incipient panic. In the hope of containing his mounting agitation, and in search of sleep, he doubles his nightcap of laudanum and dreams of being in a crowd. In a nightmare he becomes the lion's victim:

> sleep [however] did not afford me respite from thought and misery; my dreams presented a thousand objects that scared me. Towards morning I was possessed of a kind of nightmare; I felt the fiend's grasp in my neck and could not free myself from it; groans and cries rang in my ears.[171]

This image captures the moment a mass flight turns into a panic. The groans and cries Frankenstein hears about him mark the onset of everyone getting in each other's way as their separate survival imperative breaks the common movement and direction of the flight. At this point in the dream Frankenstein is awoken by his father. He experiences intense reassurance, almost as a child would, in the feeling of security which his father's presence imparts. In the story's 1831 edition in particular, the son here speaks for all the burkophobia fears of the late 1820s:

> My father, who was watching over me, perceiving my restlessness, awoke me; the dashing waves were around: the cloudy sky above; the fiend was not here: a sense of security, a feeling that a truce was established between the present hour and the irresistible, disastrous future imparted to me a kind of calm

170 Canetti, 1989, 352.
171 *Frankenstein*, 155.

> forgetfulness, of which the human mind is by its structure peculiarly susceptible.[172]

These words, however, also belong to the story's proleptic legislation script. They are a barometer of the insecurities felt by people in the large post-1832 dissection constituency. The key figure here is the father. Frankenstein's dream occurs on the voyage from Ireland, where his father recently vouched for his son's identity in a claiming procedure no different in kind from the impending bureaucratic ritual in the workhouse. But as Frankenstein awakes from his nightmare here – and sees his father – his words spell out the human dimension of these procedures as they were to affect people living in, or in fear of, the workhouse in the post-1832 world. Richardson observes that the law:

> did not envisage an obligation to inform survivors when a death had occurred – and since it permitted corpses to be taken when only forty-eight hours had elapsed, there was a likelihood that relatives' absence could be construed as 'indifference'. The clause [permitting the requisition of 'unclaimed' corpses for dissection] was a mandate for official disregard both of mourned and mourners' feelings.[173]

Frankenstein's father is drawn ever further into a world in which relatives turn into corpses; and soon after Elizabeth's death the weight of perplexity and grief precipitates his own death. Throughout the story, he witnesses nothing but an inexplicable undermining or reversal of his family's original happiness and middle-class estate. The Frankenstein family fate is a metaphor for the 'Condition-of-England' in 1831, when England stood on the verge of revolution.

Canetti's typology of mass behaviour includes the 'reversal' crowd. The psychic nature of this crowd is indicated by a sentence, and a question, in an eighteenth-century letter:

---

172 *Ibid.*

173 Richardson, 1989, 207.

> 'Dear Friend, the wolves have always eaten the sheep; are the sheep going to eat the wolves this time?' This sentence, which comes from a letter which Madame Jullien wrote to her son during the French Revolution, contains the essence of reversal. So far a few wolves have held down many sheep. Now the time has come for the many sheep to turn against the few wolves. It is true that sheep are not carnivorous, but, in its very absurdity, the sentence is full of meaning. Revolutions are times of reversal; those who have been defenceless for so long suddenly find teeth. Their numbers have to make up for the experience in viciousness which they lack.[174]

Nor is the Creature in *Frankenstein* a carnivore; following Rousseau, in the state of nature he observes a vegetarian diet. But find teeth he certainly does, as Frankenstein is all too aware the moment he galvanises his creation into existence. The meaningful absurdity noted above is matched in Frankenstein's consternation at the 'birth' of a huge Creature whose teeth, 'a luxuriance',[175] are fully formed. Frankenstein's eyes go straight to the 'teeth of pearly whiteness'.[176] 'To be without teeth,' remarks Canetti, 'is contemptible and there is a touch of asceticism in refusing to show those that one has'.[177] In some comments on the early nineteenth-century history of dentistry, Richardson notes[178] the large sums of money dentists were prepared to pay resurrectionists for human teeth; the traffic in 'canines' was a commercial sideline to the larger trading. She reports 'a crass appeal to self-interest' made in 1819 by Macartney, Professor of Anatomy at Trinity College, who countered a proposal by a charitable institution to defend a large pauper graveyard:

> I do not think the upper and middle classes have understood the effects of their own conduct when they take part in impeding

174 Canetti, 1981, 66.
175 *Frankenstein*, 58.
176 *Ibid.*
177 Canetti, 1981, 261.
178 Richardson, 1989, 67

> the process of dissection . . . very many of the upper ranks carry in their mouths teeth which have been buried in the hospital fields.[179]

The Creature's impressive set of teeth assimilates Frankenstein to the dentistry business in the 1820s, but with this emphasis: the first encounter stages a symbolic reversal of the 'very many' toothless corpses lying in the nation's hospital fields.

## Laughter

The Creature bares his teeth on a number of occasions. He disregards the polite etiquette which holds the open display of the teeth down to a minimum. As De Quincey's commentary on acute human fears shows, in the social panic no such rules apply and biting becomes the last-ditch avoiding action. The connection of the teeth to terror, however, is the reverse of defensive. Here we take up the subject of laughter in the anatomy literature – in the graveyard scene in *Frankenstein* and elsewhere. Canetti observes:

> *Laughter* has been objected to as vulgar because, in laughing, the mouth is opened wide and the teeth are shown. Originally laughter contained a feeling of pleasure in prey or food which seemed certain. A human being who falls down reminds us of an animal we might have hunted and brought down ourselves. Every sudden fall which arouses laughter does so because it suggests helplessness and reminds us that the fallen can, if we want, be treated as prey. If we went further and actually ate it, we would not laugh. We laugh *instead* of eating it. Laughter is our physical reaction to the escape of potential food.[180]

In this account, laughter is a display of power and a surveillance operation. Richardson[181] has drawn attention to the role of

---

179 *Ibid.*, 106.
180 Canetti, 1981, 261.
181 Richardson, 1989, 144, 184.

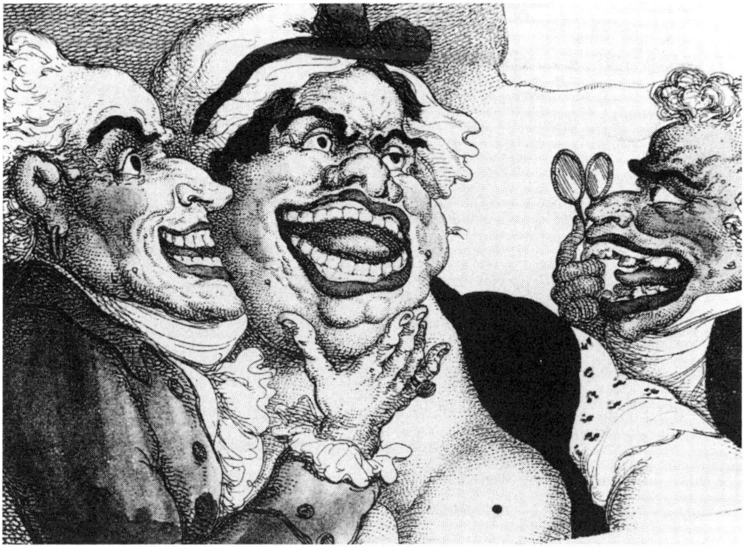

When Nicholas Dubois de Chemant brought his porcelain dentures to England in the 1790s they were eagerly sought after by the gentry. This contemporary cartoon is by Thomas Rowlandson.

laughter – and its power to reveal hypocrisy – in the Anatomy Act debate. The events in Edinburgh exposed the unacceptable face of *laissez-faire*'s eye for prey; and indeed many representations of surgery in the pre-anaesthetic era impose metaphors of butchery, cannibalism and repletion. For example, in the wake of the Edinburgh burkers, Thomas Love Peacock in a humorous passage described an Anglican divine's latent talents (in De Quincey's sense) saving him from the burkers. His assailant, who succeeds in burking someone else, is described in Frankensteinian terms:

> 'Oh, the creature!' exclaimed the Reverend Doctor Folliott, 'he has made a subject for science of the only friend he had in the world.' . . . 'if my old reading, and my early gymnastics . . . had not imbued me with . . . holy rage, I should be, at this moment, lying on the table of some flinty-hearted anatomist,

> who would have sliced and disjointed me as unscrupulously as I do these remnants of the capon and chine.[182]

In another image of ingestion, Rowlandson's cartoon sees gargantuan aristocrats parading their new porcelain teeth. For them, there is no distinction between eating and laughing.

The Creature's laughter in *Frankenstein* erupts when his creator is finally alone in his family's graveyard. As Frankenstein summons his crowd, he kneels. The defencelessness of this posture belies his belligerent rhetoric. The Creature, lying in wait, responds:

> I was answered through the stillness of the night by a loud and fiendish laugh. It rang on my ears long and heavily; the mountains re-echoed it, and I felt as if all hell surrounded me with mockery and laughter. Surely in that moment I should have been possessed by frenzy and have destroyed my miserable existence but that my vow was heard and that I was reserved for vengeance.[183]

As Victor Sage observes, in gothic fiction horror enters first by the ear.[184] The laughter here rings out from the social abyss and echoes across the mountains. It serves notice that more terror of this order is easily within the Creature's power. As the density and the range of this laughter indicates, Frankenstein is surrounded by a crowd. The Creature is laughing in contempt; and in him the hosts of the dead are laughing at Frankenstein.

The nocturnal graveyard scene reproduces certain aspects of the honeymoon attack on Elizabeth. In Como Elizabeth cries out – with 'a shrill and dreadful scream' – as the Creature strikes. After Edinburgh, the Anatomy Act was designed to avert the worst kind of human fear. Canetti observes:

> There is nothing that man fears more than the touch of the unknown. He wants to *see* what is reaching towards him, and to be able to recognise or at least classify it . . . Even clothes

182 Peacock, 1982, 193–4.
183 *Frankenstein,* 169.
184 Sage, 1988, 193.

> give insufficient security: it is easy to tear them and pierce through to the naked, smooth, defenceless flesh of the victim. All the distances which men create around themselves are dictated by this fear . . . The fear of burglars is not only the fear of being robbed, but also the fear of a sudden and unexpected clutch out of the darkness.[185]

This description applies to the never-forgotten hand which reaches towards Frankenstein when he first flees from the 'monster' in the dark. Darkness indeed was the very medium of the burkophobia fears – the dread of the dark which was felt nationwide after Edinburgh was focused by the fact that Burke and Hare took their last victim on Hallowe'en night. As Burkophobia spread, the scandal threw the shadow of murder across medicine's everyday objects: the terror was epitomised by the fear of suffocation by medicinal pitch plasters, which were widely thought of as burking instruments.[186] In *Frankenstein* the Creature is veiled by the night when, in the manner of a burglar, he enters the honeymoon villa. As he leaves Elizabeth's aristocratic-pauper body on the 'bridal bier', he offers a third category of corpse to the surgeon: a newly solemnised bourgeois body. Canetti's account of fear applies particularly to the

---

[185] Canetti, 1981, 15.

[186] In *Middlemarch* (1871–72) George Eliot recalls the burkophobia era and the fear of pitch-plaisters. Her commentary on what the Middlemarchers think of Dr Lydgate beautifully captures the public perception of the medical men in the late 1820s: 'Mrs Dollop became more and more convinced by her own asseveration, that Doctor Lydgate meant to let the people die in the Hospital, if not to poison them, for the sake of cutting them up without saying by your leave or with your leave; for it was a known "fac" that he had wanted to cut up Mrs Groby, as respectable a woman as any in Parley Street, who had money in trust before her marriage – a poor tale for a doctor, who if he was good for anything should know what the matter was with you before you died, and not want to pry into your inside after you were gone. If that was not reason, Mrs Dollop wished to know what was; but there was a prevalent feeling in her audience that her opinion was a bulwark, and that if it were overthrown there would be no limit to the cutting-up of bodies, as had been well seen in Burke and Hare with their pitch-plaisters – such a hanging business as that was not wanted in Middlemarch!' (*Middlemarch,* Ch. 45).

distanciated bourgeois body, for 'the touch of the unknown' is what enables an individual to feel separate and to fear being absorbed into a crowd. Frankenstein comments on his childhood that 'it was my temper to avoid a crowd',[187] and he retains this disposition as an adult. The laughter in the graveyard shows the Creature exploiting Frankenstein's avoidance of close human contact in order to visit him with the same order of fear which Elizabeth experiences at the rape and murder climax of the wedding-night. His laughter enters by the ear rather than the sight: the threat behind it defies immediate classification. Frankenstein's recourse is to invoke his own crowd in the scheme of his vengeance – indeed, the Creature's surrounding laughter provokes his rhetoric. As the laughter subsides, the Creature, 'apparently close to my ear', announces himself 'satisfied'.[188] The encounter in the graveyard forces an admission of the crowd-character of class identity.

In my discussion of *Barnaby Rudge* in Chapter 4 we saw Francis Place in 1832 exploiting laughter in a successful bid to gain the labour aristocracy exemption from the dissection threat. Canetti argues that Hobbes got laughter only half right:

> As Hobbes said, laughter expresses a sudden feeling of superiority, but he did not add that it only occurs when the normal consequences of this superiority do not ensue. His conception contains only half the truth. Perhaps because animals do not laugh, he did not see that our laughter is originally an animal reaction. But neither do animals deny themselves obtainable food if they really want it. Only man has learnt to replace the final stage of incorporation by a symbolic act. It is as though the whole interior process of gulping down food could be summed up and replaced by these movements of the diaphragm which are characteristic of laughter.[189]

When he played the Hobbesian card and cued his audience to

---

[187] *Frankenstein*, 42.

[188] *Ibid.*, 169

[189] Canetti, 1981, 261–2.

laugh at 'the poor', Place showed a utilitarian willingness to exploit the spirit of the age. The first plans for anatomy reform, as we have seen, were protected by discretion. 'Secrecy', Canetti tells us, 'lies at the very core of power',[190] as does the act of lying in wait for the prey. When Robert Peel bound Bentham over to secrecy and discretion in the first instance[191] he was aware that the mooted legislative move effectively marked down the prey long before it could be clearly aware of the fact. The third edition of *Frankenstein* appeared when the move for a legislative solution was out in the open, prompted by Burke and Hare.

In the scheme of digestion as a central process of power, after the open terror of the seizing everything takes place unknown in the dark recesses of the body. The seizing is only the brief, visible phase of a longer, unseen process of assimilation.[192] *Oliver Twist* belongs to the post-legislation archive of the anatomy literature. There are hints that the criminal ways of Fagin and Sikes derive from their earlier occupation as bodysnatchers. The legislation has seen to it that their services are no longer required. This emerges when Sikes first appears in the story:

> 'What are you up to? Ill-treating the boys, you covetous, avaricious, in-sa-ti-a-ble ole fence?' said the man, seating himself deliberately. 'I wonder if they don't murder you! I would if I was them. If I'd been your 'prentice, I'd have done it long ago, and – no, *I couldn't have sold you afterwards*, for you're fit for nothing but keeping as a curiosity of ugliness in a glass bottle, and I suppose they don't blow glass bottles large enough. 'Hush! hush! Mr Sikes,' said the Jew, trembling, 'don't speak so loud.'[italics added][193]

Fagin is glimpsed here as a malformed creature fit only for the medical museum. In his own person this famous criminal figure

---

190 *Ibid.*, 338.
191 Richardson, 1989, 111.
192 Canetti, 1981, 338.
193 Dickens, 1961, 122.

embodies nineteenth-century official preoccupations with human anomalies and monstrosities, and their anatomy.

Dickens' story is a fairy-tale which charts Oliver's departure and eventual safe distance from the workhouse and the dissection constituency. At one point Dickens describes Oliver convulsed with laughter. The scene takes place in Fagin's den, where the criminal ringleader is giving his charges a lesson in how to pick a pocket. Demonstrating the art, Fagin starts up a theatrical routine in which he mimics polite self-importance. In this post-legislation cameo, pickpocketing is a displaced form of body-snatching. Since 1832, incorporation has been replaced by a symbolic act – laughter:

> Sometimes he stopped at the fireplace, and sometimes at the door, making believe that he was staring with all his might into shop windows. At such times he would constantly look around him, for fear of thieves, and would keep slapping all his pockets in turn, to see that he hadn't lost anything, in such a very funny and natural manner, *that Oliver laughed till the tears ran down his face*. All this time the two boys followed him [Fagin] closely about, getting out of his sight so nimbly, every time he turned round, that it was impossible to follow their motions. At last the Dodger trod upon his toes or ran upon his boot accidentally, while Charley Bates stumbled up against him from behind; and in that one moment they took from him, with the most extraordinary rapidity, snuff-box, watch-guard, chain, shirt-pin, pocket-handkerchief, even the spectacle case [italics added].[194]

Dickens gives the last laugh of the bodysnatching era to this innocent little boy. Oliver never laughs so well or so freely again. As he draws the child's tears, Fagin, the museum piece, delivers his impersonation of the newly constituted 'two nations' social order. In a flash, the thieves take everything, as Dickens anatomises the appurtenances of respectability.

The long timetable of the anatomy question contains a famous

---

194 *Ibid.*, 93–4.

remark which makes a contribution to the theory of laughter. It concerns the mother of the author of *Frankenstein*. Horace Walpole once refered to Mary Wollstonecraft as 'a hyena in petticoats'.[195] Walpole's resort to zoological abuse says a good deal about how he and many of his contemporaries felt when confronted by Wollstonecraft's derision. It indicates an unwillingness to regard her as fully human. Canetti uses the hyena to illustrate human laughter:

> The only animal to make a sound really resembling human laughter is the hyena. This sound can be induced by placing food before a captive hyena and then withdrawing it quickly before the animal has time to snatch it. Here it is worth remembering that, in freedom, the hyena's food consists of carrion. It is easy to imagine how often food must have been snatched away from under its eyes by other animals after its own appetite had been aroused.[196]

The experiment first withdraws the hyena from the state-of-nature and then returns it there. Walpole's notorious epithet puts Wollstonecraft – and her sexuality in particular – on the line of demarcation between the state-of-nature and society. Mary Wollstonecraft gave Horace Walpole cause to feel threatened. In retaliation, he turned her into a category-confusion, 'a hyena in petticoats'.

The post-childbirth deathbed of Mary Shelley's mother provides a bleak portrait of the state of medicine in the late eighteenth century. In 1797, when Wollstonecraft died, it was not known that microbes caused disease. At the hands of a Dr Poignand, a physician and man-midwife, the 'hyena in petticoats' underwent an unnecessary and fatally damaging surgical removal of her placenta which resulted in infection and fever. According to Godwin's biographer, another medic was summoned, a Dr Clarke, who instructed that Mary was to be given 'as much wine as her stomach

---

195 *The Letters of Horace Walpole*, 1905, vol. 15, letter 2956.
196 Canetti, 1981, 262.

would tolerate'.[197] In his description of her death William St Clair describes the tragic irony of the situation:

> Mary was given the most modern care available. But there was no cure for infection. Certain religious writers were later to imply that it was not unfitting that Mary Wollstonecraft should die in childbirth, a suitably primitive punishment for one who presumed to challenge the ordained place of women in society. But it was the philosopher who had proclaimed that man would become immortal who was the Promethean figure in the tragedy. If Mary's childbirth had been left to nature, if Godwin had been less concerned, less efficient, less well-connected, or less speedy in fetching the doctors, then she might have lived. But with the heaped ironies which the gods enjoy on such occasions, the more the victims struggled the more certain was their fate. During Mary's dying days Godwin spent anguished hours forcing her to drink the wine, vaguely aware that he was partaking in a superstitious ritual of substituting red wine for her lost red blood. At intervals Mary was made to give suck to the puppies employed to draw off her excess milk.[198]

On the model of her first pregnancy, she had planned to be up the next day, in defiance of the post-birth confinement routine which was considered appropriate for genteel women in her day. Before the birth, Wollstonecraft vetoed the presence of a doctor, with Godwin's reluctant assent. Instead, she requested, and obtained, an experienced midwife. However, when the alarm was raised about the retained placenta, the decisions quickly passed out of her hands.

## The hare

In the course of the chase in *Frankenstein* the hunted Creature, in a gesture of mocking encouragement to his pursuer, leaves

---

[197] St Clair, 1989, 178.
[198] *Ibid.*

Frankenstein 'a dead hare'[199] for his refreshment. This gesture is charged with a political allusion. 'The French Revolution', observes Canetti, 'is usually considered to have begun with the storming of the Bastille. It actually began earlier with a massacre of hares.' [200] In May 1789 the States General, meeting at Versailles, debated the abolition of feudal rights, including the nobility's hunting rights. On 10 June, a month before the storming of the Bastille, the Bretons carried out some of the articles of their *cahiers de doléance* with a massacre of hares, some four to five thousand head of game. In his account of the reversal crowd Canetti comments on the sequence apparent in these events: 'Before they dare attack the wolves, the sheep turn against hares. Before the reversal directed at superiors, they turn on the lowliest available quarry.'[201] Frankenstein, in other words, is offered fare which corresponds to those targeted by the impending anatomy legislation. He has already admired 'the quantity of game' in Windsor forest.[202] The French Revolution was greatly feared by many people in England. The storming of the Bastille marked the beginning of a reversal of power which saw the populace take over the right to inflict capital punishment and the right of mercy. The act of administering justice passed to the crowd. The English workhouses – the source of the corpses after 1832 – were popularly called 'Bastilles'. The reference to tyranny in the name contains a reminder that oppression can be overturned. As he comes across the hare, Frankenstein confronts the Creature's words: 'My reign is not yet over – you live, and my power is complete'[203] – carved in stone. The hare mockingly offered to Frankenstein is a metonymy of the reversal crowd.

The hostile chase towards the end of the story shows Frankenstein reducing to a cadaverous figure, 'a mere skeleton'. But his essential mood throughout the chase remains constant. The hunt,

---

199 *Frankenstein*, 171.
200 Canetti, 1981, 67.
201 *Ibid.*
202 *Frankenstein*, 136.
203 *Ibid.*, 171.

Canetti comments, 'bears a striking affinity to the processes of another mental illness, namely mania'.[204] Mania is 'a paroxysm of desire for prey'.[205] The sighting, overtaking and seizing of the quarry is paramount; the incorporation is not so important. When a sighting of the Creature is reported to Frankenstein, Walton observes a change, 'a new spirit of life' animating 'the decaying frame of the stranger' and 'the greatest eagerness to be upon deck.'[206] Canetti observes that:

> The maniac's transformations have a tremendous ease about them; they share the linear and roving character of the hunter's and also the disconnectedness of his aims, which change each time he fails to attain what he wants, though he nevertheless persists with the hunt. The maniac also resembles the hunter in his elation; wherever he may find himself, his mood is always intense and determined; he always has *an* aim.[207]

The hare is offered to Frankenstein to sustain him in the chase. As a trace of the elusive prey, the offering symbolises the Creature's capacity to effect transformations which provoke and protract Frankenstein's obsessional pursuit. Walton observes the manic glint in his friend's eyes, 'an expression of wildness, and even madness'.[208]

Frankenstein's experience of the hunt for 'the chamois',[209] however, is a compound of mania with its opposite: melancholy. Not long after the first encounter, he develops a conviction of being marked down, more hunted than hunting. This feeling surfaces in gloomy premonitions and intermittent suicidal moods. It becomes concentrated when he assumes that he personally is the target of the Creature's wedding-night assignation. The word Frankenstein repeatedly uses in this connection is 'melancholy'.

204 Canetti, 1981, 401.
205 *Ibid.*
206 *Frankenstein*, 34.
207 Canetti, 1981, 401.
208 *Frankenstein*, 33.
209 *Ibid.*, 167.

Walton also uses this term about him.[210] Canetti describes melancholy as the complement of mania. It commences, he says:

> when flight-transformations are abandoned because they are all felt to be useless. A person in a state of melancholia feels that pursuit is already over and he has already been captured. He cannot escape; he cannot find fresh metamorphoses. Everything he attempted has been in vain; he is resigned to his fate and sees himself as prey; first as prey, then as food, and finally as carrion or excrement. The process of depreciation, which makes his own person seem more and more worthless, is figuratively expressed as feelings of guilt. Guilt was originally the same as debt (in German there is still only one word for them both). If one is in debt to someone one is to that extent in his power. Feeling guilty and thinking of oneself as prey are thus basically the same.[211]

Canetti comments on the destruction of defenceless creatures:

> our behaviour . . . betrays the contempt we feel for a being which is utterly defenceless, which exists in a completely different order of size and power from us, with which we have nothing in common, into which we never transform ourselves and which we never fear except when it suddenly appears in crowds . . . The destruction of these tiny creatures is the only act of violence which remains unpunished even *within* us. Their blood does not stain our hands, for it does not remind us of our own . . . In brief they are outlaws.[212]

The same outlaw logic applies to the hare which the Creature leaves for Frankenstein as a token of his earlier graveyard laughter. The offering makes a potent political point because, alongside the reference to France, a memory and a continuing perception of the English Bloody Code[213] – the country's repressive penal system

---

210 *Ibid.*, 34.
211 Canetti, 1981, 401–2.
212 *Ibid.*, 239–40.
213 See n. 44, Ch. 4.

– informs the Creature's gesture here in *Frankenstein*. The hare is a demonstration of the Creature's improvisory powers of metamorphosis, his ability to evade capture and punishment. The consensus among historians is that the Bloody Code collapses in the 1830s for various reasons – but it is arguable that after 1832, with the Anatomy Act in operation in English 'Bastilles', the spirit of the old code remained in place, but hidden away.

In the latter part of the story, Frankenstein, in contrast, is dominated by a feeling that he himself cannot effect any kind of transformation. An illustration of this feeling occurs in the Orkneys, after he has destroyed his work, and the Creature's trust in him. One day, when he hears the door creak, Frankenstein is overcome by a feeling of powerlessness:

> I trembled from head to foot; I felt a presentiment of who it was . . . But I was overcome by the sensation of helplessness, so often felt in frightful dreams, *when you in vain endeavour to fly from an impending danger*, and was rooted to the spot [italics added].[214]

The 'monster' in the mind here reduces Frankenstein to a paralysed fixity. His first encounter with the Creature is in effect reproduced here, but this time flight and escape is impeded. As his fear of his Creature grows, his inability to transform himself is the source of his melancholy.

One other image links Frankenstein's melancholy with his fear of being eaten by the Creature:

> My father . . . turned his thoughts towards the best method of eradicating the remains of my melancholy, which every now and then would return by fits, and with *a devouring blackness* overcast the approaching sunshine. At these moments I took refuge in the most perfect solitude [italics added].[215]

The 'devouring blackness' appears elsewhere as 'dark melancholy',

---

214 *Frankenstein*, 117.

215 *Ibid.*, 128–9.

and on the wedding-day, as the sun sinks towards the horizon, the groom and bride both succumb to 'reflection upon melancholy subjects'.[216] This imagery supports Canetti's emphasis that:

> it is clear that *all* the phases of this [digestion-power] process, and not only the external and half-conscious ones, must have their correspondence in the psyche. The symptoms of melancholy are especially illuminating in this context.[217]

The anatomy of melancholy in *Crowds and Power* has an application to Frankenstein's apprehension of the 'devouring blackness'. Canetti focuses the melancholic's relation to food:

> The melancholic does not want to eat and, as a reason for his refusal, may say that he does not deserve to. But the real reason is that he sees himself being eaten and, if forced to eat, is reminded of this. His own mouth turns against him; it is as though a mirror were held before him and he saw a mouth in it and saw that something was being eaten. But this something is himself. The terrible penalty for always having eaten is suddenly and ineluctably before him. This transformation into something which is eaten is the last, the transformation which ends all flight. It is to avoid it that, in whatever shape offers, everything living flees.[218]

The hare offered to Frankenstein by the Creature is the invitation and the reminder: 'eat and be refreshed'.[219] The key to Frankenstein's feelings is apparent when Elizabeth observes her fiance's advanced 'emaciation'[220] when he finally returns to her. His loss of appetite effectively commences at the outset of the first encounter, when Frankenstein sees – and flees – the Creature's open mouth.

Mania and melancholy are alternating shadows inside Frankenstein's psyche. There is mania in his single-handed endeavours in

---

216 *Ibid.*, 162

217 Canetti, 1981, 246

218 *Ibid.*, 402.

219 *Frankenstein*, 171.

220 *Ibid.*, 159.

the laboratory of 'filthy creation', but Frankenstein's melancholy deepens as he remains silent about the Creature's existence. After Justine's execution his guilt is irreversible. The 'devouring blackness' is present from the moment he contracts – and begins to shrink from – his promise to the Creature. The monstrous anatomy he half-creates is aborted – indeed torn to pieces – after dark, and its remains are dumped in the sea just as thick cloud obscures the moonlight. At midnight aboard the ship sailing from Ireland, Frankenstein recalls 'the night in which he [the Creature] first lived'[221] – and this prompts his admission of the regular laudanum fix. But mania colours his apprehensions as well. As I have noted, the first, and unsuccessful, legislative move for the bodies in 1829 was dubbed the 'Midnight Bill'. It is remarkable how often the time stands at midnight in *Frankenstein*. The hour is 'near midnight',[222] Walton notes, when cracks in the ice and the visibility difficulties around the ship cause Frankenstein to fear an irretrievable loss of the prey.

## The Ship-of-State

In his essay 'The Politics of Health in the Eighteenth Century' Foucault comments on a development which was well advanced by the time *Frankenstein* appeared:

> Medicine, as a general technique of health even more than as a service to the sick or an art of cures, assumes an increasingly important place in the administrative system and the machinery of power – a role which is constantly widened and strengthened throughout the eighteenth century. The doctor wins a footing within the different instances of social power . . . [He] becomes the great adviser and expert, if not in the art of governing, at least in that of observing, correcting and improving the social 'body' and maintaining it in a permanent state of health.[223]

---

221 *Ibid.*, 154.
222 *Ibid.*, 34.
223 Foucault, 1980, 176–7.

There is an episode in *Frankenstein* which shows the doctor exercising to the full his new authority in society.

It occurs when Frankenstein rises from his sickbed to address the ship's crew, who have made a representation to Captain Walton to return home. The passage requires a long quotation:

> His eyes sparkled, and his cheeks flushed with momentary vigour. Turning towards the men, he said, 'What do you mean? What do you demand of your captain? Are you, then, so easily turned from your design? Did you not call this a glorious expedition? And wherefore was it glorious? Not because the way was smooth and placid as a southern sea, but because it was full of dangers and terror, because at every new incident your fortitude was to be called forth and your courage exhibited, because danger and death surrounded it, and these you were to brave and overcome. For this it was a glorious, for this it was an honourable undertaking. You were hereafter to be hailed as the benefactors of your species, your names adored as belonging to brave men who encountered death for honour and the benefit of mankind. And, now, behold, with the first imagination of danger, or, if you will, the first mighty and terrific trial of your courage, you shrink away and are content to be handed down as men who had not strength enough to endure cold and peril; and so, poor souls, they were chilly and returned to their warm firesides. Why, that requires not that preparation; ye need not have come thus far and dragged your captain to the shame of a defeat merely to prove yourselves cowards. Oh! be men, or be more than men. Be steady to your purposes and firm as a rock. This ice is not made of such stuff as your hearts may be; it is mutable, and cannot withstand you, if you say it shall not. Do not return to your families with the stigma of disgrace marked on your brows. Return as heroes who have fought and conquered and who know not what it is to turn their backs on the foe'.
>
> He spoke this with a voice so modulated to the different feelings expressed in his speech, with an eye so full of lofty design and heroism, that can you wonder that these men

> were moved? They looked at one another and were unable to reply.[224]

This speech shows Frankenstein assuming a proto-Carlylean 'heroic' leadership role in an effort to undermine the crew's resolve to return home. Walton has feared a 'mutiny';[225] but five days later he accedes to the crew's case, even acknowledging an 'injustice'.[226] It is important to be clear about the nature of the crew's action as it becomes the object of Frankenstein's derogatory – and manic – rhetoric. The men do not actually strike; they make an orderly representation and indicate their will as a corporate group: they do not want to press ahead with the ship's enterprise. The crewmen form what Canetti calls a prohibition crowd, a stationary crowd which is created by a collective, self-imposed refusal. The chief modern example is the strike:

> There is something deeply serious and worthy of respect about such an organisation and, when the ferocity and destructiveness of crowds are mentioned, one cannot help remembering the responsibility and dignity of these structures sprung spontaneously from crowds . . . As long as it remains true to its nature, [a prohibition crowd] . . . is averse to destruction.[227]

The threat to power represented by a strike is the interdict placed on the workplace; the protection of entry invests the space with the aura of common possession. Seen in this light, the crowd scene aboard the ship in *Frankenstein* is informed by the Ship-of-State analogy, and Frankenstein's speech inevitably has the national reform debate in its subtext. In the story's 1831 edition, the negotiation of the differences on board without a 'mutiny' would have formed a marked contrast to an often violent national argument.

For Frankenstein the orator, the crewmen's action offers an

---

224 *Frankenstein,* 178.
225 *Ibid.*, 177.
226 *Ibid.*, 179.
227 Canetti, 1981, 65.

opportunity to mythologise, and efface, class relations. His speech deserves a longer analysis than I shall give, but a summary of its nature as political rhetoric is essential to an understanding of the hypocrisy generated by the anatomy question. The long harangue is an exercise in mesmeric leadership, mythic masculinity and charisma politics (it is notable that the men are reduced to silence). The principal consideration for the men, apparently, is the reputation and standing of the captain. Contrary to his promise that everyone aboard will achieve renown, Frankenstein knows that it is only leaders, and not the men they lead, who are accredited with victories. The vein of flattery in the speech shows Frankenstein maintaining – or constructing – certain socially useful fictions. Canetti argues that myths of national identity often incorporate symbols which share the same attributes as crowds. The symbols figure 'in the conceptions and feelings nations have about themselves'.[228] Nationalistic claims are 'always latent . . . becoming active in times of war.'[229] It is decisive, in this regard, that Frankenstein invokes the sea as being at the heart of the glorious challenge, especially the sea in its aspect as danger and terror. As he addresses the crew, Frankenstein mounts an appeal to a characteristic national faith and an idealised male community. The consideration shown to Walton and the construction of an external enemy are the points in his rhetoric where crowd symbolism is present. As Canetti observes:

> Everybody knows what the *sea* means to an Englishman; what is not sufficiently known is the precise form of the connection between his relationship to the sea and his famous individualism. The Englishman sees himself as a captain on board a ship with a small group of people, the sea around and beneath him. He is almost alone; as captain he is in many ways isolated from his crew.[230]

---

[228] *Ibid.*, 199.
[229] *Ibid.*, 198.
[230] *Ibid.*, 199–200.

This description applies to Captain Walton, the Englishman, in *Frankenstein*. Frankenstein implies, as he addresses the men, that the captain in his individualism is essentially alone with the sea. Walton, at the outset of the story, indicates his solitude and isolation from the crew in his private correspondence. Frankenstein's oratory reminds the crew that the captain rules the waves; the speech tacitly enlists the mens' devotion and discipline ('fortitude' and 'courage' are euphemisms) into an assumption of rule. The vast sea is to be ruled, and the ship, as Canetti observes, 'is personified in its captain'.[231] A command to the crew is actually a command to the sea, which must obey. In the imperial overtones of this conception, the sea's frequent obedience is a sign of whom it obeys. But this assumption of rule is not explicit as Frankenstein speaks. Instead, he dwells on the collective activity of the venture. The warm fireside is not where the national essence is enacted. The sea offers more expansive and testing forms of essential identity; the fireside, in contrast, is a complementary scene of unchanging securities and fixtures.

In an interview in 1989 the social historian E. J. Hobsbawm replied to this question:

> QUESTIONER: How did the ruling orders in society cope with the problem of appearing to hand over the semblance of power to the masses and yet hang on to it themselves?
>
> E. J. HOBSBAWM: They had to become hypocritical.[232]

Hobsbawm here is referring to the problems besetting liberal politicians, and his comment refers to rather later nineteenth-century developments in British national life. His point about hypocrisy concerns a state of affairs in which politicians said one thing publicly to the masses, but kept their reservations to themselves, as rhetoric became divorced from thought. Hobsbawm's

---

231 *Ibid.*

232 The interview was on BBC *Timewatch*, 'An Age of Empire', broadcast on 8 Feb. 1989.

larger argument, however, is that patriotic tradition and ritual were invented by the liberal bourgeoise precisely to stop social class, and its potential for conflict, becoming the basis of British politics. The latent code in Frankenstein's speech is of course patriotism, the gender dimension of which is Frankenstein's desire to keep men, and a male ethos, firmly at the helm in English society. As he speaks the story's 'Ship-of-State' episode stages a rehearsal of post-1832 developments in the British state.

The speech is laden with the rhetoric of a well-maintained and robust body politic. The metaphors Frankenstein uses to promote the patriotic cause are of moral strength legitimately directed. And Walton's patriotic discourse stands alongside Frankenstein's; it too draws on the sea as England's national symbol. When it comes to personal qualities, the ship's captain admires one man in particular. The following passage is Walton's endorsement of the English national character in the figure of his lieutenant:

> My lieutenant, for instance, is a man of wonderful courage and enterprise; he is madly desirous of glory: or rather, to word my phrase more characteristically, of advancement in his profession. He is an Englishman, and in the midst of national and professional prejudices, unsoftened by cultivation, retains some of the noblest endowments of humanity . . . finding that he was unemployed in this city, I easily engaged him to assist in my enterprise.
>
> The master is a person of an excellent disposition, and is remarkable in the ship for his gentleness and the mildness of his discipline. This circumstance, added to his well known integrity and dauntless courage, made me very desirous to engage him . . . . I cannot overcome an intense distaste to the usual brutality exercised on board ships: I have never believed it to be necessary; and when I heard of a mariner equally noted for his kindness of heart, and the respect and obedience paid to him by his crew, I felt myself peculiarly fortunate in being able to secure his services.[233]

---

[233] *Frankenstein*, 29.

This impressive character reference constructs an idealised version of England's political state on the eve of 1832. In reality there was nothing 'mild' about the Anatomy Act and the New Poor Law. The Ship-of-State in *Frankenstein* is a mythic ship where the commanding and the commanded enjoy ultimately negotiable relationships and, up to a point, a common perception of an enemy. Walton does not immediately accede to the men's demands. His gambit follows his observation of the effects of Frankenstein's eloquence on the men. He offers a promise to turn back, but privately hopes that Frankenstein's words will cause reflection and renewed courage among the men. Walton has authority, but not charisma. 'The men', he notes, 'unsupported by ideas of glory and honour, can never willingly continue to endure their present hardships'.[234] Voiced as it is in private correspondence, this reflection, in the context of Hobsbawm's thesis, sums up many of the dilemmas that were to confront the political masters of the post-1832 body politic. Frankenstein's speech offers an uneasy prognosis, and on the strength of it Walton turns back.

[234] *Ibid.*, 179.

CHAPTER 9

# Frankenstein's mask: England 1831–32

I have argued that the killings in *Frankenstein* are an enactment of the burking violence which was exploited after the Burke and Hare scandal to press the case for legislative anatomy reform. Frankenstein's decision to remain silent about his creation means that, from the time of Justine's trial and execution, he wears a mask. As the violence escalates, the 'monster' is the secret that stands behind it. The mask, therefore, is loaded with terror and, where Elizabeth is concerned, uncertainty.

## The mask

In his account of mummery Canetti distinguishes three related terms, mask, figure and transformation. All three terms are in play in *Frankenstein* in some episodes we will now read. The true mask, Canetti argues, inspires terror:

> The mask is distinguished from all other end-states of transformation by its rigidity. In place of the varying and continuous movement of the face [the mask] presents the exact opposite: a perfect fixity and sameness . . . To fixity of form is added fixity of distance. What gives the mask its interdictory quality is the fact that it never changes. Everything behind the mask is mysterious . . . no one must know what lies behind it. A mask expresses much, but hides even more. Above all it *separates*. Charged with a menace which must not be precisely known – one element of which, indeed, is that it *cannot* be known – it comes close to the spectator, but in spite of this proximity, remains clearly separated from *[her]*. It threatens *[her]* with the

> secret dammed up behind it. Unlike a face, there are no passing changes in it which can be interpreted, and so [*she*] suspects and fears the unknown that it conceals.
>
> The real use of the mask is not in isolation but in ceremonies, and if it then behaves in a familiar and expected manner it can also have a reassuring effect. Here it stands between the dangerous power which is behind it and the spectator. If properly treated it can keep this danger away from *[her]*. It can gather the danger into itself and contain it, only allowing it to overflow in one manner – the manner corresponding to its own shape. Once the spectator has established a relationship to the mask, [*she*] can behave in an appropriate way. It is a figure with its own idiosyncrasies of behaviour. Once these have been learnt, once one knows how much distance it demands, it acts as a protection against the the dangerous power contained within itself [gender pronouns altered to denote Elizabeth].[1]

Richardson observes that the anatomy legislation's 'synchronicity with the Reform Act meant that it sank almost without trace in the press of the day'.[2] With Frankenstein's marriage to Elizabeth, Mary Shelley's story rehearses the political settlement in 1832 which sees the Anatomy Act becoming law behind the Reform Bill crisis, and masked by it. As I shall now show, every aspect of Canetti's description of the mask appears in *Frankenstein* as the marriage ceremonial impends.

In one key image, the Creature himself adopts the body posture which in due course draws attention to Frankenstein's mask just after Justine's trial. In the catalyst to the social terror, the Creature *kneels* as he begs for accommodation in the de Lacey cottage – in vain, as it turns out. 'Kneeling', comments Canetti,[3] 'is always in some sense the prelude to a last moment', and Justine, who is innocent of murder, falls to her knees in entreaty to Elizabeth and Frankenstein in the prison-chamber scene prior to her execution.

---

1 Canetti, 1981, 435–6.

2 Richardson, 1989, 265.

3 Canetti, 1981, 457.

This episode freezes Frankenstein behind his mask of silence; it prefigures Elizabeth's bondage to his silence before their wedding ceremony. The prison-chamber scene is remarkable for its combination of innocent disbelief and radical bemusement on Elizabeth's part. It commences with her statement to Frankenstein:

> 'Alas!' said she. 'How shall I ever again believe in human goodness? Justine, whom I loved and esteemed as my sister, how could she put on those smiles of innocence only to betray? Her mild eyes seemed incapable of any severity or guile, and yet she has committed a murder.'[4]

It proceeds to Elizabeth's question to Justine:

> 'Rise, my poor girl,' said Elizabeth; 'why do you kneel if you are innocent? . . . I believed you innocent, notwithstanding every evidence, until I heard that you yourself had declared your guilt.'[5]

Justine replies. She tells Elizabeth and Frankenstein of the duress employed to extract her confession; and even in her own extremity here she continues to mourn for William. As Justine's execution impends, what follows next is a paradoxical last *and* first recognition scene:

> 'Oh Justine! Forgive me for having for one moment distrusted you. Why did you confess? But do not mourn, dear girl, Do not fear. I will proclaim, I will prove your innocence. I will melt the stony hearts of your enemies by my tears and prayers. You shall not die! You, *my playfellow, my companion, my sister,* perish on the scaffold! No! I never could survive so horrible a misfortune' [italics added].[6]

In a reversal of Frankenstein's attitude, from the first, to his Creature, Elizabeth remains true to Justine right to the end. As

---

[4] *Frankenstein*, 80.
[5] *Ibid.*
[6] *Ibid.*, 81.

Elizabeth addresses Justine, Frankenstein stands by, solitary and masked. The word 'stony' applies equally to his petrification. Justine's prostration here flatters the mask as Frankenstein commits himself to wearing it.

The apprehension the mask inspires eventually communicates itself to Elizabeth. She writes to Frankenstein in some perplexity, and an incipient unease, on the subject of their marriage betrothal. Her letter rehearses a repertoire of roles – in quest of recognition and relationship – that is virtually identical to the roles which surface in the exchange above with Justine:

> You well know, Victor, that our union had been the favourite plan of your parents ever since our infancy. We were told this when young and taught to look forward to it as an event that would certainly take place. We were *affectionate playfellows* during childhood, and, I believe, *dear and valued friends* to one another as we grew older. But as *brother and sister* often entertain a lively affection towards each other without desiring a more intimate union, may not such also be our case? Tell me, dearest Victor. Answer me, I conjure you, by our mutual happiness, with simple truth – Do you not love another?
>
> I, who have so disinterested an affection for you, may increase your miseries tenfold by being an obstacle to your wishes. Ah! Victor, be assured that your *cousin and playmate* has too sincere a love for you not to be made miserable by this supposition. Be happy, my *friend*; and if you obey me in this one request, remain satisfied that nothing on earth will have the power to interrupt my tranquillity . . . and if I see but one smile on your lips when we meet, occasioned by this or any other exertion of mine, I shall need no other happiness.
>
> Elizabeth Lavenza
>
> Geneva, May 18. 17–
> [italics added][7]

---

7 *Ibid.*, 157–8.

Elizabeth is always conscious of Frankenstein's distance as well as his supposed closeness to her, but here the question of propinquity presses to a crisis. The letter rehearses uncertainties and ambiguities which express Elizabeth's apprehension of a mask. Consistent with Canetti's emphasis on ceremony, it shows Elizabeth recounting and nominating several status-roles – 'playmate', 'sister', 'cousin', 'friend' – in an effort to establish *relationship* to the mask; she is, after all, explicitly requesting reassurance. Elizabeth cleaves to the sign she needs: 'if I see but one smile on your lips when we meet'.[8] Furthermore, as the prison scene shows, experience has made Elizabeth sensitive to apparent masks: thinking she confronts the murderer, she cannot credit Justine 'putting on' innocent smiles.

In *Frankenstein* the paradigm face – as opposed to a mask – belongs to Caroline Beaufort, the kneeling figure in the portrait above the mantelpiece. Caroline, as a mother and an aunt, has 'the brightness of a beloved eye'[9] and 'her countenance expressed affection even in death'.[10] It is she, on her death-bed, who secures a promise of the marriage between Frankenstein and Elizabeth; it is she who admits Justine into the household. In one brief – but mediated – glimpse, the Creature sees Caroline Beaufort as she is best known to the family: he sees the miniature portrait of her. Looking at Caroline, he is looking at the face of benevolent paternalism in the years preceding 1832. But as he looks at her he has just throttled her youngest son William:

> As I fixed my eyes on the child, I saw something glittering on his breast. I took it; it was a portrait of a most lovely woman. In spite of my malignity, it softened and attracted me. For a few moments I gazed with delight on her dark eyes, fringed by deep lashes, and her lovely lips; but presently my rage returned; I remembered that I was forever deprived of the delights that such beautiful creatures could bestow and that she

---

8 *Ibid.*,
9 *Ibid.*, 47.
10 *Ibid.*

> whose resemblance I contemplated would, in regarding me, have changed that air of divine benignity to one expressive of disgust and affright.[11]

The glimpse occurs, that is to say, precisely as he qualifies for the dissection reserved for the murderer in the pre-1832 era. Caroline Beaufort's portrait momentarily draws Frankenstein's 'monster' into a non-judgemental gaze which he reciprocates until his self-awareness breaks the illusion. In the next few moments he places the portrait in the folds of Justine's dress. This passage shows the Creature imagining Caroline's condemnation of him as her youngest son's killer – and therefore her verdict on him effectively sanctions the subsequent verdict on Justine. The execution of the innocent Justine is the event in *Frankenstein* which above all marks the end of benevolent paternalism in early nineteenth-century England.

The Creature's imaginative engagement with Caroline's portrait has the power of epiphany: in the artefact of the face he sees the face itself in its mobility and readiness for transformation. The same warm face, as Frankenstein knows, is apparent in Justine, who physically reminds Elizabeth of their mutual aunt – and the icon of this face damns the hapless child at her trial. Elizabeth, however, is to look in vain for a face. She must confront the thing she fears most, Frankenstein's mask:

> I wrote to Elizabeth. My letter was calm and affectionate. 'I fear, my beloved girl,' I said, 'little happiness remains for us on earth; yet all that I may one day enjoy is centred in you. Chase away your idle fears; to you alone do I consecrate my life and my endeavours for contentment. I have one secret, Elizabeth, a dreadful one; when revealed to you it will chill your frame with horror, and then, far from being surprised at my misery, you will only wonder that I survive what I have endured. I will confide this tale of misery and terror to you the day after our marriage shall take place, for, my sweet cousin, there must

11 *Ibid.*, 123.

be perfect confidence between us. But, until then, I conjure you, do not mention or allude to it. This I most earnestly intreat, and I know you will comply.'[12]

The bride is enjoined to silence; the interdictory quality of the mask – its changelessness[13] – remains intact for the duration of the ceremonial. The danger Elizabeth stands in at this point has long been signalled by the promise – *I will be with you on your wedding-night* – which hauntingly mocks the power of ceremony to defuse the threat behind the mask.

I have argued that the Creature as a crowd-body 'reclaims' Elizabeth's plebeian corpse on her wedding-night. However, it is no less true that, as Frankenstein's aristocratic bride, Elizabeth is sexually abused, throttled and left for the surgeon in retaliation for her class betrayal. Canetti's observations on the way the 'shape' of the danger can be contained in ceremony are relevant here. As the promise *I will be with you* extends to the wedding night – and as the Creature steals from behind Frankenstein's mask – he imposes an obscene inversion of the true purpose of the ceremony, the creation of a safe relationship between the spectator and the mask. The problem of 'relationship' commences with Frankenstein's first rejection of his Creature, the encounter which is the *locus classicus* of the anatomy literature. As I argued in Chapter 5, the wedding-night completes the ritual of the 'gallows wedding' which confronts Frankenstein throughout the story in his role as the surgeon. As the Creature claims Justine and Elizabeth as versions of his eternal bride, the 'gallows wedding' is his reply to early utilitarian ideology. In the 1831 context, however, another development in England intersects the Creature's representation, as Mary Shelley herself observed when *Frankenstein* reappeared that year.

---

12 *Ibid.*, 159.

13 Canetti, 1981, 435.

## 'The burnings, the alarms'

Commenting on the third edition of her story, the author referred to the 'Swing' rick-burning demonstrations which flared across southern England in 1831: '[t]he burnings, the alarms, the absorbing politics of the day render booksellers almost averse to publishing at all' (Letters).[14] It cannot be known what Mary Shelley had specifically in mind when she added the phrase 'the alarms' to her remarks. But, as I suggested in my opening chapter, the copycat murders committed in the wake of Burke and Hare in 1831 would have warranted the observation. The following passage from the Creature's narrative sees the 'monster' commencing his 'everlasting war' on society with an act of arson. It follows the catastrophic outcome of the kneeling encounter with the de Lacey family, and occurs a short time after that family has fled the cottage in fear:

> As the night advanced, a fierce wind arose from the woods and quickly dispersed the clouds that had loitered in the heavens; the blast tore along like a mighty avalanche and produced a kind of insanity in my spirits that burst all bounds of reason and reflection. I lighted the dry branch of a tree and danced with fury around the devoted cottage, my eyes still fixed on the western horizon, the edge of which the moon nearly touched. A part of its orb was at length hid, and I waved my brand; it sank, and with a loud scream I fired the straw, and heath, and bushes, which I had collected. The wind fanned the fire, and the cottage was quickly enveloped by the flames, which clung to it and licked it with their forked and destroying tongues.
>
> As soon as I was convinced that no assistance could save any part of the habitation, I quitted the scene and sought for refuge in the woods.[15]

*Crowds and Power* contains an account of crowd symbols or metaphors often used for the crowd. While not made up of men, these

---

[14] Cited in Shelley, 1992, 14.

[15] *Frankenstein*, 120.

are '*felt* to be a crowd.'[16] The symbols 'shape the precise contours of the human crowd among the material crowd'.[17] In his account, the Creature uses the plural forms – 'flames' and 'tongues' – to invoke the connection between fire and crowds. Fire is the prime crowd symbol. It seems to be alive, and is treated as if it were. This passage in *Frankenstein* is a representation in which the attributes of fire delineate the attributes of the crowd: contagious, insatiable and sudden.

The passage employs the symbolism in a way that reaches far into some of the key meanings carried by the Creature's own narrative. The propensity to incendiarism is the most dangerous trait of the crowd. Fire is the dominant symbol here in the story, but four others are present which Canetti lists: rain, wind, the forest and, in collected form, the heap. The dispersal of the cloudburst emphasises that this truly is a fire which no miracle from God can extinguish. The heap, the final remains of the cultivation around the cottage, is not lit until the moon touches the edge of the horizon. Until the dramatic moment of ignition comes, the Creature appears to fire-dance 'in fury' in order, it seems, to summon the suddenness and the full velocity of the fire – and to transform himself into it. The emotions in play in this furious dancing have their source, nevertheless, in the acquisition of human culture which has taken place during the Creature's existence in the hovel adjacent to the cottage. This passage sees the Creature using his most human acquisition – his speech – as he addresses Frankenstein. The dance movement appears to be the only form of movement that is adequate to his experience of rejection from the whole scheme of human culture as represented by the de Lacey family and cottage settlement.

His utter isolation is the key to this spectacular act of arson. Earlier in the Creature's narrative the firewood from the forest was the gift from the unknown, benign stranger; it came from the lonely figure who longed for the company and the warm eyes

---

[16] Canetti, 1981, 87–109.
[17] Muscovici, in Hulse (ed.), 1987, 51.

of others. The forest, however, adds the suggestion of another potentiality in the Creature which surfaces when he refers to the 'spark'[18] of his existence: the fact, as Canetti notes,[19] that arson originates in the burning of forests. The heap here is not from the forest in the first instance, but comprises every vestige of the garden cultivation which differentiates culture from nature, and in this fire everything perishes. In his entry on fire Canetti comments that: 'It seems appropriate to speak here of the significance of impulsive incendiarism in relation to the individual who commits it, an individual who is really isolated and outside the sphere of any religious or political faith.'[20] Canetti proceeds to a case that is described by Kräpelin, the principles of which have an exact application to this episode in the Creature's address to Frankenstein. It concerns a lonely person and it establishes 'the connection between fire and the crowd, even in isolated individuals'.[21] Cases of this kind are 'not as rare as one might think':[22]

> arson is a fixed idea, and he feels driven to it as though by an invisible power . . . He certainly likes watching fire, but he also likes confessing, and confessing very circumstantially. He must, early in his life, have experienced fire as a means of attracting people; the commotion around a fire was probably his first experience of a crowd, and it was easy later for fire to take the place of the crowd . . . He has a double relationship with arson. Isolated at an early stage by his lamentable history, he has had . . . no opportunity of mingling with crowds.[23]

The Creature comments that he 'waited with forced impatience until the moon had sunk to commence my operations'.[24] In the continuing case:

---

18 *Frankenstein*, 117.
19 Canetti, 1981, 90.
20 *Ibid.*, 92.
21 *Ibid.* The case in question concerns a woman. To avoid confusion I have replaced 'she' with 'he'.
22 *Ibid.*
23 *Ibid.*, 92.

> . . . he wants, first of all, to be part of the crowd staring at the fire – a fire which is reflected in all eyes and under whose powerful compulsion all eyes turn in the same direction. When the initial blaze is over and the crowd threatens to disperse and escape him, he keeps it alive by suddenly transforming *himself* into the fire. This he achieves very simply: he confesses that he caused it. The fuller and more detailed his story, the longer he will be stared at, the longer he himself will remain the fire.[25]

The equivalent confession is made in the passage under review, within the Creature's own narrative and in Frankenstein's company. Thus 'the double relationship with arson' commences in his creator's eyes: 'His self-accusation results from his feeling that everyone is watching him. He likes this feeling and, through it, transforms himself into the fire that people are watching.'[26]

The Creature's final transformation into fire, as projected to Walton, comes at the end of the story: in the flames of his funeral pyre amid the isolation of the cold polar gloom. When they meet beside Frankenstein's corpse, Walton charges the Creature with arson.[27] However, in a significant phrase, the Creature indicates to Walton that his funeral pyre consummates 'the series of my being'.[28] The cottage fire is therefore only the first of a series of threatening configurations of the Creature in Frankenstein's mind in which no distinction exists between fire and crowd. With the exceptions of the final apotheosis and the cottage fire, the Creature's actions always spell death to somebody, as Walton now knows. In the forest ceremony here, where the Creature identifies himself with fire, the scream at the lighting of the straw heap is the war-cry, the start of his 'everlasting'[29] reign of terror. This moment precedes the narrative which Frankenstein divulges to

---

24 *Frankenstein*, 120.
25 Canetti, 1981, 92.
26 *Ibid.*
27 *Frankenstein*, 183.
28 *Ibid.*, 184.
29 *Ibid.*, 118.

Walton; and it is narrated in the Creature's own words. The other fires in 'the series' belong to Frankenstein's perception of the crowd, and hence, as I shall now show, they carry his accentuations and anxieties.

In *Cholera 1832* R. J. Morris discusses the relationship between class, power and the social experience of the epidemic. There are two items in Morris' analysis which help to identify the play of masks and transformation in *Frankenstein*. He reports that the chief medical officer of Sunderland, Dr W. Reid Clanny: 'spent his spare hours before the arrival of cholera in Sunderland counting flashes of lightning, hoping to find a clue to the causes of the disease.'[30] A contemporary scientist, a Dr Adam Neale, was 'even more apocalyptic'.[31] On 17 August he sighted a spectacular thunderstorm passing from Dover to Liverpool:

> a body of vapour of extraordinary magnitude, arising apparently out of the earth, accompanied by a very loud rumbling noise. It resembled the smoke of a conflagration and had a fiery appearance. It continued ascending for the space of about three minutes, all of the time accompanied by the noise above mentioned.[32]

The crowd symbols of wind and fire are well in evidence here. Dr Neale's vision returns us to my commentary in Chapter 8 on the new access, via the microscope, to animalacular objects. Neale, subscribing to the contagion theory of the cholera, 'believed that the disease was carried by clouds of minute insects too small for the eye to detect, helped along by favourable winds and an imbalance in terrestial electricity.'[33] Morris adds an observation which appropriately glosses Frankenstein's own arrogant dismissal of older cosmologies of knowledge. As Neale contemplated the vapour's appearance:

---

30 Morris, 1976, 171–2.
31 *Ibid.*, 172.
32 *Ibid.*
33 *Ibid.*, 170.

Here, he thought, was the means by which Divine Providence had disseminated those minute insects. The failure of the rational empirical traditions of science allowed a more primitive thought pattern to emerge. There was an archetypal fittingness in the correlation between violent disruptions of nature, thunder, lightning and volcanoes, and the violent disruption of the human body by cholera. It was a correspondence of natural, social and personal events which would have satisfied the readers of Aquinas and Shakespeare not just as analogy but as explanation.[34]

## The midnight figure

Dr Adam Neale's unwitting contribution to the genre of monster-imagery is apt for a number of reasons which bear on one decisive moment in Frankenstein's apprehensions. An equivalent spectacle occurs when Frankenstein resolves to visit the spot where William was murdered. He does so at midnight, amid storm and lightning. Several crowd symbols are apparent in the lightning spectacle:

> I saw the lightnings playing on the summit of Mont Blanc in the most beautiful *figures*. The *storm* appeared to approach rapidly . . . It advanced; the heavens were clouded, and I soon felt the *rain* coming slowly *in large drops*, but its violence quickly increased . . .
>
> I quitted my seat and walked on, although the darkness and storm increased every minute and the thunder burst with a terrific crash over my head. It was echoed from Saleve, the Juras, and the Alps of Savoy; *vivid flashes of lightning dazzled my eyes*, illuminating the lake, *making it appear like a vast sheet of fire*; then for an instant everything seemed of a pitchy darkness, until the eye recovered itself from the preceding flash. The storm . . . appeared at once in various parts of the heavens . . .
>
> While I watched the tempest, so beautiful yet terrific, I

---

34 *Ibid.*

> wandered on with a hasty step. This noble war in the sky elevated my spirits; I clasped my hands and exclaimed aloud, 'William, dear angel! This is thy funeral, this thy dirge!' As I said these words, I perceived in the gloom *a figure* which stole from behind a clump of *trees* near me; I stood *fixed, gazing intently*; I could not be mistaken. A flash of lightning illuminated the object and discovered its *shape* plainly to me; its gigantic stature, and the deformity of its aspect, more hideous than belongs to humanity, instantly informed me it was the wretch, the filthy daemon to whom I had given life. What did he there? Could he be (I shuddered at the conception) the murderer of my brother? No sooner did the idea cross my imagination than I became convinced of its truth; my teeth chattered, and I was forced to lean against a tree for support. The *figure* passed me quickly, and I lost it in the gloom. Nothing in human shape could have destroyed that fair child . . . *He* was the murderer! I could not doubt it. The mere presence of the idea was an irresistible proof of the fact . . . I remained *motionless*. The thunder ceased, but the *rain* still continued . . . I revolved in my mind the events which I had until now sought to forget: the whole train of my progress towards the creation, the appearance of the work of my own hands alive at my bedside, its departure [italics added].[35]

The symbols are present in the combining formations of fire, water (including rain), a hint of the forest and the wind. In respect of the sheer volume of noise – something which Neale also noted – the wind is the crowd:

> The strength of wind varies, and, with it, its voice. It can whine or howl, and, loud or soft, there are few sounds of which it is not capable. It thus affects men as something living, long after other natural phenomena have become inanimate. Apart from

[35] *Frankenstein*, 72–3. Lightning of course plays a spectacular part in the many film versions of *Frankenstein*. The lightning sequence in *The Bride of Frankenstein* (Universal, 1935) is famous.

> its voice, the most striking thing about wind is its direction; in order to name it, it is essential to know which quarter it comes from. Since man is entirely surrounded by air, the buffetings he receives from wind are felt as something peculiarly physical. One feels entirely contained in wind, it gathers everything to itself and, in a storm, everything that it seizes is driven along together.[36]

As it gathers everything to itself, the wind resembles a growing crowd. In the 'resurrectionist' cameo of the Irish episode, as I showed in Chapter 8, it is the sea wind which brings Frankenstein to the attention of the Irish crowd. And even in the isolated Orkneys Frankenstein's memory of the winds and water in Switzerland – which are in evidence in the lightning passage – remains to haunt his apprehension of the likely direction of the Creature en route to claim his companion.

Adam Neale's agglomeration of insects is an illustration of the 'Lilliput-effect' which I discussed in the previous chapter: the confrontation between an observer and dense crowds of tiny things. The significant orientation here, as I have noted, is the observer's position of detachment from the hosts of infinitesimal creatures surrounding him. These configurations are experienced as something outside of the self, and do not transform the spectator who confronts them. The scheme applies to Frankenstein in the passage under review:

> He preferably watches them from a distance. As long as they do not threaten him, and thus force him to define his position in relation to them, he enjoys their fluidity and ease of movement. But sometimes they reach a point where even a semblance of orientation becomes impossible; where *everything* around is fluid and transitory he naturally begins to feel very uncomfortable himself.[37]

In the lightning scene, the Creature's sudden proximity and

---

36 Canetti, 1981, 100.
37 *Ibid.*, 420.

shadowy elusiveness mimes this fluidity of movement. The same transitory scheme is retained in the memory as Frankenstein remains haunted by the precise moment of the Creature's departure after the first encounter. Each intermittent sighting – as here in the lightning – is a version or a reproduction of the first spectacle, the creation galvanised into life. This sighting, however, as the omnipresent 'idea' lodges in his mind, marks Frankenstein's own orientation with uncertainty, and it prepares the ground for his soon-to-be-assumed mask of silence:

> I paused when I reflected on the story I had to tell. A being whom I myself had formed, and endued with life . . . I remembered also the nervous fever with which I had been seized just at the time that I dated my creation, and which would give an air of delirium to a tale otherwise so utterly improbable . . . These reflections determined me, and I resolved to remain silent.[38]

Secrecy isolates. It is the final defence against questions; and it removes any opportunity for self-transformation.

In this respect the significant detail in the lightning passage is Frankenstein's state of fixity. It is as 'I stood *fixed*, gazing intently' that the figure steals into view. And as the figure strides the mountains in departure, he leaves Frankenstein 'motionless' and in full recall of the events in his 'workshop of filthy creation'[39] up to the Creature's first appearance and disappearance. In Canetti's discussion of crowd-processes in *Crowds and Power* there is an astonishingly comparable 'workshop' which, if taken in the context under review, indicates the nature and the limits of transformation.

He quotes a case treated by Bleuler, a schizophrenic's own report of a delirium attack:

> What I had suddenly to see there made my hair stand on end. *Forests, rivers and oceans* with every kind of dreadful animal and human figure, such as no human eye ever saw before, whirled

---

[38] *Frankenstein*, 73.
[39] *Ibid.*, 56.

> by incessantly, alternating with workshops of every trade, in which horrible spirit figures were working.[40]

and comments:

> The 'forests, rivers and oceans' which appear here are already known to us as crowd symbols, but, as though they were here only in the process of *becoming* symbols, they are not yet quite detached from the crowds for which they often come to stand later. They are still alive 'with every kind of dreadful animal and human figure, which no human eye ever saw before'. The propagation of new creatures, and in such numbers, by the combination of existing ones is the work of transformation. Again, the delirious patient is not himself drawn into these transformations; all the more marked, therefore, are the combinations and permutations in his world; and all these new creatures are immediately present in vast numbers.[41]

The ocean is the omnipresent context of Frankenstein's narrative. At the end of the tale Walton observes in Frankenstein a man marked by 'solitude and delirium'.[42] As the midnight spectacle passes, Frankenstein, recalling his 'workshop', dates the onset of his 'nervous fever' – 'which would give an air of delirium to a tale otherwise so utterly improbable'[43] – with his 'filthy creation'.[44] In common, then, with Bleuler's case:

> It is remarkable how this particular patient makes the familiar entities of the forest, river and ocean, in which new life has a natural origin, alternate with the 'workshops of every trade'. He equates production with transformation, a notion which many primitive peoples share with him.[45]

---

40 Canetti, 1981, 425.
41 *Ibid.*
42 *Frankenstein*, 175.
43 *Ibid.*, 73.
44 *Ibid.*, 56.
45 Canetti, 1981, 425.

As it reminds Frankenstein of his creation labours, the lightning passage can help us to see his notorious workshop as nothing other than the production workshop of early nineteenth-century capitalism. The Creature is a product of and belongs to Frankenstein; but he seeks his own progeny, and in this he is dispossessed by the broken promise of a mate. As we saw in the previous chapter, alongside the Creature's persuasive appeal to his own future virtue there remains Frankenstein's uneasy contemplation of increasing numbers of proletarians. Canetti observes:

> When the concept of a dispossessed proletariat was first advanced and began to take effect, it retained the full optimism of increase. No one supposed for a moment that, because their lives were miserable, there ought perhaps to be fewer of them. People relied on production; through its increase the proletariat too would increase. Their productivity should serve themselves. Proletariat and production should grow together. This is the very connection which invariably manifests itself in the activities of primitive increase packs.[46]

And hence in the continuing commentary on Bleuler's patient:

> The various trades [and] . . . all their products are immediately present in huge numbers; one cannot help feeling that the workshops are actually only there in order to bring into existence vast masses of things in the quickest possible way. It is the processes of work as abstractions that we see here, together with their results; they are carried out by obscure spirit-figures.[47]

The bodysnatching era ends in 1832 as the political and social foundations are laid for a full market economy.

The equivalent 'spirit-figures', as this transition occurs, are Burke and Hare. In the bodysnatching period, at the moment of its greatest scandal, there surfaces within officialdom an apprehension in which these two men appear in a script with a potential cast

---

[46] *Ibid.*, 225.

[47] *Ibid.*, 425.

of thousands. In his book *Burke and Hare* Owen Dudley Edwards summarises the findings of a committee which met in 1829, at Robert Knox's request, to investigate the allegations against him:

> The committee forthrightly stated that they knew of no evidence 'that Dr Knox or his assistants knew that murder was committed in procuring any of the subjects brought to his rooms, and the Committee firmly believe that they did not'. They agreed that suspicion might have been aroused by the brevity of the interval between death and delivery, the 'absence of external marks of disease' and the views of Knox and other anatomists that most people engaged in the body traffic were of a 'generally abandoned' character.[48]

The latter point prompts Edwards to this observation:

> (This, incidentally, suggests that all resurrectionists were embryo Burkes and Hares, which raises an interesting point about public ethics – were Burke and Hare, as so often stated, unique in their infamy, or were they potentially two of thousands? The committee, in its aside, was opening up a fear which may have been widespread.) But since nobody knew that Dr Knox or anyone else had ever had suspicions excited by Burke and Hare, the committee found no evidence that they had been. No marks on the bodies were known to have given a presumption of death by violence as against disease, and dissection naturally made further investigation difficult.[49]

As the 'workshops of every trade' alternate with alive crowds in Bleuler's report, so too do the crowd symbols in the lightning episode in *Frankenstein* assist Frankenstein's full recall of 'the workshop of filthy creation' – and hence they summon officialdom's worst nightmare: masses of Burkes and Hares. The mental spectacle confronting Frankenstein for the remainder of the night is hedged by one relevant qualification: 'I considered the being whom I had

---

[48] Edwards, 1980, 130–1.
[49] *Ibid.*

cast among mankind . . . *nearly* in the light of my own vampire, my own spirit let loose from the grave and forced to destroy all that was dear to me' (italics added).[50] Guilt by near association was the sum of the unproven case against Knox. This is the observation in *Frankenstein*, perhaps above any other, which states the Anatomy Act's Foucaultian contribution to the 'discipline and punish' technology of 1832. As De Certeau has commented, the vampire metaphor informs Foucault's story of modern discipline. *Discipline and Punish* tells the story of 'how the humanitarian and reformist projects' of early capitalism 'are "vampirized" by disciplinary procedures [which increasingly organise] the social realm itself'.[51]

In 1832 the political writer Edward Gibbon Wakefield published a volume entitled *Householders in Danger from the Populace*. The populace, in Wakefield's idiom, is the 'rabble' and he lists its 'specimens' in an inventory: 'costermongers, slaughters of dead cattle, drovers, *dealers* in dog's meat and *dead bodies*, cads, bricklayers, chimney sweepers, nightmen, and scavengers' (italics added).[52] In the same year Wakefield had pondered in print the alternatives to the resurrectionist trade,[53] so this cannot have been a casual reference to dealers in dead bodies. With the word 'scavengers' included, this loaded construction of the crowd succinctly spells out the surgeons' aims in the 1820s in terms of their nightmare: their failure to achieve a status less criminal and above the 'rabble'. Not by accident was Astley Cooper nicknamed 'The King of the Resurrectionists' in the eighteen-teens and -twenties. The same nightmare of indistinction is enacted in *Frankenstein* as the 'monster' – as a crowd – answers to Frankenstein's requirements with corpses from the well-to-do community.

But it is a reduction of my argument to see the Creature in *Frankenstein* as merely a projection of Burke and Hare. The story's vocabulary supplies a term which repeatedly sets the 'figure' of

---

50 *Frankenstein*, 73.
51 De Certeau, 1986, 22. The full statement is quoted in my first chapter.
52 Quoted in Hopkins, 1982, 213.
53 Richardson, 1989, 190.

the Creature in a contrast with Frankenstein's mask. For example, as the wedding-night shows, the story links the terms 'mask' and 'figure'. Frankenstein has mystified his uncomprehending bride with a secret, as the Creature after her murder also knows: 'I saw at the open window *a figure* the most hideous and abhorred . . . he pointed towards the corpse of my wife.'[54] This sentence is the story's version of Wakefield's eye-catching title. The same 'figure' – 'nothing in human shape' – is momentarily discerned by Frankenstein in the midnight spectacle. Canetti distinguishes the 'figure' from the mask:

> The product of transformation is . . . the *figure.* This is an entity that is not susceptible to further transformation and which manifests itself only after transformation has been completed . . . It is not a natural object, but the creation of man; it is his escape from the ceaseless flux of transformation . . .
>
> These figures . . . are twofold – the shape of an animal *and* a human being . . . What actually is it that they represent? . . . [the] earliest *figures* are representations of the *process* of transformation. From the unending flux of possible transformations, *one* is picked out and given permanent form. The very process of transformation, or rather a particular instance of it, is secured forever and thus, in comparison with all those which are excluded, is filled with special significance . . . It is what one may call a *free* figure. Its two aspects are equal in importance; neither is ranked higher than the other and neither is hidden behind the other . . . Originally it expressed both the process of transformation and its result.
>
> The mask is distinguished from all other end-states of transformation by its rigidity. In place of the varying and continuous movement of the face it presents the exact opposite: . . . a fixity and sameness.[55]

In the lightning spectacle, the 'figure' Frankenstein sees does not

---

54 *Frankenstein,* 164.
55 Canetti, 1981, 432–3.

only pass by quickly; its attributes are themselves unfamiliar. His sightings of his creation, as he often remarks, are serial versions of the first sighting. Only when the whole game is up does the Creature abandon his social invisibility and board the ship. The 'figure' glimpsed in the trees, however, will turn up again later in writing on forest bark and – in a metamorphosis made permanent – in cameo as words carved on stone.[56] When the Creature boards the Ship-of-State, Walton sees 'a mummy' beside Frankenstein's coffin, a term which applies to animals as well as humans: 'As he hung over the coffin, his face was concealed by long locks of ragged hair; but one vast hand was extended, in colour and apparent texture like that of a mummy . . . [he was uttering] exclamations of grief and horror.'[57] This is the final 'claiming' ritual in the story. The extended hand is the same hand which originally sought in vain 'to detain' Frankenstein in the first encounter, where the word 'monster' first appears. This 'monster' has it in him to grieve for his maker, and is about to renounce the role of the survivor. The dual animal-human 'figure' is capable of becoming either animal or human at will, an ambiguity which is apparent in the moral ambiguity of the *Creature* – truly called – who can just as easily save life as take life. After the encounter in the lightning Frankenstein reflects:

> I well knew that if any other had communicated such a relation to me, I should have looked upon it as the ravings of insanity. Besides, *the strange nature of the animal* would elude all pursuit, even if I were so far credited as to persuade my relatives to commence it [italics added].[58]

The proposition weighs with the surgeon, and on goes the mask. Canetti comments that the mask

> is a *conclusion*; into it flows all the ferment of the as yet unclear and uncompleted metamorphoses which the natural human face

---

56 *Frankenstein*, 170.
57 *Ibid.*, 181.
58 *Ibid.*, 73.

> so miraculously expresses, and there it ends. Once the mask is in position there can be no more *beginnings*, no groping towards something new. The mask is clear-cut; it expresses something which is definite, and neither more nor less than this. It is *fixed*; the thing it expresses cannot change.[59]

The secret dammed up behind Frankenstein's mask is the Anatomy Act as it passes into law in 1832 behind and effectively obscured by the final drama of the Reform debate.

At the end of the bodysnatching decade, all people without property in England were denied a specific transformation: they were denied the vote, and with this denial the dissection constituency was created. The third edition of *Frankenstein*, and the 'lightning' scene not least, is prescient as regards the immediately pending historical moment. As a sympathetic eye-witness recorded, Bentham's dissection – 'that hour in which the principle of utility triumphed' – was illuminated by lightning:

> None who were present can ever forget that impressive scene. The room is small and circular, with no windows, but a central skylight, and was filled, with the exception of a class of medical students and some eminent members of that profession, by friends, disciples, and admirers of the deceased philosopher, comprising many men celebrated for literary talent, scientific research, and political activity. The corpse was on the table in the centre of the room, directly under the light, clothed in a night-dress, with only the head and hands exposed. There was no rigidity in the features, but an expression of placid dignity and benevolence. This was at times rendered almost vital by the reflection of the lightning playing over them; for a storm arose just as the lecturer commenced, and the profound silence in which he was listened to was broken, by loud peals of thunder, which continued to roll at intervals throughout the delivery of his most appropriate and affecting address. With the feelings which touch the heart in contemplation of departed

[59] Canetti, 1981, 434.

> greatness, and in the presence of death, there mingled a sense of the power which that lifeless body seemed to be exercising in the conquest of prejudice for the public good, thus co-operating with the triumphs of the spirit by which it had been animated.[60]

The medical profession needed to change public perceptions of dissection as well as its own conditions of practice. The anatomy legislation, as Bentham designed it, supplied the surgeons with their materials and enabled them to withdraw from public controversy.

The dissection of the human body is an unmasking, a search for causes. Mary Shelley's story in its third edition unmasks hypocrisy as it draws to the surface the darker legislative face of middle-class hegemony at a watershed moment in English national life. 'The British working class of 1832', E. P. Thompson contends,[61] comprised 'perhaps the most distinguished popular culture England has known.' The famous 'monster' in *Frankenstein* contests officialdom's criminalisation of poverty by legislative fiat. He is given his own voice. His account of himself – even in Frankenstein's eyes – does credit to an identity which is above degradation to an animal. After Justine's execution, Frankenstein raises the spectre of the serial killings to come. The crowd symbolism in the earlier lightning spectacle establishes the 'race of devils' projection as a subliminal thought in Frankenstein's mind before it precipitates his decision to dishonour his political bargain with his creation. There is never the suggestion, however, except in Frankenstein's mind subsequently, that the Creature will not honour his side of the famous promise. In the event, all that is needed to halt the violence is the keeping of the promise which would raise the Creature out of the impending dissection constituency.

There are remarks made by Mary Shelley herself which lend partial support to the proposition in my preceding sentence.

---

60 Lewes, 1848, 46–7.
61 E. P. Thompson, 1963, 914.

Johanna Smith, the modern editor of the third edition of *Frankenstein*, sketches Mary Shelley's own equivocal stand on the Reform debate by reference to the author's letters in 1831: 'To one correspondent she says, "it looks as if the autocrats would have the good sense to make the necessary sacrifices to a starving people"'.To another she writes:

> *Progressiveness* is certainly finely developed just now in Europe – together with a degree of *tyrant quellingtiveness* which is highly laudable – it is a pity that in our country this should be mingled with a *sick destructiveness*; yet the last gives action to the former – and without [it], would our Landholders be brought to reason? Yet it is very sad – the punishment of the poor men being not the least disaster attendant on it.[62]

I quoted a part of this letter in my first chapter where I recommended that we should trust the tale, not the teller. But I submit that only now, having read the story, can we appreciate the full import of that last sentence as it applies to the Anatomy Act. If it could ever be ascertained that the Anatomy Act was not in Mary Shelley's mind here – and this cannot be ascertained – it would not effect a claim that her language spells out the ideological climate in which the punitive anatomy legislation was being publicly debated with a view to the statute book. Her attitude here is equivocal, a compound of 'tyrant quelling' and a deep fear of the lower orders.

How she may have been inclined to interpret her own story thirteen years after its first appearance is an intriguing question, to which we cannot know the answer. It is true, of course, that the events in Edinburgh in 1828 could not have been part of her original scheme of intention. As the world knows, Mary Shelley put a monster into the story; but soon afterwards her social and political culture added another one. The historical monster in *Frankenstein* is the 1832 Anatomy Act, the lineaments of which were assembled after the story appeared in 1818. The resurrectionist

62 Quoted in Shelley, 1992, 15.

culture Mary Shelley grew up in in the eighteen-teens is present in her story in Victor Frankenstein's famous nocturnal visits to graveyards. But history recasts *Frankenstein* after Burke and Hare – and again after Bishop and Williams, and again after the Anatomy Act. In this book I have tried to read the script which history put into the tale of *Frankenstein*. Nevertheless, the transformations we have observed occur in the story she wrote in the eighteen-teens, and this is the astonishing thing about it. A small number of minor changes found their way into the third edition, but they do not bear on the metamorphosis. *Frankenstein* testifies to the spirit of the age with a penetration which is not matched elsewhere in the anatomy literature. There are genuinely prescient elements – and developments – in the story over the decade in question. I maintain that this best-seller fast became public discourse in the late 1820s and can be read as such.

CHAPTER 10

# Conclusion

> 'The higher and middling orders are the natural representatives of the human race. Their interest may be opposed, in some things, to that of their proper contemporaries, but it is identical with that of the innumerable generations which are to follow.' – Macaulay, returned as the Member for Leeds, December 1832, and an advocate of the Anatomy Act.[1]

The Anatomy Act received Royal Assent on 1 August 1832. In its most significant clauses it repealed the dissection provisions of the 1752 Murder Act and requisitioned instead the institutionalised dead for dissection. The medical profession was granted automatic access to all unclaimed inmates of workhouses and hospitals. The legislation effectively ended the graverobbing trade by putting it out of business. In addition it caused a decline in voluntary bequests of bodies – a practice which had been on the increase before the Anatomy Act – because many people came to believe that the new law provided an adequate supply (though in fact, as the nineteenth century progressed, it did not). Towards the end of the century, however, the continuing shortage brought the social bias in the existing arrangements into renewed focus and an argument for a fairer bequest system found more acceptance socially. In England after the Second World War a system of free donation was adopted, reflecting the widespread increase in actual donations. But throughout the nineteenth and early twentieth centuries the Anatomy Act imposed upon the world of poverty a punishment which previously had been reserved for murderers. In her study of 1832, Richardson quotes E. P. Thompson's

[1] Quoted in E. P. Thompson, 1980, 905.

observation that the architects of the Reform Bill delivered 'a definition of class of almost arithmetical exactitude . . . the line was drawn with the crudity of an indelible pencil.'[2] She adds: 'The Anatomy Act drew a similar line in a similar place, demarcating and isolating the propertyless as its victims.'[3]

In this book I have focused the remarkable historical adjacency of the third edition of *Frankenstein* to the immediately ensuing political settlement and have interpreted Mary Shelley's story as an allegory of that watershed year. Victor Frankenstein's broken promise to his Creature, from the working-class standpoint, presages all the worst fears that were to follow from the double political bill of 1832. And after the betrayal of the promise, as informed contemporaries could have observed, the mounting violence in the story delivers a supplementary narrative of the copycat burking scandals which were to carry the argument in Parliament for the Anatomy Act. As the classic of the bodysnatching era in its intensive phase, *Frankenstein* truly belongs to the 1820s, the decade which spans its first, second and third editions.

In Chapter 8 I quoted Thompson's claim that 'there is a sense in which the Chartist Movement commenced . . . at the moment when the Reform Bill received Royal Assent'.[4] The legislation on anatomy is not mentioned in *The Making of the English Working Class*, but Ruth Richardson's study of this lesser known dimension of 1832 is an essential supplement to Thompson's compendious narrative. In my reading of *Frankenstein* I have ventured upon an interdisciplinary dialogue with the historians of 1832. I have introduced, from before and after the legislation, a larger sample of 'anatomy literature' which bears out the force of Thompson's general observation with one main emphasis: the punitive terror promoted by the Anatomy Act was the true face of the Reform Bill.

---

2 *Ibid.*, 909.

3 Richardson, 1989, 262.

4 E. P. Thompson, 1980, 909.

## Two nations, two funerals: 'the punishment of the poor men' in Mrs Gaskell's *Mary Barton*

I want to conclude my survey of the anatomy literature by showing how Mrs Gaskell's *Mary Barton* focuses the aftermath of 1832 in a way which confirms Mary Shelley's insight in 1831 that 'the punishment of the poor men' will be 'not the least disaster' ensuing from the final turbulent phase of the national Reform debate. Gaskell's story of the 'Hungry Forties' provides a valuable fictional portrait of the effect of the 'class legislation'[5] of the early 1830s on the working-class community – and, as we will see, her story at a crucial juncture invokes the spectre of Frankenstein's Creature. Richardson makes no reference to *Mary Barton* in her study of the effects of the anatomy reform, but her account contains much that illuminates Gaskell's story.

The historians of the anatomy debate point out that actions and attitudes in everyday life can implicitly relate to dissection, but appear to involve other things. For example, anxieties about being able to support a family and remain financially secure generally are concerns which intersect with the dreaded prospect of a pauper's funeral, or a move into the workhouse. Richardson notes that emigration and prostitution were often resorted to as attempts to avoid the workhouse,[6] and the latter strategy has an application to Esther, Mrs Barton's sister in *Mary Barton*. Likewise, illness and unemployment,[7] and the uncertain cycle of seasonal employment, were factors that affected the ability to sustain regular payments to friendly societies – the sole securities of a great many people in their efforts to be able to afford a decent burial. The social historians of the 1830s sometimes appear uninformed of the dissection threat which motivated these payments. Michael Thompson's comments on work in *The Rise of Respectable Society*, in the context of the friendly society habit, are a useful lead into

[5] The phrase is contemporary, as Richardson notes (1989, 271).

[6] *Ibid.*, 279.

[7] *Ibid.*, 276.

Mrs Gaskell's portrait of the Davenport family in *Mary Barton*, and to much else in the text, but a reference to the ultimate fate in the workhouse is lacking:

> It can be argued . . . that the crucial steps towards forming a broad-based respectable working class were made in the mid-Victorian years, with the later accelerated expansion building on these foundations; and further, that these crucial steps were less a response to rising disposable incomes, since there was no marked rise, than a deliberate re-ordering of family budgets to make room for 'respectability' or 'security' payments.[8]

After Ben Davenport's death in *Mary Barton* the issue of lapsed payments comes up. Through no fault of his own Davenport could not sustain regular employment: 'It was agreed that the town must bury him; he had paid to a burial club as long as he could; but by a few weeks' omission, he had forfeited his claim to a sum of money now.'[9] Richardson notes that 'lapse rates were high, and many societies depended for their profit upon them remaining so'[10] – and she reports the fact that the Manchester Unity of Oddfellows secured a sixfold increase in its membership in the decade after 1832.[11] In Gaskell's account the Mancunian John Barton sustains a club membership which enables him to afford the funeral arrangements for his wife when she dies in premature labour; but alongside this fact the storyteller notes that Barton's bereavement weakens the bonding of the family and draws him closer to political associations. *Death, Dissection and the Destitute* points to exactly what is at stake in the Davenport funeral episode I shall consider shortly:

> The calculated shabbiness and indignity of the pauper funeral served to enhance the attraction and meaning of the pomp and display undertakers provided for their more fortunate clients. A

---

8 F. M. L. Thompson, 1988, 203.
9 Gaskell, 1967, 67.
10 Richardson, 1989, 277.
11 *Ibid.*, 275.

> carefully constructed negative image of the respectable funeral, it provided a simultaneous fillip for economic concepts of respectability, and of social failure. The religion of parsimony deconsecrated the bodies of the poor, and disinherited them from that potential future the leaden coffin and impressive monument so comfortingly assured. Dissection added a penumbra of fear to death on the parish – casting fundamental doubt upon the likelihood that any pauper would even reach the flimsy coffin and the unmarked grave.[12]

The unmarked grave in *Mary Barton* awaits Esther, who does reach it. As we saw in Chapter 7, the leaden coffin formed the subterranean defence against the resurrectionists and surgeons, for those with enough money to afford it. The patent coffin was registered in 1818,[13] the year *Frankenstein* first appeared. In *Oliver Twist* the undertaker Mr Sowerberry uses a snuff box which is a miniature model of this famous coffin design. By the time of Dickens' story the patent coffin was a commerical relic of the recent past:

> 'I have taken the measurements of the two women that died last night, Mr Bumble,' said the undertaker.
>
> 'You'll make your fortune, Mr Sowerberry,' said the beadle, as he thrust his thumb and forefinger into the proffered snuff-box of the undertaker which was an ingenious little model of a patent coffin . . .
>
> 'Think so?' said the undertaker in a tone which half admitted and half disputed the probability of the event. 'The prices allowed by the board are very small, Mr Bumble.'
>
> 'So are the coffins,' replied the beadle, with precisely as near an approach to a laugh as a great official ought to indulge in.[14]

As Richardson comments,[15] the medical profession's requirements,

---

12 *Ibid.*
13 *Ibid.*, 81.
14 Dickens, 1961, 48.
15 Richardson, 1989, 274.

prior to the 1832 legislation, turned the afterlife into a saleable commodity.

Ben Davenport's living, and dying, predicament bears a residual resemblance to Tom Paine's historic recognition in *Rights of Man* of the funeral requirements of the needy: 'Also twenty thousand pounds to be appropriated to defray the funeral expenses of persons, who, travelling for work, may die at a distance from their friends. By relieving the parish of this charge, the sick stranger will be better treated.'[16] Ben Davenport in the 1840s is a late version of Paine's 'sick stranger', for he is not actually among friends in Manchester. As Uglow notes, the city dwellers in *Mary Barton* 'have fled for work in the city and many live in dread of being flung back on the harsh new Poor Law of the country parish.'[17] Davenport is one of these. He is a newcomer to the city by three years, and he fears being returned to his parish in Buckinghamshire; since losing his work with the Carsons he regularly 'tramps' in search of employment. Here in the 1840s context, it is not personal acquaintance but class solidarity which quickly bonds Barton to Davenport and his family when they learn of his typhus affliction. Wilson asks Davenport's intermittent employer, Mr Carson, for an infirmary order. The employer does not even know who Davenport is; his minimal gesture is to hand out an outpatient order.

Throughout the passage which describes Davenport's funeral the middle-class narrator remains external to the event, but well in touch with the sensitivities of the moment. The sequence requires a full quotation to register the extent of the social contrast which it presents. Mary improvises a dress for the poverty-conscious widow from the dress she wore at her mother's funeral:

> So when the funeral day came, Mrs Davenport was neatly arrayed in black, a satisfaction to her poor heart in the midst of her sorrow. Barton and Wilson both accompanied her, as she led her two elder boys, and followed the coffin. It was a

---

16 Paine, *Rights of Man*, 1976, 268.

17 Uglow, 1993, 194.

> simple walking funeral, with nothing to grate on the feelings of any; far more in accordance with its purpose, to my mind, than the gorgeous hearses, and nodding plumes, which form the grotesque funeral pomp of respectable people. There was no 'rattling the bones over the stones', of the pauper's funeral.[18]

The quotation in the last sentence is a remarkable element in this description, for it is actually a semi-quotation and in effect a stifled reference to the dreaded fate of dissection. It is from T. Noel's Victorian poem 'The Pauper's Drive'. The lines are quoted and usefully glossed in *Death, Dissection and the Destitute*:

> Rattle his bones over the stones,
> It's only a pauper whom nobody owns.

Richardson comments that this was a well-known refrain, and adds: 'Of course, "owns" is another word for "claim" in this context'.[19] The passage under review appears to suppress Noel's lightly veiled reference to the pauper's ultimate fate in Victorian England: the line is cut off and the rhyme tantalisingly withdrawn. Mrs Gaskell marks her presence in the description by the 'to my mind' interpellation, but her judicious tone has its limits: the allusion to dissection stands, but remains literally unspeakable.

The other funeral in *Mary Barton* is glimpsed in the course of John Barton's expedition to London, the disillusioning effects of which precipitate his decision to become a Chartist. Barton recalls the petitioners' fatigue in a congested Oxford Street, and his state of mind:

> I were like a child, I forgot a' my errand in looking about me . . . we were dusty and tired, going a step now and a step then. Well, at last we getten into a street grander nor all, leading to th' Queen's palace, and there it were I thought I saw th' Queen. Yo've seen th' hearses wi' white plumes, Job?'
>
> Job assented.

---

18 Gaskell, 1967, 67.

19 Richardson, 1989, 375.

> 'Well them undertaker folk are driving a pretty trade in London. Wellnigh every lady we saw in a carriage had hired one o' them plumes for the day, and had it niddle nodding on her head. It were th' Queen's drawing room, they said, and th' carriages went bowling along toward her house, some wi' dressed up gentlemen like circus folk in 'em, and rucks o' ladies in others. Carriages themselves were great shakes too. Some o' th' gentlemen as couldn't get inside hung on behind, wi' nosegays to smell at, and sticks to keep off folk as might splash their silk stockings. I wondered why they didn't hire a cab rather than hang on like a whip-behind boy; but I suppose they wished to keep with their wives, Darby and Joan like.[20]

The enchantment of power causes Barton to forget his purpose. This is Barton with a petition in his hand, not the weapon of violence that comes later and which is prompted by the rejection of his case to Parliament on this very day. Barton's journey to London is an important moment in the story's representation of the social hopes that were invested in the struggle for political rights. Karl Polanyi's 'Condition-of-England' metaphor is relevant here, but it needs the additional emphasis, as Richardson argues, that the anatomy legislation was to all intents and purposes an advance clause to the New Poor Law. The two politicians Polanyi invokes were firm supporters of the Anatomy Act:

> When the Chartist Movement demanded entrance for the disinherited into the precincts of the State, the separation of economics and politics ceased to be an academic issue and became the irrefragable condition of the existing system of society. It would have been an act of lunacy to hand over the administration of the New Poor Law with its scientific methods of mental torture to the representatives of the self-same people for whom the treatment was designed. Lord Macaulay was only consistent when he demanded in the House of Lords . . . the unconditional rejection of the Chartist petition in the name of

---

[20] Gaskell, 1967, 94; 'rucks', a great quantity.

> the institution of property on which all civilisation rested. Sir Robert Peel called the Charter an impeachment of the Constitution.[21]

In the passage under review, Barton is drawn into the spectacle that reduces him to a mesmerised infant; he recalls how the slow spectacle kept the men waiting for a long time on their way to the Parliament, and how, attempting to cross the street, he was 'pushed' and 'struck' by the police, and then laughed at by the officers. Shortly afterwards the Parliamentarians refuse to hear the petition. Here, at the pinnacle of social power, the nodding plumes are a heraldic item deriving from the older funerary rituals of the nobility,[22] and are retained in the paraphernalia of the 'respectable' funerals to which Mrs Gaskell refers. Richardson comments: 'Respectable funerary display was a powerful articulation of social aspiration and attainment. It demonstrated at one and the same time wealth and – in stark contrast to the pauper's funeral – distance from the workhouse.'[23] There is much else in *Mary Barton* that qualifies the text as anatomy literature. The problematic representation of Chartism in this text has been much discussed,[24] but it has not been observed that Barton's political conversion has its roots in the working-class death culture which was threatened in a premeditated way by the 1832 anatomy reform. As *Mary Barton* shows, the culture of improving medical care promoted by the legislation did not extend to its victims, the poor in mid-Victorian society. It is Barton who unselfishly supplies what money he has to seek medical assistance for Davenport, but his money only buys a delusory hope at the hands of the quack culture: 'Barton left the shop with comfortable faith in the physic given him; for men of his class, if they believe in physic at all, believe that every description is equally efficacious.'[25] This is also

---

21 Polanyi, 1941, 220.
22 Richardson, 1989, 272–3.
23 *Ibid.*, 273.
24 See Williams, 1977, and Baldick, 1987.
25 Gaskell, 1967, 58.

metaphor, of course, for Mrs Gaskell shares Thomas Carlyle's fear of Chartism as dangerous political quackery.[26] Before he resorts to violence, however, John Barton attends two kinds of funeral in the social scale. After the stifled reference to Noel's poem, Mrs Gaskell takes the widow's part as Davenport's funeral proceeds:

> Decently and patiently was he followed to the grave by one determined to endure her woe meekly for his sake. The only mark of pauperism attendant on the burial concerned the living and the joyous, far more than the dead, or the sorrowful. When they arrived in the churchyard, they halted before a raised and handsome tombstone; in reality a wooden mockery of stone respectabilities which adorned the burial ground. It was easily raised in a very few minutes, and below was the grave in which pauper bodies were piled until within a foot or two of the surface; when the soil was shovelled over, and stamped down, and the wooden cover went to do temporary duty over another hole. But little they recked of this who now gave up their dead.[27]

The Frankensteinian 'monster' of Chartism was created, not born, in the year of the Great Reform Bill. This dignified funeral is the rejection scene in *Frankenstein* transposed into the quotidian world of the victims of 1832, the politically defenceless communities of the late 1840s.

The explicit allusion to *Frankenstein* – 'that monster of many human qualities, ungifted with a soul'[28] – occurs in *Mary Barton* as the rhetorical prelude to Barton's conversion. 'John Barton', comments Mrs Gaskell, 'became a Chartist, a Communist, all that is commonly called wild and visionary. Ay! but being visionary is something. It shows a soul, a being not altogether sensual; a creature who looks forward for others, if not for himself.'[29] Here, as she records the moment of conversion, Gaskell is at the outer

---

26 See Carlyle, 'Chartism', *Selected Writings*.
27 Gaskell, 1967, 67–8.
28 *Ibid.*, 219.
29 *Ibid.*, 220.

limit of a genuine sympathy for Barton, prior to her rejection of him as a Frankensteinian monster of violence. In this story John Barton turns to Chartism because he 'looks forward for others': he seeks to free his class from what Mary Shelley in 1831 judged correctly would be 'the punishment of the poor men' in the command culture of England's post-1832 era. In *Crowds and Power* Canetti describes freedom with an emphasis which justifies mass resistance to oppression:

> Only commands which have been carried out leave their sting in the obeyer. Commands which have been evaded need not be stored; the 'free' man is not the man who rids himself of commands after he has received them, but the man who knows how to evade them in the first place. But the man who takes longest to rid himself of them, or who never achieves it, is undoubtedly the least free.[30]

These words are the political epitaph of the thousands of people who fell victim to the Anatomy Act before it was repealed when the Welfare State was set up after the Second World War.[31] Where the 1830s and 1840s are concerned, Karl Polanyi sums up the spirit of the age: 'In England after 1832 it became the unwritten law of the Constitution that the working class must be denied the vote. The Chartist leaders were jailed; their adherents, numbered in millions, were derided by a legislature representing a fraction of the population, and the mere demand for the ballot was often treated as a criminal act by the authorities. Of the spirit of compromise allegedly characteristic of the British system – a later invention – there was no sign.'[32]

---

[30] Canetti, 1981, 355.

[31] As noted, the Welfare State arrangements introduced a system in which bequest of one's body for medical research replaced the Anatomy Act's requisition of pauper corpses.

[32] Polanyi, 1944, 221.

# Select bibliography


Abernethy, J., *Hunterian Oration* (London, 1819).

Arendt, H., *The Human Condition* (Univ. of Chicago, London, 1958).

Aries, P., *The Hour of Our Death* (Penguin, Harmondsworth, 1987).

Austen, J., *Sense and Sensibility* (Penguin, Harmondsworth, 1986).

Bailey, B., *The Resurrection Men* (Macdonald, London, 1991).

Baldick, C., *In Frankenstein's Shadow* (Oxford UP, Oxford, 1987).

Ball, J. M., *Bodysnatchers* (Dorset Press, New York, 1989).

Barnouw, D., 'Mind and Myth in *Masse und Macht*', *Modern Austrian Literature*, 16, 1983, 65–79.

Barrell, J., *The Infection of Thomas De Quincey* (Yale, New York and London, 1992).

Barrell, J., & J. Bull (eds.), *English Pastoral Verse* (Penguin, Harmondsworth, 1982).

Bennet. B. T., *The Letters of Mary Wollstonecraft Shelley* (John Hopkins UP, Baltimore, 1980, 1983, 1988).

Bennett, T., *et al., Popular Culture and Social Relations* (Open UP, Milton Keynes, 1986).

Bentham, J., *Bentham's Works* ed. J. Bowring (New York, 1962).

Blake, W., *Complete Works* (Oxford UP, London, 1966)

Bourdieu, P., *Distinction,* trans. R. Nice (Routledge & Kegan Paul, London, 1984).

Bowerbank, S., 'The Social Order *vs.* the Wretch: Mary Shelley's Contradictory-Mindedness in *Frankenstein*', *English Literary History,* 46:3, 1979, 418–31.

Bronfen, E., *Over Her Dead Body* (Manchester UP, 1992)

Canetti, E., *Crowds and Power* (Penguin, Harmondsworth, 1981).

Canetti, E., *The Human Province* (Andre Deutsch, London, 1985).

Canetti, E., *The Conscience of Words & Earwitness* (Picador, London, 1987).

Carlyle, T., *Selected Writings* (Penguin, Harmondsworth, 1987).

Cole, H., *Things for the Surgeon* (Heinemann, London, 1964).

Cooper, D., *The Lesson of the Scaffold* (Allen Lane, London, 1974).

De Certeau, M., *Heterologies* (Manchester UP, Manchester, 1986).

De Certeau, M., *The Practice of Everyday Life* (Univ. of California, Berkeley and Los Angeles, 1988).
Deleuze, G., & F. Guattari, *A Thousand Plateaus* (Athlone Press, London, 1988).
De Quincey, T., *On Murder Considered As One of the Fine Arts* (Blackwoods, 1827, 1839); repr. in *Selected English Essays*, ed. W. Peacock, (Oxford UP, London, 1918).
Dickens, C., *Oliver Twist* (Signet, London, 1961).
Dickens, C., *Barnaby Rudge* (Penguin, Harmondsworth, 1987).
Dickens, C., *David Copperfield* (Penguin, Harmondsworth, 1988).
Dickens, C., *Great Expectations* (Penguin, Harmondsworth, 1985)
Durey, M., *The Return of the Plague* (Gill & Macmillan, Dublin, 1979),
Durey, M., 'Benthamites and Bodysnatchers', *London Journal*, 2, 1976, 200–225.
During, S., *Foucault and Literature* (Routledge, London, 1992).
Edwards, O. D., *Burke and Hare* (Mercat Press, Edinburgh, 1980).
Evans, E. J., *The Great Reform Act of 1832* (Routledge, London, 1983).
Feldman, P. R., & D. Scott-Kilvert, *The Journals of Mary Shelley*, 2 vols (Oxford, Clarendon Press, 1987).
Fido, M., *Bodysnatchers* (Weidenfeld & Nicolson, London, 1988).
Fiske, J., *Understanding Popular Culture* (Unwin Hyman, London, 1989).
Foucault, M., *Madness and Civilization* (Tavistock, London, 1967).
Foucault, M., *Discipline and Punish* (Penguin, Harmondsworth, 1979).
Foucault, M., *Power/Knowledge*, ed. C. Gordon (Harvester, London, 1980).
Foucault, M., *The Birth of the Clinic* (Routledge, London, 1989).
Freeborn. R., 'Frankenstein's Last Journey', *Oxford Slavonic Papers*, New Series, vol. xviii, 1985, 102–119.
Friedman, L. D., 'Sporting with Life: *Frankenstein* and the Responsibility of Medical Research', *Medical Heritage*, 1:3, May/June, 1985, 181–5.
Garrett, C., *Respectable Folly* (John Hopkins UP, Baltimore and London, 1975).
Gaskell, E., *Mary Barton* (Everyman, J. M. Dent & Sons, London, New York, 1967).
Gatrell, V. A. C., *The Hanging Tree* (Oxford UP, New York, 1994).
Gittings, J., *John Keats* (Penguin, Harmondsworth, 1968).
Godwin, W., *Essay on Sepulchres* (London, 1809).
Godwin, W., *Enquiry Concerning Political Justice* (Penguin, Harmondsworth, 1985).

Golby, J. M., & A. W. Purdue, *The Civilisation of the Crowd* (Batsford, London, 1984).

Goldburg. M. A., 'Moral and Myth in Mrs Shelley's *Frankenstein*', *Keats-Shelley Journal*, 8, 1959, 27–38.

Gonzalez-Crussi, F., *Notes of An Anatomist* (Picador, London, 1986).

Gilbert, S. M., & S. Gubar, *The Madwoman in the Attic* (Yale UP, London, 1979).

Grigson. G. (ed.), *Southey's Selected Verse* (Faber, London, 1970).

Harland, R., *Superstructuralism* (Methuen, London, 1987).

Harrison, J., *The Second Coming* (Routledge & Kegan Paul, London, 1979).

Harrison. R., *Bentham* (Routledge & Kegan Paul, London, 1983).

Harrison, M., *Crowds and History*, (Cambridge UP, Cambridge, 1988).

Hartley, J., *Understanding News* (Methuen, London, New York, 1985).

Hay, D., *et al., Albion's Fatal Tree* (Penguin, Harmondsworth, 1977).

Hazlitt, W., *Selected Writings*, ed. Jon Cook, (Oxford UP, Oxford, New York, 1991).

Hazlitt, W., *New Writings by William Hazlitt* (Martin Secker, London, 1925).

Helman, C., *Body Myths* (Chatto & Windus, London, 1991).

Heller, L. E., '*Frankenstein* and the Cultural Uses of Gothic' in Smith, *Frankenstein*, 312–41.

Hewlett. D., *John Keats* (Hutchinson, London, 1970).

Hindle, M. (ed.), *Caleb Williams* (Penguin, Harmondsworth, 1988).

Hindle, M. (ed.), *Frankenstein* (Penguin, Harmondsworth, 1992).

Hobsbawm, E. J., & G. Rudé, *Captain Swing* (Penguin, Harmondsworth, 1985).

Hogg. T. J., *Life of Shelley*, ed. H. Wolfe, 2 vols (J. M. Dent, London, 1933).

Hood. T., *The Poetical Works* (Oxford, 1906).

Hopkins, J. K., *A Woman To Deliver Her People* (Univ. of Texas, Austin, 1982).

Howe, P. P., *The Complete Works of William Hazlitt* (Dent & Sons Ltd, London, 1931).

Hulse, M. (ed.), *Essays in Honour of Elias Canetti* (Andre Deutsch, London, 1987).

Ignatieff, M., *A Just Measure of Pain* (Penguin, Harmondsworth, 1978).

Ingpen, R., *Shelley in England* (Kegan Paul, London, 1917).

Lawrence, D. H., *Selected Literary Criticism* (Mercury, London, 1961).

Levine, G., & U. C. Knoepflmacher (eds.), *The Endurance of Frankenstein* (Univ. of California Press, Berkeley, 1982).

Lewes, G. L., *Dr Southwood Smith: A Retrospect* (Blackwood & Sons, 1848).

Lindop, G., *The Opium-Eater: A Life of Thomas De Quincey* (Oxford UP, Melbourne, 1985).

Linebaugh, P., 'The Tyburn Riot Against the Surgeons', in D. Hay *et al.*, 1977, 65–117.

Litten, J., *The English Way of Death* (Robert Hale, London, 1991).

Low, D., *Thieves' Kitchen* (Alan Sutton, Guernsey, 1987).

Mackenzie, W. J. M., *Power, Violence, Decision* (Penguin, Harmondsworth, 1975).

Mandeville, B., *An Enquiry into the Causes of the Frequent Executions At Tyburn* (Augustan Reprint Soc., vol. 105, 1964).

Marmoy, C. F. A. 'The Auto-Icon of Jeremy Bentham at University College, London', *Medical History*, vol. 11(2), 1958.

Mellor, A., *Mary Shelley: Her Life, Her Fiction, Her Monsters* (Methuen, London, 1988).

Moers, E., 'Female Gothic', in Levine and Knoepflmacher, *The Endurance of Frankenstein*, 77–87.

Montag, W., '"The Workshop of Filthy Creation": A Marxist Reading of *Frankenstein*', in Smith, *Frankenstein*, 300–12).

Moretti, F., *Signs Taken for Wonders* (Verso, London, 1983).

Morris, R. J., *Cholera 1832* (Croom Helm, London, 1976).

Mort, F., *Dangerous Sexualities* (Routledge & Kegan Paul, London, 1987).

Owen, A., *The Darkened Room* (Virago, London, 1989).

Paine, T., *Rights of Man* (Penguin, Harmondsworth, 1976).

Peacock, T. L. *Crotchet Castle* (Penguin, Harmondsworth, 1982).

Piel, E., 'Putting An End to Power', in Hulse, *Essays in Honour of Elias Canetti*, 146–166.

Poe, E. A., *Selected Writings* (Penguin, Harmondsworth, 1980).

Polanyi, K., *The Great Transformation* (Octagon Books, New York, 1980).

Poovey, M., *The Proper Lady and the Woman Writer* (Univ. of Chicago, Chicago and London, 1984).

Porter, R., *English Society in the Eighteenth Century* (Penguin, Harmondsworth, 1982).

Porter, R., *Disease, Medicine and Society in England 1550–1860* (Macmillan, London, 1987).

Porter, R., *Mind Forg'd Manacles* (Penguin, Harmondsworth, 1990).

Porter R., & D. Porter, *In Sickness and In Health* (The Bath Press, Avon, 1988).

Porter, R., & D. Porter, *Patient's Progress* (Polity Press, Cambridge, 1989).

Powers, K. R., *The Influence of William Godwin on the Novels of Mary Shelley* (Arno Press, New York, 1980).

Poynter, F. N. L., & K. D. Keele., *A Short History of Medicine* (Scientific Book Club, London, 1961).

Richardson, R., *Death, Dissection & the Destitute* (Penguin, Harmondsworth, 1989).

Richardson, R., & B. Hurwitz, 'Jeremy Bentham's self image: an exemplary bequest for dissection' in *British Medical Journal*, vol. 295, 18 July 1987.

Risse, G. B., *Hospital Life in Enlightenment Scotland* (Cambridge UP, Cambridge, 1986).

Rousseau, J.-J., *Reveries of a Solitary Walker* (Penguin, Harmondsworth, London, 1981).

Rule, J., *Albion's People* (Longman, Harlow, 1992).

Sage, V., *Horror Fiction and the Protestant Tradition* (Macmillan, London 1988).

Sales, R., 'Poor Relations: Writing in the Working Class 1770–1835' in *The Penguin History of Literature: The Romantic Period* ed. D. B. Pirie (Penguin, London, 1994).

Sandwith, F., *Surgeon Compassionate* (Cox & Wyman, Reading, 1960).

Schiebinger, L., 'Skeletons in the Closet' in C. Gallagher, & T. Lacqueur, *The Making of the Modern Body* (Univ. of California, 1987)

Scott, W., *The Journal of Sir Walter Scott* ed. W. E. K Anderson (Oxford, Clarendon Press, 1992).

Sharpe, J. A., *Judicial Punishment in England* (Faber & Faber, London, 1990).

Shelley, M., *Frankenstein*, ed. J. Smith (Bedford Books, Boston, 1992).

Sheridan, A., *Michel Foucault: The Will to Truth* (Tavistock, London and New York, 1980).

Skillen, A., *Ruling Illusions* (Harvester, Sussex, 1977).

Small, C., *Ariel Like A Harpy* (Gollancz, London, 1972).

Sontag, S., *Illness As Metaphor* (Penguin, Harmondsworth, 1983).

Sontag, S., *Aids and Its Metaphors* (Penguin, Harmondsworth, 1990).

Southwood Smith, T., 'The Uses of the Dead to the Living', *The Westminster Review* 2, 1824, 59–97.

St Clair, W., *The Shelleys and the Godwins* (Faber & Faber, London, 1989).

Stallybrass, P., and A. White, *The Politics and Poetics of Transgression* (Methuen, London, 1986).

Sterrenburg. L., 'Mary Shelley's Monster: Politics and Psyche in Frankenstein', in Levine and Knoepflmacher, *The Endurance of Frankenstein*, 143–71.

Swift, J., *Gulliver's Travels* (Everyman, Dent, London, 1966).

Thompson, E. P., *The Making of the English Working Class* (Penguin, Harmondsworth, 1980).

Thompson, F. M. L., *The Rise of Respectable Society* (Fontana, London, 1988).

Thorpe, A., *Ulverton* (Minerva, London, 1993).

Tomalin, C., *Shelley and His World* (Penguin, Harmondsworth, 1992).

Townsend, J., *A Dissertation on the Poor Laws* (Univ. of California, London, 1971).

Turner, B. S., *Medical Power and Social Knowledge* (Sage, London, 1991).

Vasbinder, S. H., *Scientific Attitudes in Mary Shelley's 'Frankenstein'*, (UMI Research Press, Ann Arbor, Michigan, 1976).

Veeder, W., *Mary Shelley & Frankenstein: The Fate of Androgyny*, (Univ. of Chicago, Chicago and London, 1986).

Volosinov, V. V., *Marxism and the Philosophy of Language* trans. L. Matejka and I. R. Titunk (Seminar Press, New York, 1973).

Wakefield, E. G., *Householders in Danger from the Populace* (London, 1832).

Williams, R., *Culture and Society* (Penguin, Harmondsworth, 1977).

Wilson, J., 'Noctes Ambrosianae XIX', *Blackwood's Magazine*, March 1828.

Wollstonecraft, M., *Maria* (Pickering, London, 1989).

Wordsworth, W., *Poetical Works* (Oxford UP, London, 1967).

# Index

Page numbers in italics indicate illustrations